Ambulatory Surgical Nursing

A Nursing Diagnosis Approach

Sharon Summers, R.N., Ph.D.
Associate Professor, School of Nursing
University of Kansas Medical Center, Kansas City, KS

Diane Whitaker Ebbert, R.N., M.S., C.N.O.R.
Clinical Nurse Specialist
University of Kansas Medical Center, Kansas City, KS

Ambulatory Surgical Nursing

A Nursing Diagnosis Approach

J. B. Lippincott Company   Philadelphia
New York   London   Hagerstown

Sponsoring Editor: Dave Carroll
Cover Designer: Susan Blaker
Production Supervisor: Robert D. Bartleson
Production: P. M. Gordon Associates
Compositor: Compset, Inc.
Printer/Binder: R. R. Donnelley & Sons

6   5   4   3   2   1

Library of Congress Cataloging-in-Publication Data

Summers, Sharon.
    Ambulatory surgical nursing : a nursing diagnosis approach /
Sharon Summers, Diane Whitaker Ebbert.
      p. cm.
    Includes bibliographical references and index.
    ISBN 0–397–54799–4
    1. Surgical nursing.   2. Nursing diagnosis.   3. Surgery,
Outpatient.   I. Ebbert, Diane Whitaker.   II. Title.
    [DNLM: 1. Ambulatory Surgery—nursing.   2. Nursing Diagnosis.
3. Surgical Nursing.   WY 161 S955a]
RD99.S92   1992
610.73′677—dc20
DNLM/DLC
for Library of Congress   91–22786
                                                  CIP

Contributors

Jo Ann Schmitting Dubin, R.N., A.D.
Private Practice (Ronald Dubin, M.D.)
Middlesboro, KY

Nancy Dudgeon, R.N., B.S.N., C.P.A.N.
Head Nurse, Post Anesthesia Care Unit
University of Kansas Medical Center
Kansas City, KS

Diane Whitaker Ebbert, R.N., M.S., C.N.O.R.
Clinical Nurse Specialist
University of Kansas Medical Center
Kansas City, KS

Mary Kopp, R.N., M.N.
Assistant Director
Kansas State Nurses' Association
Topeka, KS
(Formerly Staff Nurse, Outpatient Surgery
St. Francis Hospital
Topeka, KS)

Nancy R. Lackey, R.N. Ph.D.
Postdoctoral Fellow
Oncology and Family
University of Utah
Salt Lake City, UT
(Formerly Associate Professor
School of Nursing
University of Kansas Medical Center
Kansas City, KS)

Jo Ann Lierman, R.N., M.N., Ed.S.
Assistant Professor
School of Nursing
University of Kansas Medical Center
Kansas City, KS

Elizabeth Monninger, R.N., Ph.D.
Professor and Director
School of Nursing
Southern Oregon State College
Ashland, OR

Remember Renfro, R.N., B.S.N.
Ophthalmic Surgical Coordinator
Midwest Eye Associates
Topeka, KS

Dolores Sabia, R.N., B.S.N.
Director, Center of
    Outpatient Surgery
Baptist Medical Center
Kansas City, MO

Sharon Summers, R.N., Ph.D.
Associate Professor
School of Nursing
University of Kansas
    Medical Center
Kansas City, KS

Joan Toot, R.N., B.S.N.
Staff Nurse, Same Day
    Surgery Unit
Lawrence Memorial Hospital
Lawrence, KS

Linda Woolery, R.N., M.S.N.
Informatics Nurse Specialist
Children's Mercy Hospital
Kansas City, MO

Preface

Ambulatory surgery is seen as one of the major shifts in patient care from traditional hospitalization to the ambulatory surgical unit (ASU). The major driving force in this shift is the high cost of patient care and reduced reimbursement by third-party payers. Although the shift from hospital-based to ASU-based care has been convenient for the patient and the physician, nursing has had little time to adapt to this changing mode of practice and to prepare for this new role. Moreover, although nurses have assumed these new roles in the ASU, there is little information included in the literature to guide this practice transition.

The purpose of this book is to provide staff nurses with information to help guide practice in this new role of ambulatory surgical nursing. Included in this book are a variety of patient assessment forms and a nursing diagnosis approach to patient care. The use of nursing diagnosis is currently included in both standards of professional practice and institutional accreditation criteria, and like the new role of ambulatory surgical nursing, is presented to help staff nurses incorporate nursing diagnosis into their practice. This book, although it was written primarily with the staff nurse in mind, can also be used to teach student nurses about this role transition.

The book is structured around five application sections: organizations, nursing practice, patient education, clinical experience, and futuristic issues. Within these five sections are 17 chapters designed to provide information for staff nurses who assume the role of the ASU nurse.

Chapter 1 describes the historical evolution of ambulatory surgical care and the evolution of the ASUs seen today. Chapter 2 describes ASU design and management for either free-standing or hospital-based units. Chapter 3 describes the use of computers to streamline patient care and facilitate general management of the ASU.

An indepth discussion of nursing diagnosis, a frequently overlooked portion of the nursing process, is presented in Chapter 4. Chapter 5 describes how nursing care plans can be structured, based on nursing diagnosis, to document the role of the professional nurse in the care of the ASU patient.

Chapter 6 compares the traditional roles of the perioperative nurse and the new role of the ASU nurse. Chapter 7 describes patient education strategies that are conducive for the ASU setting.

Chapters 8 through 12 illustrate care strategies, based on nursing diagnosis, for patients typically seen in the ASU. The case studies presented include patients admitted to the ASU for inguinal herniorrhaphy, cataract removal, dilatation and curettage, carpal tunnel repair, and laser cholecystectomy. Chapter 13 presents a discussion of nursing practice issues that impact the ASU, as well as some practical solutions for resolving those issues. Chapter 14 discusses the nutritional aspects of ASU patient care. Future directions in ASU nursing care, including preoperative home instruction, are discussed in Chapter 15. Chapter 16 presents a discussion of why nursing students need to have ASU experience incorporated into their nursing education curriculum. Finally, Chapter 17 presents nursing education strategies, providing guidelines for a two-week course that includes didactic and clinical practice in the ASU with an emphasis on nursing process and nursing diagnosis.

It is hoped that this text will serve as a helpful resource for nurses in incorporating the nursing process into practice as more surgical patients are cared for in the ambulatory surgical setting. Included in the case study chapters are indepth discussions of the nursing process, lengthy assessment forms, and elaborate care plans so that the reader has an overview of nursing-diagnosis–based care. Readers can then adapt certain nursing process applications to meet their individual practice needs. This text may also be used to guide educators in planning perioperative learning experiences for students in the ASU setting, and to assist students in learning the perioperative role of the nurse in the ASU.

We wish to thank our families for their understanding during the authoring and editing of this manuscript. We also wish to thank the contributors for their scholarly contributions to this text. Thanks are also extended to Boni Davenport for her word processing efforts in preparing both the draft and final forms of this manuscript.

S.S. & D.E.

Kansas City, 1991

Contents

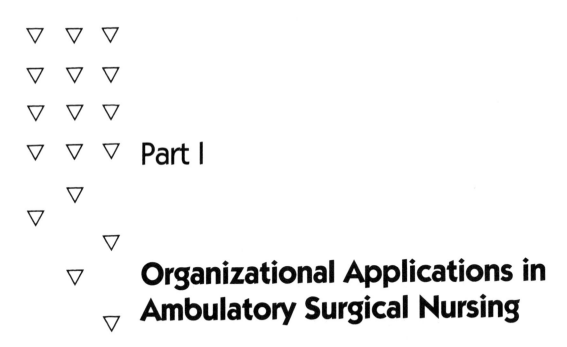

Part I

Organizational Applications in Ambulatory Surgical Nursing

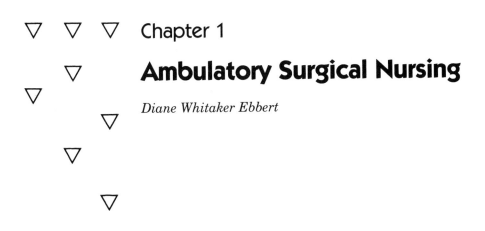

Chapter 1

Ambulatory Surgical Nursing

Diane Whitaker Ebbert

Ambulatory surgery is not a new concept, but the rapid growth, expansion, and acceptance of this alternative method of health care is relatively new, having occurred primarily in the last decade. It has been estimated that, in the early 1990s, as many as 60% of surgical cases will be performed in ambulatory surgery units (ASUs), and some believe that number will approach 80% by the year 2000.[1] As those numbers continue to grow and increasingly complicated procedures are performed in the ASU, the need for nurses specialized in perioperative care will also increase. In addition to the skills necessary to implement the nursing process with these patients, these nurses will need to be well versed in the business of ambulatory surgery, understanding its evolution, how units are set up, its organizational structures, and the manner in which patients access the system.

This chapter answers the following four questions:

1. Historically, how did the ambulatory surgery setting evolve?
2. What are the common terms used to define ambulatory surgery settings?
3. What are the four most common settings for ambulatory surgery?
4. What criteria are used for selection of ambulatory surgery patients?

Historical Evolution

Traditionally, surgical procedures have been performed on patients entering the hospital one day to one week prior to their surgery, allowing time for preoperative testing and preparation. These patients had a good understanding of their procedure and remained in the hospital for the duration of their recovery. Although minor surgical procedures would occasionally be performed on an outpatient basis, most major surgical procedures were performed on an inpatient basis.

Although ambulatory surgery reached its current level of acceptance only within the past 10 years, it has been performed throughout this century. Nicholl was one of the first to document the results of procedures performed on ambulatory patients,[2] reporting that the 8,988 outpatient surgical procedures performed at the Glasgow Royal Hospital for Sick Children were as successful as those performed on an inpatient basis.

In 1919, the Down-Town Anesthesia Clinic in Sioux City, Iowa was opened by Ralph Waters for dental and minor surgical procedures. Within two years, the concept had gained such popularity that the facility was enlarged.[3] At the time, many must have doubted the statement made about the facility that "the future for such a venture, I believe, is bright."[3]

Lahti reported the basic principles of ambulatory surgery in 1968.[4] Lahti's research supported the finding that, over the prior 30 years, the postsurgical hospitalization period had steadily declined.[4] In studying the course of 1,000 patients, Lahti found that patients expecting to be ambulatory immediately after surgery and to be discharged early were more relaxed, less fearful, and required less postoperative medication than their inpatient counterparts. This research led to the conclusion that there was no reason to prolong hospitalization for the typical patient beyond the time necessary to recover from anesthesia.

Lahti's study was timely. Until the early 1970s, the prevailing opinion was rooted in the fantasy of "health care, regardless of the cost." Modern technology had provided the necessary knowledge and instruments not only to improve, but also to prolong life. This factor, coupled with a rapidly aging population, quickly accounted for greater numbers of health care dollars, thereby increasing the cost of health care delivery. For a period of time, consumers were sheltered from the reality of health care costs by third-party reimbursements, Medicare, and Medicaid.

When the financial burden became too great to bear, there was a call for a revolution in health care delivery. Health maintenance organizations (HMOs), paid provider organizations (PPOs), and a plan for prospective payment based upon diagnosis-related groupings (DRGs) were introduced to control the cost of health care delivery without sacrificing quality care. As a result of these endeavors, hospitals and physicians were forced to become competitive, creative, and efficient providers of health care in order to survive.

The modern era of ambulatory surgery, as we know it today in the United States, began with the establishment in 1968 of a free-standing facility, The Dudley Street Ambulatory Surgical Center in Providence, Rhode Island. The Phoenix Surgeries in Phoenix, Arizona opened in 1970.

Ambulatory surgery today is also a part of the health care revolution.

Multiple factors have contributed to the successful growth of ambulatory surgery, as detailed in the following list.

Cost efficiency

Early patient ambulation

Improved surgical technology

Development of new anesthetic drugs

Changes in third-party reimbursement policies

Patient satisfaction

Acceptance by health care providers

One of the most significant factors in the growth of ambulatory surgery is cost reduction. Ambulatory surgical patients frequently require less laboratory and preoperative work-up than do typical inpatients. Moreover, these patients are under medical supervision for shorter periods of time and, therefore, require less medication than do patients admitted to the hospital. In addition, ambulatory surgical procedures are shorter in duration, allowing for quicker turnover and higher patient volume, resulting in more efficient use of time, facilities, and services. Although the costs for supplies and use of the operating room may be the same or similar to those incurred by an inpatient, the ambulatory surgery patient avoids the escalating costs of an unnecessary inpatient hospital stay.

We live in a mobile society, and patients today, unlike 20 years ago, believe that they can undergo surgery, recover in the comfort and convenience of their own home for a day or two, and then return to work. Ambulatory surgery results in less disruption in patients' lives and reduces the psychological stress often associated with hospitalization.

New developments in medical technology have made procedures that previously were considered appropriate only for inpatients accessible to outpatients. For example, laser technology has given rise to a whole new gamut of procedures that can safely and comfortably be performed on outpatients, including laser cholecystectomy, laser mastectomy, and uterine endometrial ablation. Improved surgical techniques have also increased the number and types of procedures that are now considered appropriate for ambulatory surgery.

The development of rapid-acting anesthetic agents with short durations of action has contributed greatly to the increase in ambulatory surgery. Many short-acting narcotics and nonnarcotics have been produced. These medications have been found to have minimal prolonged side effects, such as nausea, vomiting, and drowsiness, but still provide the patient with an adequate anesthetic. Other tranquilizers, antiemetics, and hypnotics have been found useful for the ambulatory surgery patient, often reducing the need for strong analgesics.[5]

In the early 1970s, insurance companies and other third-party reimbursers were not supportive of ambulatory surgery and, in many cases, would only cover the cost of a procedure if it was performed on an inpatient basis. These companies have now come to recognize the benefits of avoiding hospitalization if at all possible. Now it is not unusual for insurance companies to pay a larger percentage of the bill when appropriate procedures are performed on an outpatient basis than they would if these services were provided to inpatients.

Patient satisfaction has also been a major factor in the growth of ambulatory surgery. Ambulatory surgery units and centers are designed to meet the needs of this specialized group of patients. Patients are not exposed to hospital "red tape," rules, and policies, allowing them a greater sense of control over their surgical experience.

Ambulatory surgery has been warmly embraced by most health care professionals. For surgeons, the ASU is a convenient, safe choice for performing procedures. Because ambulatory surgical patients are carefully selected, the preoperative work-up usually requires less time and paperwork, which frees the surgeon for other responsibilities. For nurses, ambulatory surgery provides an opportunity to perform in a new and expanded nursing role. Care is focused not only on preparation for and performance of the operative procedure, but also on the preparation and education of patients before they return home to direct their own recovery phase. To best provide this care, nurses must be productive, efficient, independent, and cross-trained in all areas of perioperative nursing, which provides a distinct challenge to the self-motivated nurse.

▽

Common Terminology

The growth of ambulatory surgery has been paralleled by the development of various terms used to describe the process. As mentioned earlier, traditionally, surgery had been performed in the hospital on an *inpatient* basis most commonly using general anesthesia. Occasionally, minor surgery would be performed under local anesthesia, outside the hospital (in a doctor's office), with immediate discharge of the patient. These procedures were referred to as *outpatient surgery*. The 1960s and 1970s began an era of *ambulatory surgery*.[5] Procedures were performed under general anesthesia and, after a period of postoperative recovery and observation, patients were discharged from the hospital the same day. Many believed surgical care to be clearly differentiated into these three classes.[5] In reality, the terms outpatient and ambulatory surgery have been used interchangeably to denote that surgery is performed without admission to the hospital. In some areas, the terms minor and major precede that of ambulatory surgery to distinguish between the use of local and general anesthesia, respectively. Other terms frequently used to describe ambulatory surgery include same-day surgery, one-day surgery, and outpatient surgery. For the purposes of all discussions in this book, ambulatory surgery refers to surgery performed on patients who arrive at the health care facility, have surgery, and return home on the same day.

▽

Common Settings for Ambulatory Surgery

Ambulatory surgery is performed in a variety of settings. The four most common settings are hospital-affiliated facilities, office-based or free-standing facilities, and the physician's office.

Hospital-Affiliated Facilities

Hospital-affiliated programs can be subdivided into three categories. Hospital-based programs using shared resources are often called *hospital integrated* programs, whereby hospitals establish formal ambulatory surgery programs utilizing their current facilities. The existing preoperative holding area, operating rooms, and postanesthesia care unit are used by both inpatients and ambulatory surgery patients. This type of program demands minimal capital outlay by the hospital. Because the overall schematic organization is already in place, the time required for start-up of the program is relatively limited. A disadvantage of this type of program is that patients are mainstreamed. Outpatients who may be awake upon their arrival to the postanesthesia care unit may be in close proximity to a very ill inpatient who requires mechanical ventilation, which may increase the outpatient's stress level. These programs can also be very demanding of nurses who must constantly be shifting their frame of reference between inpatients and outpatients, each of whom has unique needs.

Another hospital-affiliated program is the self-contained ambulatory unit, referred to as a *hospital autonomous* program. Such programs are newly constructed or remodeled units dedicated to ambulatory surgery. The units are self-sufficient, are usually located in the hospital or on the hospital grounds, and are connected to the hospital. Because the units are designed specifically to be convenient, safe, comfortable, and efficient, they generally evoke increased satisfaction among patients and personnel. The disadvantage of a hospital autonomous unit is the initial escalating cost of its construction. However, once in place, this type of unit is usually quite cost-effective because it is designed to provide a single service that is offered repeatedly several times per day.

A variation of the hospital models just mentioned is a particularly integrated system. One or more of the areas (preoperative holding, operating room, or postanesthesia care unit) may be shared by both inpatients and outpatients. The most common unit of this type has its own admission area, preoperative preparation area, and postanesthesia care unit, but the operating rooms are shared with inpatients. One disadvantage of this type of program is that the sharing of operating rooms can often result in delays for the outpatient if an emergency case arises.

The third hospital-affiliated program is the *hospital satellite,* which is located away from the hospital. This type of surgical unit is autonomous, but is sponsored and operated by the hospital or as a joint venture among hospitals. These units provide hospitals with an opportunity to serve a different market and generate additional revenue. The location away from the hospital, although advantageous in terms of attracting a different clientele, can also be a disadvantage in the event of an emergency that requires the services of the main hospital.

Physicians' Offices

It has been reported that 20% of ambulatory surgery is performed in physician's offices or clinics.[6] The procedures performed in this setting vary according to specialty, but usually do not require a great deal of equipment, specially trained staff, or a hospital setting. The advantages of this setting are its low cost, efficient use of the surgeon's time, and its availability/accessibility for patients. The disadvantages include the lack of back-up for emergency situations, the limit as to the types of procedures that can safely be performed, and the potential lack of quality control. The number of cases performed in physician's offices may significantly increase in the future owing to new policies being instituted by insurance companies.[7] As more surgeons incorporate ambulatory surgery into their office practice, specific policies, procedures, and criteria for quality assurance will need to be developed.

Free-Standing Clinics

Free-standing clinics refer to ambulatory surgery centers that are autonomous—that is, independently owned and operated without any hospital affiliation. They are in business solely for providing ambulatory surgery services. The prototype for this type of center was opened in 1970 by Drs. Wallace Reed and John Ford in Phoenix, Arizona. The number of such facilities continues to grow. A high degree of patient and physician satisfaction with the free-standing centers has been reported.[8] A contributing factor to this satisfaction may be that the decision-making process in the smaller scale, free-standing facility is much more streamlined than that found in the hierarchical organization of a full-service hospital. These free-standing units also are more cost-effective than many hospitals because basic hospital costs do not have to be prorated in the charges to patients.[5] Morale among employees may also be enhanced by the small size of the center. Moreover, smaller settings provide more convenient parking and access for delivering and picking up patients. Studies have indicated that free-standing centers are the most convenient and cost-effective means of providing ambulatory surgical service. They do, however, have the disadvantage of a lack of hospital back-up in an emergency situation,[8] although this seems to be more of a potential problem than an actual one because free-standing centers screen potential patients carefully for any systemic problems that might lead to potential complications. Indeed, keen assessment skills, together with the appropriate selection of patients and procedures, and adequate preoperative preparation, are necessary for the success of any ambulatory surgery facility.

▽

Patient Selection

For many years, candidates for ambulatory surgery were considered to be those who were young, healthy, and undergoing a one- to two-hour procedure. Addressing the issue of patient selection, the American Society of Anesthesiologists developed a classification system for patients based on risk. Patients meeting the criteria for class I (healthy) or class II (having well-controlled mild to moderate systemic disease, such as type II diabetes, hypertension, or moderate obesity) were considered to be suitable candidates for ambulatory surgery.[7] However, ambulatory surgery is no longer reserved for the young and healthy. These days, it is not unusual for class III patients (those with more severe systemic disease, such as insulin-dependent diabetes, coronary artery disease with a history of angina or previous infarction, or moderate pulmonary insufficiency) to undergo surgery in the ASU. In some cases in which admission to the hospital may pose an increased risk, even class IV patients (those with severe, already life-threatening diseases) are undergoing ambulatory surgery.

▽

Procedure Selection

Surgical procedures performed in ambulatory surgery settings range from lesion biopsies to laser cholecystectomy. The most common procedures performed on an outpatient basis are dilatation and curettage, cataract extraction, inguinal herniorrhaphy, fallopian tube occlusion (laparoscopy), tonsillectomy, plastic surgical procedures on the nose, and arthroscopy.[1] Ideally, outpatient procedures should result in minimal bleeding and metabolic derangement, and should not involve major intervention in the cranial vault or abdominal or thoracic cavities. Moreover, they should be short to moderate in duration, associated with minimal to no complications, and should not require extensive recovery time.[7]

The appropriateness of a procedure for an ambulatory surgery setting depends, in part, upon the patient's ability to recover from the anesthetic and be discharged to perform self-care at home. If patients are unable to care for themselves and adequate postoperative care cannot be arranged, then an alternative that is frequently being used in hospital-based units is 23-hour hospitalization. Instead of being discharged home following ambulatory surgery, patients are admitted to a special unit where they can stay for up to 23 hours at a rate that is substantially less than the usual hospital day charge. These units provide patients with meals and assistance as necessary. Some require that patients bring their own medications for self-medication. Alternative care arrangements, such as the 23-hour care unit, permit a larger segment of the population to utilize ambulatory surgery settings.

▽

Preoperative Preparation

Preoperative assessment and evaluation have become increasingly critical to the ambulatory surgery setting, especially considering the trend for sicker patients to undergo more extensive procedures and to be discharged home the same day. Clearly, some patients are not candidates for ambulatory surgery; however, it is unlikely that all such patients will be identified prior to the scheduling of a procedure. Creative questions, asked during a preoperative phone call or preoperative visit, help to identify patients with special needs. This information (preferably in written form) can then be directed to the appropriate health care team member, whether it be anesthesiologist, nurse, or surgeon.

Depending on their regulating agency, ambulatory surgery settings may require that more extensive laboratory tests or histories and physicals, which are usually performed within seven days of the scheduled surgery, be available 24 hours prior to surgery. This information is helpful to the anesthesiologist, as well as to the perioperative nurse who is determining the appropriate plan of care.

▽

Summary

Ambulatory surgery and ambulatory surgical nursing have made valuable contributions to the improvement of health care. As with any organization or profession, an understanding of its history and evolution sheds light on the pathway to continued growth. This chapter has provided information on the basic background of the specialty of ambulatory surgery. Building on this information, each practitioner can help to determine the future direction of this specialty area of nursing.

References

1. Hill, G. J. (Ed.). (1988). *Outpatient surgery* (3rd ed., p. 3). Philadelphia: W. B. Saunders.
2. Nicholl, J. H. (1909). The surgery of infancy. *British Medical Journal, 2,* 753.
3. Waters, R. M. (1919). The down-town anesthesia clinic. *American Journal of Anesthesia (Suppl.), 33*(7), 71.

4. Lahti, P. T. (1968). Early postoperative discharge of patients from the hospital. *Surgery, 63,* 410–415.
5. Davis, J. E. (Ed.). (1986). *Major ambulatory surgery.* Baltimore: Williams and Wilkins.
6. Gruendemann, B. J., & Meeker, M. H. (1987). *Alexander's care of the patient in surgery.* St. Louis: C. V. Mosby.
7. Wolcott, M. W. (1988). *Ambulatory surgery and the basics of emergency surgical care.* Philadelphia: J. B. Lippincott.
8. Orkand, D. S. (1977). Report to the Society for the Advancement of Free-standing Ambulatory Surgical Care, Chicago, October 1977. *Same Day Surgery, 1,* 97.

▽ ▽ ▽ Chapter 2

▽

▽

▽

Ambulatory Surgical Unit Designs

Dolores Sabia

▽

▽

▽

Ambulatory surgery, the relative newcomer in the surgical arena, holds special requirements and opportunities for design. An attractive, comfortable environment can also allow both the nursing and medical staffs to deliver optimal, safe care. The prolific growth of all ambulatory services has pointed to various forms of basic designs. Ambulatory surgery services, once allowed only a small part of in-hospital space, has now come to the forefront, especially with hospital investors and nonmedical corporations owning and running ambulatory facilities. These operations may physically be a part of the hospital, sharing the facilities and services of the hospital; or they may be "on-campus" facilities that are housed in a separate building on hospital property; or they may be completely free-standing in the community. The purpose of this chapter is to answer the following questions:

1. What strategies are used in designing, planning, implementing, and managing an ambulatory surgical facility?
2. What are the particular ergonomic needs of nurses in patient admission, patient education, family waiting room, operating room, and recovery room areas?

▽

Strategies in Designing Ambulatory Surgery Units

The ambulatory surgical unit (ASU) requires complex design consideration owing to the inherent safety measures required for patients, visitors, and staff. Several regulatory agencies on local, state, and federal levels publish requirements and standards that must be met by ambulatory surgical facilities. The federal standards found in *Guidelines for Construction and Equipment of Hospitals and Medical Facilities* must be followed with regard to basic design.[1] These requirements provide the basic framework from which state licensing requirements and local standards are derived. It is important to be aware of regulations that are in effect in a particular locale to prevent costly design changes. Architectural firms and construction companies that have experience in designing and building ASU areas are generally well versed in noting and conforming to design requirements.

The design and function of ambulatory surgery facilities can be divided into two major areas; physical layout and clinical practice. The former involves structural considerations that are affected by architectural codes, as outlined in (1) *Guidelines for Construction and Equipment of Hospitals and Medical Facilities;* (2) *National Fire Protection Agency (NFPA) Requirements, NFPA Code 101,* which dictates construction requirements, and *NFPA Code 250,* which references building materials, and heating, ventilation, and air conditioning (HVAC) standards; and (3) federal, state, and local plumbing and electrical codes.[1-4]

The location, size, and function of the ASU should be defined clearly to maximize design possibilities. For instance, federal, state, and local codes and professional standards may dictate one design for an in-hospital ASU located on the first floor and a different design for a free-standing center located on the second floor of a medical arts building.

The types of services offered may also dictate variations in the overall physical structure. For example, a facility with services directed toward elderly patients should pay special attention to ease of access, sufficient parking for the handicapped, and the facilities and level of accessibility afforded by the reception area. If the ASU is located on the second floor, wheelchairs should be available at the entrance and an easily accessible storage area be provided so that they are not a hazard to other patients and visitors. The elevators should be near the entrance and should be large enough to accommodate more than one wheelchair. By contrast, a facility providing services to a large pediatric population may benefit from a separate activity area for children that encourages and allows therapeutic play without disturbing other patients and visitors.[5]

Once a strategic plan has been formulated and information regarding the services offered and the patient mix is available, design possibilities should be discussed.[6] Here, clinical practice must start to interact with planned construction. Close attention must be paid to every detail, and occasionally, aesthetic objectives may have to be sacrificed to ensure patient safety or to enhance delivery of care. For instance, nurses must ensure that allowances have been made for adequate storage of medical gases and equipment necessary to evaluate a patient. Limited storage means that staff must leave patients to perform necessary tasks, reducing productivity and increasing cost. Likewise, consideration must be given to the effect of the environment on the patient. For example, a preparatory area for surgery that is open and airy may reduce apprehension and present a bright, cheery environment for the patient [6]

Both free-standing and hospital-based settings are discussed, as many aspects of their overall design are similar. Several design prototypes can be altered to suit the specific needs of the ASU.[2,6] The design chosen must meet patient needs, as well as building code requirements. If a new facility is to be constructed, the design and shape of the facility will dictate the overall interior design. For example, a centrally located patient elevator that is surrounded by spacious corridors may be attractive, but it may also hinder placement of operating rooms in the facility. Likewise, it may be easiest to design physician offices and other departments around the construction of the surgical areas to optimize space for the facility.

Figures 2-1 through 2-4 illustrate several basic ASU designs. As noted, every effort should be made to keep traffic flowing in one direction. This limits contact between preoperative and postoperative patients, thereby enhancing infection control.

The overall appearance of the building forms the patient's first impression of the surgical experience. Whether the surgical facility is free-standing or hospital-based, there should be ample parking and easy access for patients. Sufficient handicapped parking must be provided and must comply with Uniformed Federal Accessibility Standards and the standards established by the American National Standards Institute (ANSI 117.1).[3] A covered patient entrance/exit that is clearly marked can help ease the access problem in a large medical complex with shared parking. If the ASU is located within the hospital, a separate entrance should be provided for its use. If possible, ASU outpatient departments should be placed on the perimeter of the hospital to separate traffic patterns. Once through the door, the patient should have a clear idea of where to go. The ASU frequently is one of the busiest units, with patients and visitors arriving and leaving throughout the day. Locating the ASU on the hospital perimeter usually limits unnecessary traffic throughout the building. A separate area must be provided for the delivery of supplies and linens. This area should be located well away from the patient entrance.

Next, the reception area should be open and airy, with special attention paid to ensuring that this area be as quiet as possible. If there are medical offices or other departments of the hospital using the same entrance, a separate reception and waiting area should be provided for the ASU. Traffic to the ASU should be isolated as soon as possible after entry to the building, as walking a lengthy corridor only heightens a patient's anxiety level.

A staff member should be available in the reception area to greet the patient and family. If registration occurs here, a quiet, private area should be available for the exchange of information. Whenever possible, the waiting area should immediately adjoin the reception desk and should provide facilities for storage of patients' personal belongings.

Access to vending machines, a coffee shop, or the hospital dining room should be provided for waiting families. A separate play area for small

Figure 2-1 On-campus ASU Shawnee Mission Medical Center Day Surgery Unit, Shawnee Mission, KS. (Reprinted with permission.)

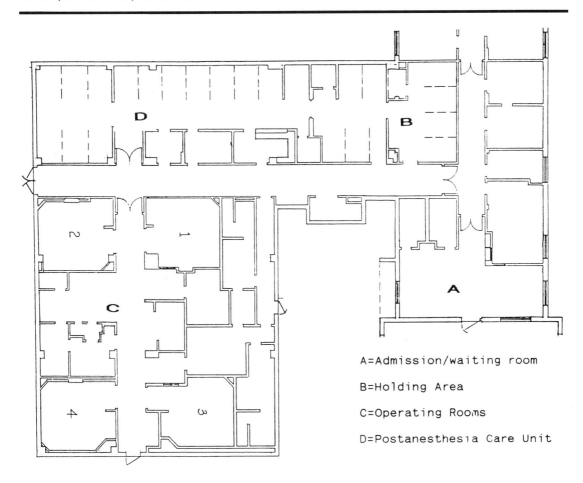

A=Admission/waiting room

B=Holding Area

C=Operating Rooms

D=Postanesthesia Care Unit

children allows the pediatric patient a welcomed distraction and helps to keep waiting brothers and sisters busy.

The appropriate design of the reception area and decisions regarding the use of materials require the help of a designer who has experience in health care and knowledge of federal and local codes.[2] An experienced designer can also help to design the unit with optimal eye appeal without sacrificing safety or comfort. Federal and local codes may dictate the use of fire-retardant materials or fabric and carpets that are antimicrobial.[1-4] At this time, the color scheme of the center may be set. The use of warm, soft colors has been shown to have a positive psychological effect on both patients and visitors.

Figure 2-2 ASU adjoining hospital: Baptist Medical Center, Kansas City, MO. Reprinted with permission.

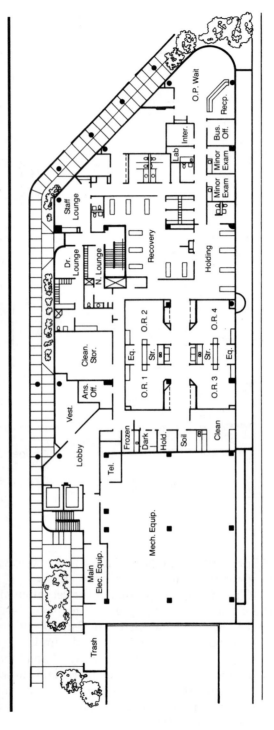

Figure 2-3 In-hospital ASU: Bethany Medical Center, Kansas City, KS (*Clo,* closet; *Toil,* toilet; *J.C.,* janitor's closet; *Sterile Stor,* sterile storage).

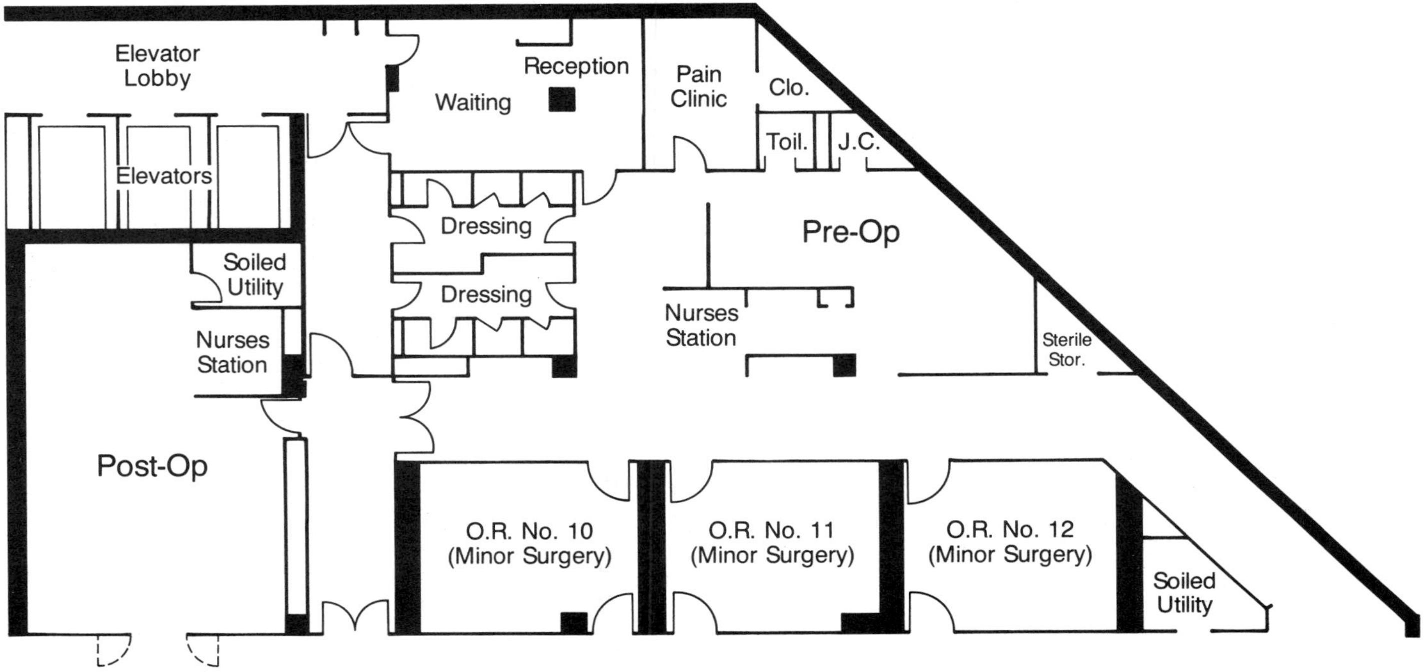

Figure 2-4 Free-standing ASU Southwestern Ambulatory Surgery Center, Pittsburgh, PA (*anest,* anesthesia).

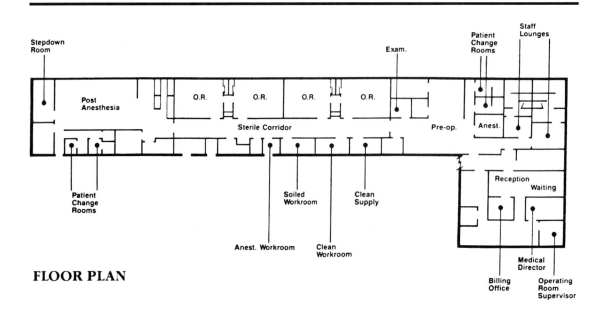

FLOOR PLAN

Ergonomic Needs of Staff

In designing an ASU, the ergonomic needs of the staff are important to consider, and the unit should facilitate efficiency with a minimum of walking. The first clinical area of the ASU is the preoperative or patient evaluation area. Construction guidelines require a preoperative patient assessment area for any facility with more than one operating room.[1-4,6] This assessment area should be convenient and accessible to the nursing and anesthesia staff. Privacy should be provided for interviewing patients. Ideally, the ASU will also contain laboratory and radiologic facilities. Special attention to regulations and codes will determine the area(s) in which x-ray services may be located. To support heavy equipment, some structural changes may be necessary, and special wall construction may be required for radiation safety.

Patient's dressing rooms should provide easy access to the preoperative holding area, and restrooms must also be provided. An optimal design accommodates patient dressing rooms, restrooms, and double-door lockers next to the holding area. Double-door lockers that are accessed from both the preoperative and postoperative areas allow patients to lock up their clothing and personal belongings while maintaining separation of preoperative and postoperative patients. Once patients have changed into hospital clothing, they should not have to enter a public corridor to progress through the ASU.

If an examination or treatment room is to be used for patient care, it should be located so that a patient can change clothes and enter, but the physician does not have to change into surgical attire. The examination room should be as spacious as possible and should include ample storage for supplies so that staff members will not have to leave the room repeatedly for procedural equipment.

There should be good lighting in the examination room. It should be noted that lighting levels or lux (footcandles) differ in different areas.[7] The American College of Surgeons' Committee on Operating Room Environment has determined the level of lighting considered appropriate for the ASU. Their recommendations are that the lighting for regular visual tasks be 100 to 200 lux and that the lighting for special visual tasks be 10,000 to 20,000 lux. The committee recommends illumination rather than task (confined area of work) illumination. Examination rooms, although not required to meet operating room lighting levels, should be well lighted. In addition, the rooms should be equipped with oxygen, a sink for handwashing, an examination table, an otoscope, and any other equipment necessary for patient assessment. The examination room should open into the preoperative area or be immediately adjacent to it so that patients are not moved through public areas.

The preoperative holding area should be spacious and bright. The number of patient units should be equal to or greater than the number of operating rooms so that while one procedure is performed, the next patient scheduled for that operating room can be prepared. The patient bedside units in the holding area should also include space for storage of linen and supplies. Each unit should have access to oxygen and a blood pressure cuff. Privacy curtains must be available in each unit to facilitate preoperative assessment and nursing care. All privacy curtains and draperies must be noncombustible or flame-retardant, and must pass both the large- and small-scale tests required by the NFPA Code 701.[1-4,6] In addition, the construction guidelines for medical facilities dictate that at least 3 feet of clearance space be provided between patient beds and the adjacent walls.[8]

A central area should be provided for the nursing staff to chart and verify surgical permits while observing patients. Additionally, if at all possible, a separate area should be available for pediatric patients. Parents must be present during pediatric nursing assessments, and the trauma of the surgical experience is minimized for the child if parents can stay with them until the time of surgery.

Immediately adjacent to the preoperative holding area is the clean corridor where all personnel wear surgical attire. Entrance to this area must be marked adequately to eliminate access by anyone not dressed in surgical attire. The overall design of this corridor is similar in many surgical facilities; access to supplies, clean utility, dirty utility, each operating room scrub sink, and traffic from staff locker rooms is usually through this corridor. This corridor must be at least 8 feet wide to accommodate the movement of patients and equipment. Standards require that no equipment be stored in the corridor that would interfere with traffic flow.[1-4,6] It is convenient, however, to provide some storage in this corridor, including space for a blanket warmer. Storage cabinets should be placed about 4 feet above the floor, allowing for placement of patient stretchers during surgical procedures. Additionally, dual scrub sinks servicing each operating room are located in the corridor; these should be recessed slightly to accommodate corridor traffic.

The corridor should be designed to provide access to all operating rooms, clean and dirty utility rooms, supply rooms, anesthesia washrooms, and an environmental services area. As this corridor acts as a hub for much of the ASU's activities, it is advisable to install emergency shutoff valves and pressure alarms for anesthetic gas lines, along with annunciator panels for the emergency call system. The guidelines for construction of medical facilities mandate a minumum area of 360 sq. ft. for all general operating rooms, as well as a minimum of 18 feet clear dimension from fixed cabinets or shelves.[1-4,6] When an operating room suite is dedicated to surgical cystoscopy or other endoscopic procedures, the total area, exclusive of cabinets and shelves, must be at least 250 sq. ft.[1-4,6]

Each operating room must be equipped with an emergency communication system and radiograph view boxes that can accommodate at least two x-ray films. Storage cabinets within the operating room should be constructed of solid surface materials with glass paneled doors. The entrance/exit to the operating room should be equipped with extra-wide doors to allow movement of patient stretchers and large equipment. A glass panel on the side wall and door are required to permit observation. Small curtains or panels should be installed to cover these window panels when necessary for patient privacy, or while certain lasers are in use. Information from the laser manufacturer will explain how and when to cover these glass panels, as lasers work with different light wavelengths which may or may not be affected by these glass panels.

Ceilings, walls, and floors must also be constructed from solid material. If ceiling tile, rather than a solid surface, is approved by state or local codes, it must have a solid, washable surface to allow for easy cleaning. Proper placement of air handlers is on the ceiling, and these must accommodate the required fifteen air exchanges per hour, five of which must be outside air. Walls may be solid or vinyl-covered, as allowed by state or local codes, but must be washable. Flooring should be conductive material with heat-sealed seams that prevent moisture seepage. Flooring material should extend up at least four inches onto wall surfaces to eliminate wall–floor seams. [1-4,6]

Special attention should be given to the placement of gas drop lines for anesthesia in order to allow for movement of anesthesia machines within the operating room. The anesthesia scavenger system should also be placed near the drop lines. Scavenging systems are required by many states and are highly recommended in the literature, as trace gases have been linked to both short- and long-term changes in cognitive and motor skills and implicated in certain types of tumors occurring in operating room personnel. Adequate vacuum lines should be available, and proper placement of nitrogen outlets in the operating room suite helps to reduce the potential hazard of long hoses running across the room in the presence of pneumatic power equipment.[1–4,6]

Attention to electrical wiring is important. For instance, if x-ray equipment is to be used, suitable lines should be installed in the rooms. Many new portable units are battery-powered and need only to be plugged into the usual 110-V lines to recharge. The use of certain basic or computerized anesthesia monitoring equipment may require special dedicated electrical wiring. Certain computerized systems also require an energy back-up to eliminate costly recalibration or replacement of parts during a power outage. A dedicated emergency generator is required for operation of the ASU. All outlets with access to the emergency power source must be marked clearly.

Lighting is of special importance in the operating rooms. As discussed earlier, rooms must be well lighted to ensure patient and staff safety.[1–4,6] Special illumination is necessary for the specific "task" of surgery. Several manufacturers supply operating room lights that are approved by Underwriters' Laboratories (UL) and that meet both federal and local codes. The newer models produce a bright, white light that is also a cool light. Another useful function of operating room lights is beam-size selection, which regulates the size (narrow to wide) of the area of illumination. These newer models can also eliminate drift, or movement of the overhead fixture.

The area between the operating rooms, or the substerile area, can be divided into two components. The first is an area for storage of equipment used in the operating rooms, along with closed cabinets to store linen and supplies. The second area is that used for cleaning of equipment. A gravity sterilizer is especially important here to allow "flashing" of instruments when necessary. Adequate counter space and a sink are helpful for the soaking of certain instruments and for handwashing. These areas must also be well ventilated to evacuate steam or fumes from soaking solutions.

An area for instrument handling should be centrally located within the clean corridor. Instruments used in the operating room should be moved quickly to the dirty utility room. Locating the dirty utility room at the center of the clean corridor minimizes the possibility of cross-contamination of instruments and saves time, as the staff does not have to walk to the ends of the corridor. The optimal layout for a dirty utility room includes a pass-through window to the clean utility room for instruments that have been decontaminated.

Usually, the equipment in the dirty utility room includes at least one sink that is wide and deep enough to hold large instruments and trays. This room should also provide enough storage area for cleaning supplies, as well as adequate counter space for holding instrument trays before processing. A separate area to handle soiled linen is required. The Joint Commission on Accreditation of Hospitals and Ambulatory Facilities requires that clean and soiled linen be kept separate at all times.[6] An area must be available to store soiled linen until it can be removed for processing. A hopper can accommodate disposal of solutions and cleaning of debris. A sonic washer large enough to hold large instruments and trays is also important in this area. This washer can lift debris that may remain on instruments after gross cleaning has been completed.

Certain manufacturers also make available a washer/sterilizer unit which performs a third step in instrument processing, utilizing detergents to surgically clean the instruments. The washer/sterilizer has both a back and front door so that objects can be placed in it from the dirty utility room and can be removed from the clean utility room. At the end of the cycle, these instruments are clean and safe for handling in the clean work area.

The clean utility room should be adjacent to the dirty utility room. As mentioned, a pass-through window obviates the need for staff to move from room to room. The clean utility room comprises two areas. The first work area is for wrapping and sterilization of instrument trays; it should also contain some cabinets for storage of supplies and wrappers. Once instrument trays are clean, they can be wrapped or processed for final sterilization.

The second area is for storing sterilized equipment and instrument trays. Sterilization equipment can consist of two types. Gravity or vacuumatic sterilizers utilize super-heated steam and a drying cycle. Although gravity and vacuumatic sterilizers are similar, the vacuum type eliminates air in all directions, and may reduce the time needed for the sterilizing cycle. The action of the vacuumatic type may also reduce wear and tear on equipment with articulating parts, thus prolonging use. Moreover, the vacuumatic type does not require turning of equipment that contains air pockets, such as basins or medicine cups. By contrast, gravity sterilizers release steam in a downward (or gravity) direction and thus have the potential disadvantage of trapping small pockets of air, thereby negating complete sterilization.

The second type of sterilizer uses a gas—ethylene oxide (ETO)—to sterilize equipment. It can be used to sterilize articles that cannot be submerged, such as those made of plastic or rubber material, cameras, and instruments with lenses. Although this type of sterilizer meets the requirements for sterilization, many additional standards govern its operation. Both the Environmental Protection Agency (EPA) and the Occupational Safety and Health Administration (OSHA) have established specific construction requirements for the housing and ventilation of

ETO.[1-4,6] New regulations also require periodic testing of areas in which ETO sterilizers are housed and operated.

As mentioned earlier, the clean corridor must also contain a janitor's closet, or environmental services area. This area holds cleaning supplies for use in cleaning operating rooms during the operation hours and for terminal cleaning at the end of the day. A sink suitable for handling large buckets of cleaning solutions, as well as a storage area for cleaning supplies, should be included in this area.

The major supply area for the ASU should be near the clean corridor. Delivered supplies should be taken out of their shipping cartons before being stored. This supply room may also accommodate some of the very large equipment used in the ASU. Locating this room near the operating room minimizes the distance and time involved in moving supplies.

After surgery, patient care is continued in the postanesthesia recovery unit. Although the ambulatory setting provides services for less complex cases and the administration time for anesthesia is usually shorter, the anesthetics used are of the same type as those used in the main hospital operating room. Therefore, both inpatients and outpatients require similar recovery facilities, the only difference being that invasive monitoring procedures are usually not necessary in the latter.

The overall design of the recovery area should facilitate the observation of all patients. A centrally located nurses' station, equipped with a sink and medication area, can help keep the nursing staff at the patient's bedside. An ample storage area for linen and supplies, along with an area for an ice machine and access to blanket warmer, should be available. At bedside, there should be access to oxygen, some supplies, a work space for charting, and cubicle curtains. Because surgical patients must be observed closely for airway maintenance and stabilization of vital signs, the emergency cart may also be kept in the recovery area. An area should also be provided for physicians to dictate or otherwise record postoperative information. It is also advisable to incorporate into the design of the recovery area a section dedicated to the care of pediatric patients. This area should be large enough to accommodate parental visitation and ideally, should be located some distance from other patient areas to minimize any disturbance caused by a crying child.

As patients progress to the second stage of recovery from anesthesia, they may be moved to another section of the main postanesthesia recovery area. This area may be located in a separate part of the main recovery area, or it may be immediately adjacent to it. As these patients are not yet discharged, nursing personnel must still be present at all times. This area should contain a patient restroom and dressing area to allow patients to prepare for discharge.

The postanesthesia recovery unit should contain enough square footage to accommodate 2.5 patient units for every operating room.[1-4,6] Affording the patient easy access to the discharge door and to parking helps to avoid any unnecessary walking. Since the Joint Commission on Accreditation of Hospital Organization (JCAHO) and state regulatory bodies require that the patient be discharged with adequate instruction for home care, a small area with seating can allow both patients and family members to review the instructions and ask any questions of the nursing staff.[6] It is preferable to discharge patients directly from the center rather than moving these patients through the reception area again.

▽

Summary

The information presented in this chapter represents a basic foundation for an ASU. It must be noted that careful attention must be paid to federal, state, and local codes. It is advisable to tour a variety of centers and to make projections regarding surgical services and patient mix before deciding on a particular design. As new technologies allow the transfer of more inpatient services to ambulatory units, additional changes may be necessary to adapt to changing client needs.

References

1. U.S. Department of Health and Human Services. (1987): *Guidelines for construction and equipment of hospital and medical facilities.* Washington, DC: U.S. Government Printing Office.
2. Erdman, M., et al. (1989). *Organizing, designing and building ambulatory health care facilities.* Madison, WI.
3. Office of the Federal Register National Archives and Records Administration (1987, July). *Code of Federal Regulation* (Labor 29, Parts 1900–1910). Washington, DC: U.S. Government Printing Office.
4. *The American Institution of Architects Committee on Architecture for Health (with assistance from the U.S. Department of Health and Human Services).* (1987). Washington, DC: The American Institute of Architects Press.
5. Patterson, J. M. (1988). Children's surgicenter keeps parents and patients together. *Health Facility Management, 1*(2), 17–18.
6. The Joint Commission on Accreditation of Health Care Organizations, 1990 (1989). *A.H.C. ambulatory health care standards.* Chicago, IL: The Joint Commission on Accreditation of Health Care Organizations.
7. Patterson, P. (1985). Designing an outpatient surgery facility. *OR Manager, 1*(3), 3.
8. O'Donavan, T. R. (1978). *Ambulatory surgical centers: Development and management.* Germantown, MD: Aspen Systems Corporation.
9. Fellows, G. E. (1987). Ambulatory surgery design. A consultant's perspective on facility planning. *AORN Journal, 46*(3), 708–724.

Bibliography

Berkoff, M. J. (1981). Planning and designing ambulatory surgery facilities for hospitals. *Journal of Ambulatory Care Management, 4*(3), 35–51.

Brickell, N. (1986). Hospital-based ambulatory surgery: History, marketing, staffing, and remodeling. *Journal of Post Anesthesia Nursing, 1*(3), 202–204.

Dachart, C. (1989). The joy of building a free-standing ambulatory surgery center. *Journal of Post Anesthesia Nursing, 4*(2), 106–108.

Ernhart, S. W. (1987). Alternative solutions for common ambulatory surgery problems. *AORN Journal, 46*(2), 1156, 1158–1161.

Howarth, P., & Kirchoff, K. T. (1986). Problems of post-anesthesia care of ambulatory surgerical patients. *Nursing Management, 17*(2), 34J–34N.

Hyna, W., & Gutmann, C. (1984). *Management of surgical facilities.* Rockville, MD: Aspen Publications.

Meshenberg, K., & Burns, L. (1983). *Hospital ambulatory care. Making it work.* Chicago: American Hospital Association.

Noon, B. E., & Davero, C. C. (1987). Patient satisfaction in a hospital-based day surgery setting. *AORN Journal, 46*(2), 306, 308, 310–312.

Radoszewski, P. H. (1986). The ambulatory surgery center nurse. *Nurse Management, 17*(1), 43–48.

Roth, R. A. (1986). Use of AORN recommended practices: Applications in ambulatory surgery. *AORN Journal, 45*(5), 991–999.

Wetchler, B. V. (1985). *Anesthesia for ambulatory surgery.* Philadelphia: J. B. Lippincott.

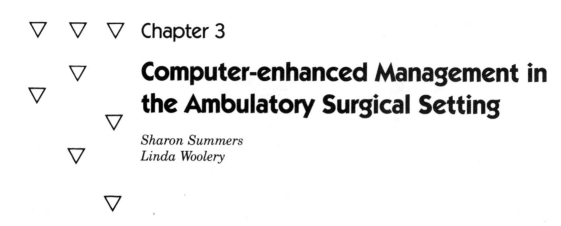

Chapter 3

Computer-enhanced Management in the Ambulatory Surgical Setting

Sharon Summers
Linda Woolery

Computer technology has become commonplace in many businesses, including health care agencies. Health care agencies have tended to use computer technology for revenue-generating processes, such as billing charges from pharmacy, laboratory, and radiologic services. A nationwide random survey of 228 hospital nurses conducted by Summers, Ratliff, Becker, and Resler[1] found that only 9 percent of the information entered into the computer by nurses was for the purpose of charting nursing care. Computer programs that can facilitate billing processes can certainly be expanded to facilitate nurses' charting of patient care. There are many textbooks currently available that contain information about computer system capabilities, and these are cited at the end of this chapter. It is not the intent of this chapter to present an in-depth discussion of computer hardware architecture or software design. However, an overview of computer applications in ambulatory surgical nursing is presented, and Figure 3–1 illustrates and defines some computer hardware. Some will argue that computer "downtime" results in chaos; however, this can be said for any electronic device, and the users need to establish routines for periodically saving information. As all computer systems evolved from paper systems, if downtime is prolonged, then paper systems can be resumed.

The use of computers to assist nurses in managing ambulatory surgical patient care is explored in this chapter by answering the following questions:

1. How can computers be used for structured preoperative teaching?
2. How can computers be used to document nursing care based on nursing diagnosis using the North American Nursing Diagnosis Association (NANDA) taxonomy?

Exhibits for Chapter 3 are located at the end of the chapter on pages 41–66.

Figure 3-1 Computer peripherals.

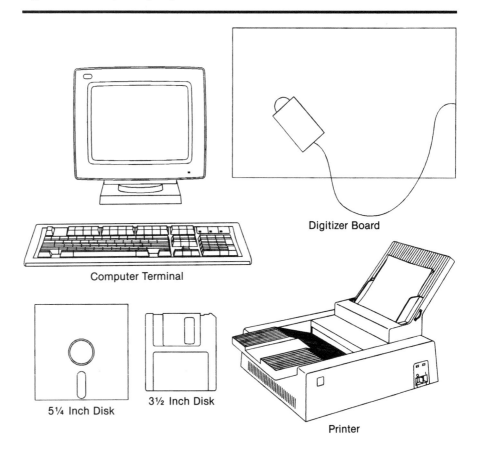

Digitizer Board

Computer Terminal

5¼ Inch Disk

3½ Inch Disk

Printer

3. How can computers assist the nurse in ambulatory surgical patient management from admission through discharge?
4. How can nurses use computers to manage staffing and scheduling, billing, purchases, and inventories?
5. What is the relationship between computerized patient data bases, quality assurance reports, and research?

▽

Computerized Preoperative Patient Teaching

There have been numerous approaches published relating to patient education techniques.[2-4] A common problem that occurs between the publication of a patient education technique and the implementation phase is the applicability to actual patient situations in different geographic areas. There is a lack of standardization of perioperative care, by both physicians and nurses, across the country, and so when patient education strategies used on the East Coast are published, they may not be applicable to the Midwest or West Coast. Another problem is the compilation of a paper file extensive enough to contain all possibilities of patient education information and to make it all available at the nurses' fingertips. A solution to both standardization and large paper files can be found using computer systems.

Computerized patient education information could consist of an electronic library containing a wide variety of patient education materials that could be tailored for each specific surgical procedure and physician preference. Instead of using printed "one form fits all" materials, the nurse could create a specific form for specific patient needs by taking pieces of information and creating a whole form. The pieces could be such items as instructions for dietary restrictions (e.g., nothing by mouth), prepping the skin with special soaps, definitions of the surgical procedures, the scheduled arrival time at the unit, and the like. The nurse could "cut and paste" these pieces electronically, enter the patient's name, and produce an individualized teaching plan. This information could then be sent to the patient at the time the surgical case was scheduled, and would include a telephone number where the patient could call for additional information. The following case study illustrates computerized preoperative patient education strategies.

Case Study

Peggy Wilson is a college graduate and the owner/manager of the Happy Hollow Day Care Center. She was seen by her doctor for the chief complaint of left wrist pain on extension that interfered with lifting small children. She was diagnosed as having a left wrist ganglion. (A ganglion is a tendon sheath pouch that usually contains synovial fluid, produces discomfort, and limits range of motion.[5])

At the time that Peggy's surgery is scheduled, the nurse could cut and paste an electronic preoperative teaching form individualized for Peggy. Although it is assumed that, as a college graduate, Peggy can read and write, consideration must be given to Peggy's busy schedule and the need for specific, factual information, such as that presented in Exhibit 3–1. Although there is much information that could be added to the preoperative patient teaching form, it should be brief, easy to read, and pertinent to the individual patient. The five-point information sheet depicted in Exhibit 3–1 can easily be assembled, printed, and mailed to Peggy, or any other patient for whom it is appropriate, when using computer-generated forms. Other uses for computers in ambulatory surgical nursing include nursing diagnosis "libraries."

▽

Computerized Documentation Using Nursing Diagnosis

As will be discussed in depth in Chapter 4, nursing diagnosis is the pivotal point in the implementation phase of the nursing process for patient

Figure 3-2 Computerized links in nursing diagnosis.

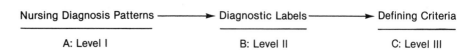

Nursing Diagnosis Patterns ⟶ Diagnostic Labels ⟶ Defining Criteria

| A: Level I | B: Level II | C: Level III |

care. Problems that prevent the implementation of nursing-diagnosis–based patient care include lack of available nursing diagnosis information for practicing nurses. As can be seen in Figure 3–2, computerized nursing diagnosis libraries could facilitate the use of nursing diagnosis by nurses. Figure 3–2A displays the first level, or main menu, computer screen for nursing diagnosis pattern selection. When a pattern is selected, the next level is accessed and the screen then would list the diagnostic label (Fig. 3–2B). Once a diagnostic label is selected, the next level, the defining criteria (characteristics), is assessed (Fig. 3–2C). When an example of an ambulatory surgical patient such as Peggy Wilson, is applied to this three-part process, it is easy to see how a nursing diagnosis could be derived.

Nursing Diagnosis: An Example

A nursing diagnosis pattern that would be applicable to Peggy's problem is *moving,* as she has pain upon extension of her left wrist. If *moving* is selected from the pattern menu, Figure 3–3, Level I, then the next level menu would relate to diagnostic labels (Fig. 3–3, Level II). If *Impaired Physical Mobility* is selected from this menu, then the next level menu would permit selection of the defining criteria (Fig. 3–3, Level III). The

Figure 3-3 Computerized links in nursing diagnosis: Example of a patient with a left wrist ganglion.

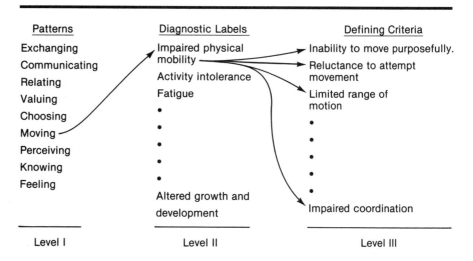

Patterns	Diagnostic Labels	Defining Criteria
Exchanging	Impaired physical mobility	Inability to move purposefully.
Communicating		Reluctance to attempt movement
Relating	Activity intolerance	
Valuing	Fatigue	Limited range of motion
Choosing	•	•
Moving	•	•
Perceiving	•	•
Knowing	•	•
Feeling	•	•
	Altered growth and development	Impaired coordination
Level I	Level II	Level III

nurse could then select the defining characteristic of limited range of motion. Selection of this nursing diagnosis could then be written as *Impaired Physical Mobility related to (R/T) limited range of motion, left wrist.* Once a nursing diagnosis is made, a standardized care plan can be selected from a care plan "library." Just as the use of nursing diagnosis can be enhanced with computerization, so can management of other aspects of the ambulatory surgical patient record.

▽

Computerized Ambulatory Patient Information Management

Computers are an effective means for managing patient information. Computer data bases provide ambulatory surgical perioperative nurses with a powerful tool for entering, storing, and retrieving large volumes of data. A well-designed ambulatory surgery computer data base enables nurses and other perioperative staff to enter a piece of patient information only once, and then that information becomes available to all other personnel (called end-users). Thus, the patient data base, which is available to the registration clerk, the nurse, the surgeon, the anesthesiologist, and all others who have authorization to access the computer information, eliminates the need for the patient to answer the same demographic questions repeatedly. For example, a patient's address, phone number, and birthdate are pieces of information that are frequently entered into a computer data base by the clerk. Once this information becomes part of the data base, members of the health care team can access this information simultaneously, thereby obviating the need for the patient to repeat the information. In order to compare and contrast computer applications in the ambulatory surgical setting, paper (hard copy) versus computer-generated charts are compared.

▽

Paper Chart System

Most nurses are all too familiar with the paper system for patient admission to the ambulatory surgical unit (ASU). The usual sequence of events begins with the completion of a series of forms by the admission clerk, including such information as a patient demographic data base, health insurance information, and laboratory data forms. The patient then is asked to sign the admission consent form. The paper charts are then assembled and the patient receives an identification bracelet/tag. Typically, the nurse completes the patient admission process by having the patient sign the surgical consent form and escorting the patient to a holding area to change into a hospital gown. The nurse then helps the patient onto a cart, assesses and records pertinent patient information on the paper chart, and sees to it that the patient is appropriately prepped, if ordered, and medicated as ordered. Part of the nurse's job is to record nursing care and to complete requisitions for all charge items.

The patient is then transported to the operating room (OR), at which time the intraoperative nurse charts all aspects of patient care, and completes all requisitions for OR supplies and equipment. During the postoperative phase, the postanesthesia nurse charts the care given to the patient, documents patient education instruction, plans for discharge, and completes requisition forms for all supplies used. Upon discharge, the nurse "signs off" on the chart, which is then returned to the admission clerk so the physician can dictate an operative note. Ultimately, the chart is transferred to the medical record department. These are the routines typically performed by nurses in the ambulatory surgical setting; they have been described by some nurses as "paper shuffling" activities, as the nurse's desk is usually cluttered with charts. The same process will now be described, using the example of the admission of Peggy Wilson, when the ASU is computerized.

▽

Computerized Chart System

When the ASU is computerized, the admission clerk enters into the computer Peggy's demographic data base and health insurance information, and then asks her to sign the electronic surgical consent form. This is done by using a digitizer board, which is a small board that allows the user to enter script information with an electronic pencil (see Fig. 3–1). Thus, the patient's script signature is entered directly into the computer. Macro keys can be used to store ASU charts and then to retrieve a new patient's chart automatically.

As Peggy's name is entered into the computer, the information is sent to the printer so that a bracelet/tag can be printed that also includes her patient identification number printed in bar code format. As the clerk completes Peggy's admission record, all requisitions are sent electronically to the laboratory, and the record is automatically sent to the computer at the nurses' station.

Peggy is then escorted to a holding area to change into a hospital gown. The nurse then helps her onto a cart and completes an assessment of Peggy. This assessment information is recorded by touching the computer screen with a light pen. The nursing diagnoses of *Impaired Physical Mobility R/T limited range of motion, left wrist* and *Fear R/T the surgical experience* are selected from the nursing diagnosis library, and a preoperative nursing care plan is selected and edited from the care plan library. A standardized care plan is then edited and personalized for Peggy; it includes typical patient education and discharge planning strategies for a patient with limited wrist mobility (Exhibit 3–2). When preparing preoperative medications, the nurse gains access to the narcotic cabinet with a magnetic card (which is far simpler than 15 nurses sharing, and thus having to search for, one narcotic key). Use of the magnetic card automatically triggers a record of the date, time, and nurse's identification number. When Peggy is prepped and medicated, appropriate information is entered into the computer by scanning both her identification bracelet/bar code tag and the bar codes on the prep kit and medication packages. When the scanned information is entered onto the electronic chart, the charges are automatically sent to the business office, and information relating to inventory adjustment is received in the central services and pharmacy departments. In addition, the narcotic record is sent to the pharmacy. This process automates record keeping and reduces the number of steps involved in tracking medications and supply charges.

Peggy is then taken to the OR and her record is electronically transferred to the computer terminal in the OR. Data from the intraoperative nursing assessment and appropriate nursing diagnoses are then added to the preoperative care plan. As the surgical procedure is completed, the intraoperative nurse charts all aspects of patient care by directly entering data into the computer using the keyboard (Exhibit 3–3). The charges are then sent to the business office electronically and the OR inventory is adjusted.

During the postoperative phase, the care plan is adjusted for Peggy's individualized needs (Exhibit 3–4). The nurse charts the care given to Peggy, electronically retrieves, prints, and documents patient education information; and electronically retrieves, prints, and documents discharge planning information for her friend who is driving her home.

All postanesthesia supply charges are sent electronically to the appropriate departments, at which time inventories are adjusted, and charges are forwarded to the business office. Upon Peggy's discharge, the nurse signs off on the chart using the digitizing board; thus, the nurse's script signature is entered into the electronic record. Physicians can access the patient's record from any computer terminal where convenience may facilitate rapid completion of the operative note. The electronic record can then be transferred to medical records and cleared from the screens in the ASU. Although this example has described documentation of the care of a single patient, computer systems are capable of capturing, generating, or retrieving numerous electronic patient records, a process that is analogous to retrieving file folders from a file cabinet.

Paper and electronic charts have been compared to illustrate the differences between the two methods of record keeping. Because many nurses are aware of the mountain of papers involved in patient care, the computerized method could offer welcome relief from this tedious task. Mountains of paperwork are also frequently encountered in the day-to-day operations of the ASU; these operations, too, can be managed efficiently by computers. Should the computer system "crash," a means by which data can be processed manually should be available, and should be well planned during computer installation.

▽

Computerized Management of the Ambulatory Surgical Unit

Computer applications for the management of ASUs are proliferating. Computer vendors sometimes consult with nurses when designing computer software, but most often, software is developed by non-nurse data programmers with little nursing input. Nurses need to become knowledgeable about computer hardware (i.e., the computer) in order to capitalize on their many uses and to make educated decisions during the selection process.

Numerous computer vendors offer products designed for the perioperative setting that could also be used in ASUs. The annual meeting of the Association of Operating Room Nurses (AORN) provides a wonderful opportunity for perioperative nurses to evaluate most, if not all, perioperative computer system vendors under one roof. Although there is only a limited capacity to evaluate a system in a busy conference booth, it is possible to eliminate some systems that would not meet institutional criteria and to select several that do meet established criteria. Table 3–1 offers a partial listing of perioperative computer system vendors. Currently, there are computer software packages (the instructions to operate the computer) available to create surgeon preference cards (Exhibit 3–7), control inventory, manage patient billing (Exhibit 3–8), create the OR record (Exhibit 3–9), generate both narrative (Exhibits 3–10 through 3–21) and graphic (Figs. 3–4 and 3–5) reports, automate surgery scheduling (Figs. 3–5 and 3–6), generate nursing reports (Fig. 3–6 and Exhibits 3–22 through 3–25), generate intraoperative records (Exhibit 3–26), generate recovery room reports (Exhibit 3–27), and discharge planning reports (Exhibit 3–28). In addition, it is possible to generate reports on periop-

Table 3-1 Perioperative Computer Vendors

Atwork Corporation
  100 Europa Drive, Suite 250
  Chapel Hill, NC   27514
  (919) 929-1313

Baxter Healthcare Corporation
  Operating Room Division
  1425 Waukegan Road
  McGraw Park, IL   60085
  (312) 473-0550

ComputOR
  3020 Bridgeway, Suite 399
  Sausalito, CA   94965
  (800) 262-7887 (outside CA)
  (800) 331-4305 (in CA)

DeRoyal Industries, Inc.
  DBS Division
  200 DeBusk Lane
  Powell, TN   37849
  (800) 331-4215

Enterprise Systems
  233 Waukegan Road, Suite East 10
  Bannockburn, IL   60015
  (312) 940-1600

Ethicon, Inc.
  (A Johnson & Johnson Company)
  PO Box 151
  Somerville, NJ   08876
  (201) 218-0707

Medical Software Systems, Inc.
  1864 S. State Street, #25
  Salt Lake City, UT   84115
  (800) 366-3677

Medinvent, Inc.
  163 Engle Street
  Englewood, NJ   07631
  (800) 447-7899

Serving Software, Inc.
  2221 University Ave., SE
  Minneapolis, MN   55414
  (800) 328-7786

Figure 3-4 A computer-generated graph depicting operating room utilization. (Reprinted by permission, ORBIT Software, Enterprise Systems, Inc., 2333 Waukegan Road, Bannockburn, IL 60015-1503.)

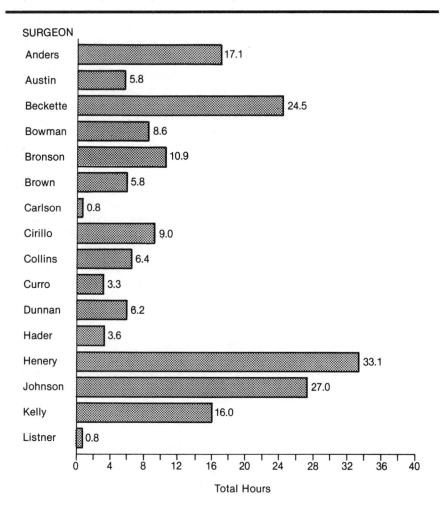

erative staff scheduling, quality assurance and risk management, and unit management, as well as nursing care plans. In addition, computerized data bases can be used to generate statistical reports regarding daily, weekly, monthly, and annual OR census data, including procedures, types of anesthesia used, daily room utilization, turnover time between cases, case mix analysis, and causes of delays.

▽

Integrated Computerized Systems

Idealistically, there is a need for OR software packages to be integrated, or designed to work together. Realistically, the nurse can expect to find

Figure 3-5 Computer-generated graph of operating room utilization organized by month. (Reprinted by permission, ORBIT Software, Enterprise Systems, Inc., 2333 Waukegan Road, Bannockburn, IL 60015-1503.)

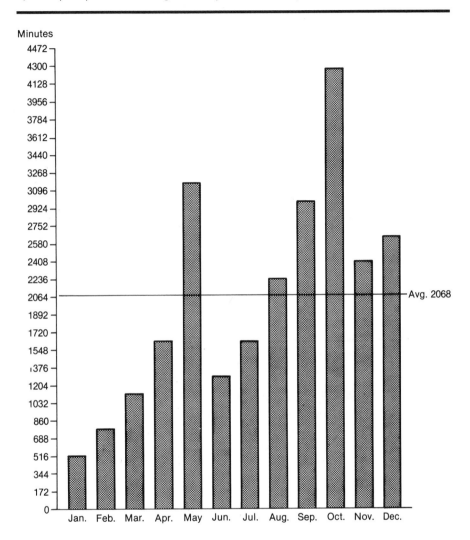

several systems or modules that combine inventory, billing, surgeon preference cards, and management reporting. Unfortunately, nursing care plans are rarely included in these packages. An example of an integrated system might be as follows.

A physician's office secretary telephones the ASU to schedule a patient for a surgical procedure. The ASU clerk then uses the integrated computer software to enter the patient's name and procedure, to schedule the surgical suite, the surgeon, the anesthetist, and the scrub and circulating nurses, and to list the equipment needed for the procedure. The

Figure 3-6 Sample of a computerized graphic report.

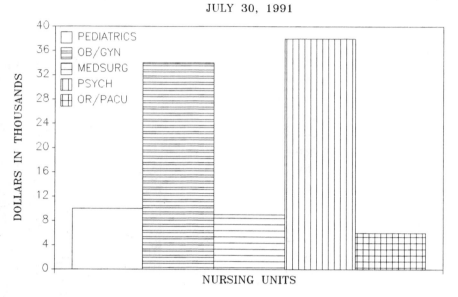

software allows for cross-checking to ensure that the surgical suite, all physicians involved , and the necessary equipment are available on the scheduled date and time, thereby eliminating double scheduling errors. The scheduling module then electronically links to the inventory module, checking for routinely used supplies. If supplies are unavailable, the inventory control person is electronically notified as to what supplies need to be ordered.

The software can automatically assemble and print the OR schedule the day before surgery. If the perioperative computer system is linked to the hospital mainframe, then the surgery schedule can be viewed on monitors throughout the institution. On the day of surgery, the circulating nurse receives a computer-generated copy of the surgeon's preference card, which is used to retrieve the inventory supplies needed for the surgical procedure. The items listed on the surgeon's preference card can be charged to the patient's account automatically. If inventory items are charged but not used, then the OR staff can credit the patient's account accordingly.

During surgery, the circulating nurse can document all surgery-related information via the computer, rather than on paper. Although a printed copy of the computerized document can be made available, chart storage is usually available on magnetic tape in the medical records department.

The advantages of on-line documentation include speed, legibility, accuracy, and completeness provided the documentation system is well designed and has benefited from adequate input from those nurses who will be using the system.

▽

Similarities Between Data Bases, Quality Assurance Reports, and Research Reports

The use of computers has been described for patient education, nursing diagnosis, patient care, and unit management. Computers are also an effective means of retrieving data bases for quality assurance reports and research projects. Data bases, quality assurance reports, and clinical research studies all require that a variety of information or data be collected. The differences in data collection for each depend on the intended purpose of the information, as will be seen in the following description of the three techniques.

A *data base* is usually defined as a collection of facts about people or things. In the ambulatory surgical setting, this could involve personnel, patients, or supplies (see Exhibits 3–10 through 3–21 and Figs. 3–4 and 3–5). In such a setting, data bases are acquired and edited daily with regard to patients and supplies. When the ASU is computerized, it is easy to retrieve data to determine the type of surgical procedures performed, the length of time required for procedures, and the names of the nurses assigned to specific patients or procedures. It is also easy to determine which supplies (e.g., 3-0 chromic sutures) are used most frequently in order to base purchases on high-volume usage.

Quality assurance reports are usually defined as standards that are established to measure how well an institution delivers care. Quality assurance reports are a form of research whereby records are reviewed to collect data about standards of professional care and justification of services. Records may be reviewed during the patient's stay or after the patient is discharged. In ASUs, quality assurance usually takes the form of a retrospective, or after-discharge, chart review. Retrospective reviews of records, however, are considered to be the weakest form of data collection because the reviewer may "read" something into the previously written account, resulting in a biased interpretation. For example, the omission of documentation by a nurse who usually documents patient care very well may prompt the reviewer to give credit for something not charted because of the reviewer's bias that this nurse always charts accurately. Data collection is usually laborious, and analysis usually consists of descriptive statistics, such as means, frequencies, and percentages.

When patient records are computerized, the data bases can be accessed for quality assurance or audits using large samples. For example, if a nurse wanted to know how many patients had undergone arthroscopic procedures during the past 12 months, the computerized data bases could be sorted by procedure (arthroscopy) and date (January to December). The computerized list of cases performed during the past 12 months could then be printed in the time it would take to review one chart. When quality assurance reports are based on computer retrieval of information, there is a decreased likelihood that bias will affect the interpretation of the patient record.

Data bases and quality assurance reports can be used in research studies just as a review of literature might be used, whereby the nurse "looks back" on past cases or problems to formulate research questions. For example, the ambulatory surgical nurse might ask the clinical research question: How well is pain controlled at home in patients who have undergone tubal ligation? Data bases and quality assurance reports could then be reviewed to determine the frequency of this procedure so the nurse could estimate the number of patients that could be asked to participate in a prospective study.

A research study is defined as the systematic collection and analysis of data where attempts are made to reduce error during data collection and analysis so that the results are an accurate measure of reality. Research studies usually begin prospectively with hypotheses or research questions, and then progress to data collection with error minimized; subsequent data analysis frequently includes both descriptive and inferential statistics. As this technique requires data collection before or at the same time as patient record formulation, research studies must be approved by institutional human subjects review boards, and forms must be created to obtain the patient's signed, informed consent to participate. The purpose of data analysis and interpretation is to answer specific research questions or to determine whether a particular hypothesis is supported by the data.

For example, a study could be designed in such a way that, as patients were admitted for tubal ligation procedures, the nurse could ask patients to participate in the study. Upon obtaining a signed consent, the nurse could also collect data, by using a diary or questionnaire, after the patient was sent home. Data collected in this manner would be strictly for the purpose of answering the research question. Data analysis and interpretation would also be for the purpose of answering the research question. As seen in Table 3–2, there are similarities in information items among the three categories.

Research can also be conducted during the delivery of routine patient care using data from a patient's chart; this type of research requires institutional approval but not informed consent. For example, a study was conducted to document the incidence of postanesthesia hypertension in normotensive patients.[7] It was not possible to determine who would become hypertensive during the postanesthesia period; therefore, the institutional human subjects committee waived informed consent while requiring the protection of patient confidentiality and anonymity.

Table 3-2 Information Included in Data Bases, Quality Assurance, and Research Reports

Data Base	Quality Assurance	Research
Name	Age	Age
Address	Sex	Sex
Age	Diagnosis	Diagnosis
Sex	Length of stay	Nursing diagnosis
Birthdate	Acuity	Acuity
Social Security number	DRG	Medications
Insurance	Insurance	Treatments
Employer	Treatments	Vital signs
Hospital number	Medications	
Diagnosis	Primary physician	
Physician's name	Consulting physicians	
	Nursing diagnosis	

Summary

This chapter has answered the five questions pertaining to computer applications in ASUs listed earlier. Computer technology can be used effectively for the purpose of streamlining the flow of patient information. Patient assessments and nursing care plans can be facilitated by easy retrieval and editing of computerized libraries. Preoperative patient education can be personalized, and discharge planning can be initiated at the time of admission. Computers can also be used to manage the administrative tasks of staffing, scheduling, billing, purchasing, and inventory control. When patient data bases, quality assurance reports, and clinical research studies are defined, it can be concluded that information in the form of data bases is at the heart of each. Further nursing diagnosis and computer applications will be presented in the various chapters throughout this text.

References

1. Summers, S., Ratliff, C., Becker, A., & Resler, M. (1988). Computerized nursing diagnosis documentation of nursing care in inpatient health care agencies. Classification of nursing diagnosis. *Proceedings of the Eighth NANDA Conference*. Philadelphia: J. B. Lippincott.
2. Dixon J., Gruyd, N., & Varricchio, D. (1975). A computerized education and training record. *Journal of Continuing Education, 6*, 20–23.
3. Redman, B. (1984). *Patient teaching*. St. Louis: C. V. Mosby.
4. Reilly, D. (1982). A computerized patient information system. *Nurse Manager 13*, 32–36.
5. Grundemann, B. J., & Meeker, M. H. (1987). *Alexander's care of the patient in surgery*. St. Louis: C. V. Mosby.

6. Saba, V., & McCormick, K. (1986). Essentials of computers for nurses. Philadelphia: J. B. Lippincott.
7. Summers, S., Dudgeon, N., & Schmitting-Dubin, J. (1988). Postanesthesia hypertension in normotensive young adult males: A pilot study. *Journal of Post Anesthesia Nursing, 3*,(5), 324–331.

Exhibit 3-1 Preoperative teaching form.

SUBJECT: Preoperative Patient Teaching

PATIENT: Peggy Wilson

SCHEDULED SURGERY: Ganglion Left Wrist

DATE: Wednesday, December 26, 1990

TIME: 8:00 a.m.

PLACE: Ambulatory Surgical Unit

You are scheduled for surgery in the Ambulatory surgical Unit at the above listed date and time. The following information is given to help provide you with the best service:

1. Do not eat or drink after midnight on Tuesday (night before your scheduled surgery). Fluids will be given to you as soon as you are awake enough to drink.

2. Please scrub your left wrist with antibacterial soap for 5 minutes the night before surgery. This will reduce the risk of infection since these soaps decrease skin surface bacteria.

3. Please plan to arrive at the Ambulatory Surgical Unit at 7:15 a.m. the morning of your scheduled surgery in order to complete the admission procedures. Parking is available across the street from the Ambulatory Surgical Unit.

4. Please arrange to have someone drive you home the day of surgery. Medications you will receive will make you drowsy and the dressing that will be applied to your left wrist will hinder driving a car.

5. Please bring your insurance card with you the day of surgery. The name of the company and your insurance policy number will help the hospital to quickly manage your billing. If you do not have insurance, be prepared to discuss financial arrangements for your bill.

Exhibit 3-2 Preoperative nursing care plan.

Patient: Peggy Wilson   Id Number:

765432

Nursing Diagnosis: 1. Impaired Physical Mobility R/T limited
                        range of motion left wrist
                    2. Fear R/T the surgical experience

Assessment	Plan	Intervention	Evaluation
B/P 128/68 P. 72, R 16 Temp 98.2 Hgb 13.2 gms	VS stable Tag and bag belongings		
Patient states she is nervous about having surgery.	Explain all procedures and provide emotional support. Inform intra-operative nurses of need for emotional support.	Procedures explained. Spent time with the patient to decrease fears. Inform intraop nurses of patient's fears.	Smiling and more relaxed.

41

Exhibit 3-4 Postoperative nursing care plan.

Patient: Peggy Wilson   Id. Number: 765432

Nursing Diagnosis: 1. Impaired Skin integrity R/T incision

2. Impaired physical mobility R/T medications

Assessment	Plan	Intervention	Evaluation
B/P 100/60 P 88, R. 12 Temp 97 O2 sat 98% Skin cool to touch DSD to lt wrist, no drainage. Responds to name		Monitor VS-----Done (see attached graphic) Warmed Blankets-Done next to skin Monitor DSD-----Done When awake,dress and ambulate	Uneventful recovery from anesthesia. Temp 98 Dressing remain dry and intact. Patient dressed, and ambulated with no problems. Education Booklet discussed with patient as to dressing remaining intact and seeing Dr. Blade in two days. Discharged at 10:30, driven away.

Exhibit 3-3 Intraoperative nursing care plan.

Patient: Peggy Wilson   ID Number:765432

Nursing Diagnosis: 1. Fear R/T surgical experience

2. Impaired skin integrity R/T incision

Assessment	Plan	Intervention	Evaluation
Peggy Wilson Dr. Blade LT Ganglion Seems calm	Verify ID Verify surgeon Verify procedure Admit to room 4 Move to table Knee strap on Provide emotional support during induction Padding and correct placement of tourniquet on limb Prep wrist, hand, and arm	-------Done ---Done -Done --Done ----Done ----Done --------Done ------Done ------Done	Procedure completed No observed problems Induction smooth Prep completed Charges completed Specimen to lab DSD to left wrist

Exhibit 3-5 Automatic scheduling of surgery. (Reprinted by permission, ORBIT Software, Enterprise Systems, Inc., 2333 Waukegan Road, Bannockburn, IL 60015-1503.)

COUNTY GENERAL HOSPITAL
OPERATING ROOM SCHEDULE
SATURDAY, OCT 01, 1988

Page 1

PROC TIME	PATIENT NAME SURGEON	PAT. AGE	SEX	ROOM NO.	PROCEDURE	ANESTHESIA
SUITE 01						
07:30 08:30	VRONSKY, ALEXI AMUNDSEN TAYLOR	49	M	315A	REPAIR DETACHED RETINA SCLERA BUCKLE AND IMPLANT LEFT EYE	GEN MATHEWS
08:30 10:30	KENT, JOHN BOWMAN MCCARTHY	89	M	301A	BELOW KNEE AMPUTATION	CHOICE HELPER
14:00 16:00	LARSON, LOIS BOHIGIAN CLEMENS	49	F	222C	SUPRACLAVICULAR MASS EXCISION MEDIASTINOSCOPY	GEN CARLSON
SUITE 02						
07:00 09:00	OLSON, SVEN ABDO HENERY	38	M	316	REPAIR DETACHED RETINA SCLERA BUCKLE AND IMPLANT LEFT EYE	GEN STEVENS OBANA
09:50 11:50	HENNEGAN, CINDY BECKETTE HANSON	40	F	223C	SUPRACLAVICULAR MASS EXCISION MEDIASTINOSCOPY	GEN CARLSON
SUITE 03						
07:30 08:30	SMITH, BOB ANDREWS	25	M	345A	ARTHROSCOPY - DIAGNOSTIC AND INTRA-OPERATIVE ARTHROSCOPY	GEN CONSTANTIN
09:00 12:00	GREEN, PERRY WILSON JOHNSON	56	M	202B	SUPRACLAVICULAR MASS EXCISION	GEN FOX
13:15 15:15	TATSUHAKI, FRANCES WILSON JOHNSON	56	M	305A	SUPRACLAVICULAR MASS EXCISION	GEN FOX
SUITE 04						
08:00 09:00	KARSTEN, JACK SPARACINO	61	M	230	REPAIR DETACHED RETINA SCLERA BUCKLE AND IMPLANT LEFT EYE	GEN BATRA
09:00 10:00	KUMMERER, GREG SPARACINO	26	M	262	REPAIR DETACHED RETINA SCLERA BUCKLE AND IMPLANT LEFT EYE	GEN BATRA
10:05 11:05	CASHMAN, THOMAS SPARACINO	67	M	239B	REPAIR DETACHED RETINA SCLERA BUCKLE AND IMPLANT LEFT EYE	GEN BATRA
11:15 11:45	GARCIA, MARIA SPARACINO	33	F	256C	CRYOPEXY LEFT EYE	GEN BATRA
12 Procedures Scheduled						

Exhibit 3-6 Automatic scheduling of surgery. (Reprinted by permission, ORBIT Software, Enterprise Systems, Inc., 2333 Waukegan Road, Bannockburn, IL 60015-1503.)

COUNTY GENERAL HOSPITAL
SURGERY SCHEDULE
FRIDAY, APR 21, 1989

TIME DUR.	SURGEON	PATIENT NAME SEX	PAT. AGE	ROOM. NO.	X	B	PROCEDURE	ANESTH.	EXTRA EQUIPMENT
7:30 AM 03:30	MILLER C VILLARS	MONTMARTE, SHEILA F	4	IP 450-2	Y	N	CHOLECYSTECTOMY; POSSIBLE CHOLANGIOGRAM; POSSIBLE COMMON DUCT EXPLORATION PATIENT IS BLIND	GEN BAILEY	
11:00 AM 03:24	MILLER C COLLINS	O'BRIEN, MAUREEN F	48	IP 530-2	N	Y	MASTECTOMY; RIGHT	GEN LATSON	
8:00 AM 01:30	MURRAY	LOHMAN, ELIZABETH F	4	IP 600	N	N	PLASTIC REPAIR OF FACIAL LACERATIONS CHILD WAS BITTEN BY A DOG.	GEN GUEDALIA	CARDIAC MONITOR
7:30 AM 08:14	TRUE LISTNER	SHADE, BRUCE M	49	IP 506-2	Y	Y	RADICAL NECK DISECTION; RIGHT POSSIBLE INSERTION OF TITANIUM BASKET	GEN PALMER	
7:00 AM 01:48	WILSON	WILLIAMS, GARY M	34	IP 4023-1	N	N	CARPAL TUNNEL RELEASE RIGHT HAND	BLOCK LOPEZ	
9:00 AM 05:00	WILSON DUNNAN	BOWMAN, ROBERT M	21	IP 123-2	Y	Y	CRANIOTOMY	GEN PERUSEK	

Exhibit 3-7 Computerized surgeon preference card.

```
DR PREFERENCE CARD FOR DR SMITH          GLOVE SIZE: 7½
************************************************************************
PROCEDURE:   APPENDECTOMY          *    POSITION:  SUPINE
_____

SUPPLIES:                          *    SUTURE:
BASIC SETUP PACK    MAJOR TRAY     *    ? 0 CHROMIC TIES
? RAYTEC                           *    ? 2-0 CHROMIC TIES
? MARKING PEN                      *    ? 3 OR 4-0 PDS RB-1
? 6650 STERIDRPE                   *    ? 0 OR 2-0 VICRYL SH X 3 ACC TO SIZE
CULTURE TUBE AVAILABLE             *    ? 4-0 VICRYL RB-1
#15 BLADES X 2                     *    ? 5-0 VICRYL CPS-3
SCRATCH PAD                        *    _____
NEEDLEPOINT                        *    PREP: BETADINE SOLUTION/ALCOHOL
? SUCTION                          *    _____
                                   *      DRESSING:
                                   *      ? ½" STERISTRIPS
                                   *      ? TELFA
                                   *      BENZOIN AMPULES
_____    *
DRUGS:                             *
ASK ABOUT ANTIBIOTICS              *
_____
    ! RETURN                              ! ACCEPT
```

Exhibit 3-8 Computer-generated record of operating room charges.

```
                    OPERATING ROOM CHARGES
***************************************************************
ENTERED BY:          PROCESS DATE: 09/11       DATE OF SERVICE: 09/07
                     PROCESS TIME: 07:59
PATIENT: BEAR, Y                               PT. BILLING #: 999999
SURGEON:

    ITEM CHARGED FOR            QUANTITY      SERVICE CODE

SKIN STAPLER                       1          03111952
WIRE SUTURE                        1          03152204
DACRON PATCH                       1          03160561
PENROSE                            1          03104544
FOLEY CATHETER                     1          03110806
                                                          >
                                                          >
```

Exhibit 3-9 Computerized record of operating room charges.

```
    OPERATING RECORD:   THIRD SCREEN   ROOM #:
    PATIENT:  BEAR, Y                MR#: 555555   BILLING #:  999999
    =====================================================================

    ESTIMATED BLOOD LOSS:   LESS THAN 10CC_____
    URINE OUTPUT:  NONE IN O.R.        __
                                                !PROBE HERE IF SURGERY
                                                 IS CANCELLED
                MEDICATIONS GIVEN:
       DRUG(S)        DOSE          METHOD              BY WHOM?      TIME
    NONE GIVEN IN O.R._____  _____   _____   _____
    _____     _____   _____   _____
    _____     _____   _____   _____
                                    _____   _____   _____
    POSTOP DIAGNOSIS   SEROUS OTITIS MEDIA         _____

    *PF5* TRANSFERRED TO: RECOVERY ROOM_____   BY:  SMITH, RN AND JONES, MD___
                                          AND BY:<_____>
    *PF6* ANY DELAYS?   NONE_____

    =====================================================================
                        *PF1* FOR FURTHER REMARKS
    *PF13* TO CANCEL AND START OVER                 PRESS ENTER TO CONTINUE
```

Exhibit 3-10 Sample surgery delay reports (sorted by surgeon). (Reprinted by permission, ORBIT Software, Enterprise Systems, Inc., 2333 Waukegan Road, Bannockburn, IL 60015-1503.)

COUNTY GENERAL HOSPITAL

RPT5515 - DELAY REPORT
Sorted By Surgeon

Page   1

Delay Code	Time	Surgeon	Anesth.	Procedure	Procedure Date Patient Type	Suite Shift	Start End	Jrnl No.
Surgeon: ANDERS								
01	00:10	ANDERS PIFFINI	VERMONT STOLLEN	D. LARYNGOSCOPY/BRONCHOSCOPY	05/04/86 IP	05 DAY	10:45 11:25	38
		Total Delays ANDERS: 1						
Surgeon: BECKETTE								
03	00:12	BECKETTE	PATTERSON	TOTAL HIP ARTHROPLASTY	05/17/86 IP	04 DAY	12:30 14:55	95
		Total Delays BECKETTE: 1						
Surgeon: BRONSON								
03	00:15	BRONSON	JONES CARLSON	ARTHROSCOPY - DIAGNOSTIC INTRA-OPERATIVE ARTHROSCOPY	05/06/86 IP	03 DAY	09:30 11:00	146
10	00:10	BRONSON CURRO	JONES FOX	RE-CRANIOTOMY RESECT POSTERIOR FOSSA TUMOR	05/01/86 IP	02 DAY	12:35 17:00	4
HL	00:15	BRONSON	PATTERSON STARR	REV OF VP SHUNT RIGHT	05/01/86 IP	08 DAY	10:10 11:40	23
		Total Delays BRONSON: 3						
Surgeon: CURRO								
SL	00:20	CURRO WILSON	STRAUS SMITH	REV VENT DRAINAGE SYSTEM RIGHT	05/02/86 IP	02 DAY	13:00 14:20	26
		Total Delays CURRO: 1						
Surgeon: DUNNAN								
02	00:10	DUNNAN	MATHEWS HELPER	EXTRACAPSULAR CATARACT EXTRACT WITH INTRA OCCULAR LENS INSERTION	05/16/86 IP	04 DAY	09:40 11:30	111
		Total Delays DUNNAN: 1						
Surgeon: HENERY								
02	01:00	HENERY	PATTERSON	CORONARY ARTERY BYPASS SAPHENOUS GRAFT	05/16/86 IP	05 DAY	14:00 20:25	133
TL	00:30	HENERY RAOUL	STOLLEN HOUSTON	D. LARYNGOSCOPY/BRONCHOSCOPY	05/01/86 IP	06 DAY	13:45 14:15	18

Exhibit 3-11 Sample surgery delay reports (sorted by service/surgeon). (Reprinted by permission, ORBIT Software, Enterprise Systems, Inc., 2333 Waukegan Road, Bannockburn, IL 60015-1503.)

COUNTY GENERAL HOSPITAL

RPT5513 - PATIENT TYPE SUMMARY
Sorted By Service/Surgeon
Printed MAR 10, 1989   Page 1

	IP		OP		AA			Total	
Surgeon	Cases	Mins.	Cases	Mins.	Cases	Mins.		Cases	Mins.
Service : CV									
ANDERS	1	245	0	0	0	0		1	245
GOLDBERG	4	1535	0	0	0	0		4	1535
HENERY	5	1780	0	0	0	0		5	1780
JOHNSON	1	115	0	0	0	0		1	115
MENG	1	375	0	0	0	0		1	375
MORANI	3	545	1	55	0	0		4	600
PIFFINI	6	1385	1	55	0	0		7	1440
SHELLY	1	375	0	0	0	0		1	375
CV Subtotals	22	6355	2	110	0	0		24	6465
Service : ENT									
CURRO	0	0	1	120	0	0		1	120
ENT Subtotals	0	0	1	120	0	0		1	120
Service : ENT/BRONCH									
BOWMAN	2	160	2	190	0	0		4	350
BROWN	0	0	2	150	0	0		2	150
CARLSON	0	0	1	45	0	0		1	45
CRUMPET	0	0	1	45	0	0		1	45
DUNNAN	0	0	1	50	0	0		1	50
HENERI	1	35	0	0	0	0		1	35
HENERY	1	30	0	0	0	0		1	30
LISTNER	0	0	3	200	0	0		3	200
MORANI	5	225	4	265	0	0		9	490

Exhibit 3-12 Surgery cancellation reports (sorted by surgeon). (Reprinted by permission, ORBIT Software, Enterprise Systems, Inc., 2333 Waukegan Road, Bannockburn, IL 60015-1503.)

COUNTY GENERAL HOSPITAL

RPT5516 - CANCELLATION REPORT
Sorted By Surgeon

Page   1

Cancellation Code Date By	Surgeon	Anesth.	Procedure	Procedure Date	O.R. Suite	Shift	Jrnl No.
Surgeon: ANDERS							
NS 05/26/89 MILLAR-HOGAN	ANDERS HENERY	HELPER FOX	CORONARY ARTERY BYPASS	06/02/89	09	DAY	118
Total Cancellations ANDERS: 1							
Surgeon: AUSTIN							
PS 05/26/89 SLATTENGREN	AUSTIN	STINE	ARTHROSCOPY - DIAGNOSTIC INTRA-OPERATIVE ARTHROSCOPY LEFT SHOULDER	05/31/89	14	DAY	127
Total Cancellations AUSTIN: 1							
Surgeon: BECKETTE							
WU 05/26/89 WALCZAK	BECKETTE	STINE	ARTHROSCOPY - DIAGNOSTIC INTRA-OPERATIVE ARTHROSCOPY RIGHT KNEE	05/30/89	13	EVE	128
Total Cancellations BECKETTE: 1							
Surgeon: HENERY							
NL 05/26/89 CARLSON	HENERY	DANIELS	EXPLORATORY THORACOTOMY OR LOBECTOMY	05/16/86	07	DAY	135
PS 05/26/89 ZEPPENFELD	HENERY	DOLLIN	EXPLORATORY THORACOTOMY OR LOBECTOMY	05/06/86	08	DAY	117
RU 05/26/89 CARLSON	HENERY	STOLLEN	PROSTATECTOMY	06/01/89	02	DAY	131
SU 05/26/89 HENERY	HENERY	DOLLIN	CORONARY ARTERY BYPASS WITH SAPHENOUS GRAFT	05/31/89	08	DAY	141
Total Cancellations HENERY: 4							
Surgeon: PIFFINI							
AU 05/26/89 SLATTENGREN	PIFFINI	STARR	CORONARY ARTERY BYPASS WITH SAPHENOUS GRAFT	06/01/89	04	EVE	138
Total Cancellations PIFFINI: 1							

Exhibit 3-13 Operating room activity statistics (sorted by procedure). (Reprinted by permission, ORBIT Software, Enterprise Systems, Inc., 2333 Waukegan Road, Bannockburn, IL 60015-1503.)

COUNTY GENERAL HOSPITAL

RPT5518 - O.R. ACTIVITY STATISTICS
Sorted By Procedure
Printed MAY 30, 1989

Procedure	Number of Procedures	Total Time	Average Time	Set-Up	Patient In Room	AVERAGE ACTIVITY TIMES Anesth	Operation	Clean-Up	Recovery Room
AORTIC BYPASS	1	3:50	3:50	0:10	4:00	4:00	3:15	0:10	0:00
APPENDECTOMY	1	1:25	1:25	0:10	1:05	1:00	0:40	0:10	0:00
ARTHROGRAM	1	1:55	1:55	0:15	1:25	1:25	1:12	0:15	0:00
ARTHROSCOPY - DIAGNOSTIC	5	10:05	2:01	0:12	1:42	1:41	1:32	0:10	0:00
CAROTID ENDARTERECTOMY	1	3:20	3:20	0:10	3:00	2:55	2:30	0:10	0:00
CESAREAN SECTION	2	2:05	1:03	0:08	0:50	0:44	0:28	0:05	0:00
CESAREAN SECTION - STAT	1	0:55	0:55	0:05	0:55	0:55	0:30	0:15	0:00
CHOLECYSTECTOMY	1	2:25	2:25	0:10	2:10	2:05	1:45	0:05	0:00
CLEFT PALATE REPAIR/EAR EXAM	1	2:35	2:35	0:20	2:05	2:05	1:55	0:10	0:00
CLOSED REDUCTION	1	1:15	1:15	0:05	1:05	1:05	0:50	0:05	0:00
COLOSTOMY	1	1:45	1:45	0:15	1:15	1:15	0:50	0:15	0:00
CORONARY ARTERY BYPASS	6	38:55	6:29	0:13	6:01	5:58	5:22	0:15	0:00
CRANIOFACIAL RECONSTRUCTION	1	12:27	12:27	0:45	11:22	11:20	9:45	0:20	0:00
CRANIOTOMY	1	2:25	2:25	0:15	2:00	1:55	1:30	0:10	0:00
CYSTOSCOPY	5	4:50	0:58	0:08	0:37	0:34	0:20	0:13	0:00
D. LARYNGOSCOPY	1	0:25	0:25	0:05	0:15	0:15	0:10	0:05	0:00
D. LARYNGOSCOPY/BRONCHOSCOPY	9	7:05	0:47	0:05	0:37	0:37	0:29	0:05	0:00
EXC GIANT NEVUS THIGH	1	2:20	2:20	0:05	2:10	2:10	1:35	0:05	0:00
EXP THORACOTOMY OR LOBECTOMY	1	1:55	1:55	0:10	1:05	1:00	0:55	0:10	0:00
EXTRACAPSULAR CATARACT EXTRACT	4	8:35	2:09	0:10	1:51	1:21	1:46	0:08	0:00
FEMORAL TIBIAL BYPASS	3	9:30	3:10	0:12	2:50	2:49	2:27	0:08	0:00
GASTROSCOPY/INST.BROVIAC PAREN	1	2:40	2:40	0:10	2:35	2:35	2:15	0:10	0:00
GASTROSTOMY, EXP & DRAIN	1	1:20	1:20	0:20	0:50	0:50	0:40	0:10	0:00
INC/DRAIN/BIOPSY INGUINAL AREA	1	0:40	0:40	0:05	0:25	0:25	0:15	0:15	0:00
INCISION/DRAIN POST AUR ABCESS	1	0:35	0:35	0:05	0:15	0:15	0:07	0:15	0:00

Exhibit 3-14 Block time utilization report (sorted by block code and surgeon). (Reprinted by permission, ORBIT Software, Enterprise Systems, Inc., 2333 Waukegan Road, Bannockburn, IL 60015-1503.)

COUNTY GENERAL HOSPITAL
BLOCK TIME UTILIZATION - REPORT 5519
SORTED BY BLOCK CODE/SURGEON

Page: 3

Surgeon	Surgeon Qualified?	Block Time Allocated	Block Time Used	Percent Block Time Used
Block Code: OB/GYN				
BRONSON	N		4:25	4.91
DUNNAN	N		2:45	3.06
HADER	N		2:00	2.22
KELLY	N		4:30	5.00
Qualified Time Totals:			0:00	0.00
Unqualified Time Totals:			13:40	15.19
Block Code Totals:		90:00	13:40	15.19
Block Code: OBGYNE				
BECKETTE	N		5:20	19.05
Qualified Time Totals:			0:00	0.00
Unqualified Time Totals:			5:20	19.05
Block Code Totals:		28:00	5:20	19.05
Block Code: OPEN TIME (UNBLOCKED)				
ANDERS			3:47	
AUSTIN			1:15	
BECKETTE			6:45	
BOWMAN			2:20	
BRONSON			3:15	
CARLSON			0:45	
CIRILLO			4:00	
COLLINS			6:25	
DUNNAN			3:25	
HADER			1:40	

52

Exhibit 3-15 Anesthesia statistics (sorted by anesthesiologist). (Reprinted by permission, ORBIT Software, Enterprise Systems, Inc., 2333 Waukegan Road, Bannockburn, IL 60015-1503.)

COUNTY GENERAL HOSPITAL

RPT5523 - ANESTHESIA STATISTICS
Sorted By Anesthesiologist
Printed JUN 01, 1989   Page 1

Anesthesia Type	Number Of Procedures	Total Minutes	Average Minutes	Minimum Minutes	Maximum Minutes
Anesthesiologist: FOX					
EPIDUR	1	60	60	60	60
GEN	2	77	39	35	42
GEN/SP	1	42	42	42	42
Anesthesiologist: HOUSTON					
GEN	6	670	112	80	170
Anesthesiologist: JACKSON					
GEN	5	535	107	15	215
Anesthesiologist: JONES					
GEN	13	1205	93	30	225
Anesthesiologist: KARSTEN					
LOCAL	1	15	15	15	15
GEN/SP	1	45	45	45	45
GEN	1	35	35	35	35
Anesthesiologist: MIKE					
BLOCK	2	0	0	0	0
Anesthesiologist: O'KEEFE					
GEN	3	105	35	15	60
Grand Totals	36	2789			

This Report Includes : All Procedures

Records Extracted By:
Anesthesiologist=
 KARSTEN, MIKE, O'KEEFE, FOX, HOUSTON, JACKSON, JONES
Records Printed: 11
Report Complete.

Exhibit 3-16 Operating room suite utilization (sorted by service). (Reprinted by permission, ORBIT Software, Enterprise Systems, Inc., 2333 Waukegan Road, Bannockburn, IL 60015-1503.)

COUNTY GENERAL HOSPITAL

RPT5525 - SUITE UTILIZATION
Sorted By Service

Page 1

Service	Number of Cases	Total Time Used	Total Time Available	Pct. Time Utilized
CV	0	0:00		0.0
ENT	2	4:00		0.0
GEN	1	1:45		0.0
GU	0	0:00		0.0
NEURO	0	0:00		0.0
ORTHO	1	1:30		0.0
PLASTIC	0	0:00		0.0
SERVICE	3	8:00		0.1
	———	———		
Grand Totals	8	17:15		
Totals for 9 Rooms Used			7420:00	0.2
Totals for 21 Rooms Available			12424:30	0.1

Exhibit 3-17 Implant listing (sorted by patient name). (Reprinted by permission, ORBIT Software, Enterprise Systems, Inc., 2333 Waukegan Road, Bannockburn, IL 60015-1503.)

COUNTY GENERAL HOSPITAL

Page 1

RPT5528 - IMPLANT LISTING
Sorted by Patient Name

Implant Description Size and Anatomical Site	Implant No. Hospital No.	Mfg. Code Catalog	Series Lot Number	Patient Name Medical Record No.	Surgeon Service	Date Suite	Journal Number
MAMMARY 250MM, LEFT BREAST	7866	DOW MI4250	2453 6781394	COOPER, CRIS 222309	CIRILLO PLASTIC	06/01/89 05	191
SPINAL ROD 12, SPINE	4322	ZIM H34782-12	16483 1759342	GOLD, EVERETT 345990	KITTNERS ORTHO	06/01/89 01	196
PACEMAKER CHEST	3443	HOWMED 234-2388-8766	6780 1326486	HEMSLEY, BLANCHE 234533	BECKETTE CV	06/01/89 09	193
SKULL PLATE 2X3, TEMPORAL	5546	AIC G22414-2	S16843 56478	RAGASE, TREY 334596	BOND NEURO	06/01/89 06	194
KIDNEY KIDNEY	1187	LD	LIVE DONOR	SCHMIDT, LINDA 344112	PIFFINI GU	06/01/89 04	197
SKULL PLATE 2X3, TEMPORAL	3667	AIC G22416-3	S16942 59987	SHIELDS, GEORGE 222590	ALLAND NEURO	06/01/89 07	192

Records Extracted By:
Manufacturer Code =
DOW
ZIM
HOWMED
AIC
LD

Records Printed: 6
Report Complete.

Exhibit 3-18 Case start time analysis (sorted by service/surgeon). (Reprinted by permission, ORBIT Software, Enterprise Systems, Inc., 2333 Waukegan Road, Bannockburn, IL 60015-1503.)

COUNTY GENERAL HOSPITAL

RPT5539 - CASE START TIME ANALYSIS
Sorted By Service/Surgeon
Printed MAR 10, 1989

Page 1

Surgeon	On Time Start Number	Percent	Early Start Number	Percent	Late Start Number	Percent	Total Number	Percent
Service: ENT/BRONCH								
BOWMAN	1	50.00	0	0.00	1	50.00	2	100.00
HENERY	0	0.00	0	0.00	1	100.00	1	100.00
MORANI	1	50.00	0	0.00	1	50.00	2	100.00
PIFFINI	1	100.00	0	0.00	0	0.00	1	100.00
RAOUL	0	0.00	0	0.00	2	100.00	2	100.00
TENDELL	0	0.00	0	0.00	1	100.00	1	100.00
Service: GENERAL								
ANDERS	1	33.33	0	0.00	2	66.67	3	100.00
BOWMAN	1	20.00	1	20.00	3	60.00	5	100.00
CIRILLO	4	100.00	0	0.00	0	0.00	4	100.00
COLLINS	0	0.00	0	0.00	1	100.00	1	100.00
HADER	0	0.00	0	0.00	1	100.00	1	100.00
HENERY	1	100.00	0	0.00	0	0.00	1	100.00
JOHNSON	1	100.00	0	0.00	0	0.00	1	100.00
MORANI	0	0.00	0	0.00	1	100.00	1	100.00
RAOUL	1	9.09	1	9.09	9	81.82	11	100.00
TENDELL	4	30.77	2	15.38	7	53.85	13	100.00
Grand Totals	16	32.00	4	8.00	30	60.00	50	100.00

Unscheduled Cases Not Included: 63

On time cases started within 5 minutes of scheduled start time.

Records Extracted By:
Service=
ENT/BRONCH, GENERAL

Exhibit 3-19 Laser usage report (sorted by surgeon). (Reprinted by permission, ORBIT Software, Enterprise Systems, Inc., 2333 Waukegan Road, Bannockburn, IL 60015-1503.)

COUNTY GENERAL HOSPITAL

RPT5543 - LASER USAGE REPORT
Sorted By Surgeon
Printed JUN 01, 1989   Page   1

Procedure	Surgeon	Patient Name / Medical Record Number	Laser Serial No.	Mode	Watts
LARYNGOSCOPY EXC. OF PAPILLOMAS WITH LASER	MORANI PIFFINI	SAMSON, CASSIE 336868	YG16374	INT	15
LARYNGOSCOPY EXC. OF PAPILLOMAS WITH LASER	MORANI PIFFINI	SIMPSON, GRETA 336868	YG16374	INT	15
REMOVAL VAGINAL WARTS	SANTORE	JAMISON, ELLEN 23908654	D-959-93	INT	15
CERVICAL CONE	TENDELL	VAN DER MEER, JANICE 08402840	A75845-Z	CONT	20

This Report Includes All Cases.
This Report Extracted From:

Records Printed: 4
Report Complete.

Exhibit 3-20 Procedure time comparison (sorted by service/surgeon). (Reprinted by permission, ORBIT Software, Enterprise Systems, Inc., 2333 Waukegan Road, Bannockburn, IL 60015-1503.)

COUNTY GENERAL HOSPITAL

RPT5551 - PROCEDURE TIME COMPARISON
SORTED BY SERVICE/SURGEON
PRINTED JUN 01, 1989

Page 2

Surgeon	PL Number	Procedure	SCHEDULED Start / End	Duration	ACTUAL Start / End	Duration	Difference Time	Percent
JOHNSON	15	CYSTOSCOPY	12:00 13:00	60	12:00 12:50	50	10	16.67
JOHNSON	10	L NEPHRECTOMY	07:30 12:30	300	07:50 12:55	305	5-	1.67-
JOHNSON		URETERAL REIMPLANT LEFT	09:00 12:38	218	09:20 12:58	218	0	0.00
JOHNSON SubTotals	Procedures: 3			578		573	5	0.87
GU SubTotals	Procedures: 3			578		573	5	0.87
Service: NEURO								
BRONSON		INSERTION OF VP SHUNT RIGHT SIDE	10:30 12:30	120	10:40 12:25	105	15	12.50
BRONSON		RE-CRANIOTOMY RESECT POSTERIOR FOSSA TUMOR	12:00 13:00	60	12:35 17:00	265	205-	341.67-
BRONSON		REV OF VP SHUNT RIGHT	10:00 11:00	60	10:10 11:40	90	30-	50.00-
BRONSON SubTotals	Procedures: 3			240		460	220-	91.67-
KELLY	22	CRANIO-CERVICAL DECOMPRESSION	08:00 12:30	270	07:55 12:25	270	0	0.00
KELLY	42	INSERTION OF VP SHUNT RIGHT	07:30 09:15	105	07:40 09:15	95	10	9.52
KELLY SubTotals	Procedures: 2			375		365	10	2.67
NEURO SubTotals	Procedures: 5			615		825	210-	34.15-
Total Procedures:	11			1478		1743	265-	17.93-

58

Exhibit 3-21 Operating room utilization by month (sorted by service/surgeon). (Reprinted by permission, ORBIT Software, Enterprise Systems, Inc., 2333 Waukegan Road, Bannockburn, IL 60015-1503.)

COUNTY GENERAL HOSPITAL

RPT5544 - O.R. UTILIZATION BY MONTH
SORTED BY SERVICE/SURGEON
PRINTED MAR 10, 1989

Page 1

Surgeon	JAN	FEB	MAR	APR	MAY	JUN	JUL	AUG	SEP	OCT	NOV	DEC	Yearly Total	Monthly Average
						NUMBER OF MINUTES								
Service: GU														
JOHNSON	0	340	170	0	510	170	0	0	0	0	680	170	2040	170.00
Service: NEURO														
JOHNSON	0	1200	0	0	0	0	0	0	0	0	0	0	1200	100.00
KELLY	0	180	0	0	0	0	90	180	0	0	0	0	450	37.50
Service: ORTHO														
TENDELL	60	120	60	60	0	0	0	0	60	0	0	0	360	30.00
Totals	------	------	------	------	------	------	------	------	------	------	------	------	------	
	60	1840	230	60	510	170	90	180	60	0	680	170	4050	337.50

Number of months used to compute average: 12

Time is calculated using Operation time.
This Report Includes All Cases
Records Extracted By:

Report Complete.

Exhibit 3-22 Procedure cost, revenue, and nursing investment (sorted by surgeon). (Reprinted by permission, ORBIT Software, Enterprise Systems, Inc., 2333 Waukegan Road, Bannockburn, IL 60015-1503.)

COUNTY GENERAL HOSPITAL
RPT5521 - PROCEDURE COST, REVENUE AND NURSING INVESTMENT
Sorted By Surgeon
Printed JUN 01, 1989

Service	Surgeon	Pref. List	Journal Number	Procedure	Cost	Revenue	Nursing Time
GENERAL	CIRILLO	54	87	EXPLORATORY LAPAROTOMY	3142.75	4327.00	6:00
GENERAL	CIRILLO	71	89	TOTAL ABD HYSTERECTOMY	2678.00	5500.00	7:10
GENERAL	CIRILLO	54	147	EXPLORATORY LAPAROTOMY	3142.75	4327.00	6:00
GENERAL	CIRILLO	71	148	TOTAL ABD HYSTERECTOMY	2678.00	5500.00	7:10
				Surgeon CIRILLO Totals:	11641.50	19654.00	26:20
GENERAL	TENDELL	4	7	EXC OF INGROWN TOENAIL LEFT NAIL	350.00	500.00	2:30
GENERAL	TENDELL	11	10	D. LARYNGOSCOPY/BRONCHOSCOPY ESOPHAGOSCOPY	523.00	1200.00	1:30
GENERAL	TENDELL	23	20	INGUINAL HERNIORRHAPHY RIGHT	1470.65	3400.00	1:30
GENERAL	TENDELL	41	21	INGUINAL HERNIORRHAPHY RIGHT/CIRC. LEFT INGUINAL EXPL	1550.00	3400.00	4:10
GENERAL	TENDELL	32	31	GASTROSTOMY, EXP & DRAIN	3300.95	6500.00	1:40
GENERAL	TENDELL		32	COLOSTOMY	3568.50	7000.00	2:30
GENERAL	TENDELL	36	45	RECTAL BIOPSY WITH FROZEN SECTIONS	1083.85	1850.00	3:15
GENERAL	TENDELL	8	61	INC/DRAIN/BIOPSY INGUINAL AREA RIGHT	1595.50	3400.00	0:50
GENERAL	TENDELL	23	68	INGUINAL HERNIORRHAPHY RIGHT	1500.25	3400.00	2:45
GENERAL	TENDELL	9	69	INGUINAL HERNIORRHAPHY LEFT	1550.00	3400.00	1:40
GENERAL	TENDELL	25	70	ORCHIDOPEXY RIGHT HERNIORRHAPHY	1277.30	1650.00	3:10
GENERAL	TENDELL	51	77	INGUINAL HERNIORRHAPHY BILATERAL	1625.25	3400.00	2:45
GENERAL	TENDELL	27	78	GASTROSCOPY/INST.BROVIAC PAREN ALIMENTATION CATH	1656.75	3500.00	6:10
GENERAL	TENDELL	45	86	REPR. PECTUS EXCAVATUM	2156.23	4500.00	8:30
GENERAL	TENDELL		142	CYSTOSCOPY			0:33
GENERAL	TENDELL		153	CERVICAL CONE			0:00
GENERAL	TENDELL	11	154	D. LARYNGOSCOPY/BRONCHOSCOPY ESOPHAGOSCOPY	523.00	1200.00	1:30
GENERAL	TENDELL	11	155	D. LARYNGOSCOPY/BRONCHOSCOPY ESOPHAGOSCOPY	3568.00	5476.00	1:30
GENERAL	TENDELL	11	156	D. LARYNGOSCOPY/BRONCHOSCOPY ESOPHAGOSCOPY	3568.00	5476.00	1:30
				Surgeon TENDELL Totals:	30867.23	59252.00	47:58

This Report Includes Primary Surgeons Only

Surgeons: TENDELL , CIRILLO
Records Printed: 23
Report Complete.

COUNTY GENERAL HOSPITAL

RPT5511 - NURSING PROFICIENCY REPORT
Sorted By Nurse
Printed   MAY 24, 1989   Page   2

Nurse	Procedure	Total Number	Total Time	Role
O'KEEFE	LIH REPAIR, EXCISION LEFT ATROPHIC COR STRUCTURES	1	0:45	S1
O'KEEFE	MAGPIE REPAIR	2	3:57	S1
O'KEEFE	NISSENFUNDOPLICATION	1	2:00	S1
O'KEEFE	PHARYNGEAL FLAP	1	1:05	S3
O'KEEFE	REMOVAL TISSUE EXPANDER EXCISION HAIRY NEVUS	1	2:50	C2
O'KEEFE	RESECT MR OU	1	0:40	S3
O'KEEFE	RIH REPAIR, LEFT INGUINAL EXPLORATION NEGATIVE	1	0:50	S1
	Nurse O'KEEFE	10	15:57	
REARDON	BIH REPAIR	2	1:30	C1
REARDON	ESOPHAGEAL DILITATION WITH CHANGE OF GASTROSTOMY	1	0:45	C1
REARDON	INSERTION CENTRAL LINE	1	0:20	C1
REARDON	LEFT ORCHIOPEXY, LIH REPAIR	1	0:55	S1
REARDON	REPAIR PECTUS EXCAVATUM	1	2:50	C1
REARDON	RT. ORCHIOPEXY	1	0:45	C1
	Nurse REARDON	7	7:05	

Exhibit 3-24 Nursing investment summary (sorted by service/surgeon). (Reprinted by permission, ORBIT Software, Enterprise Systems, Inc., 2333 Waukegan Road, Bannockburn, IL 60015-1503.)

COUNTY GENERAL HOSPITAL

RPT5512 - NURSING INVESTMENT SUMMARY
Sorted By Service/Surgeon
Printed MAY 24, 1989   Page   1

Surgeon	Number of Procedures	Total Nursing Time
Service: CV-CLOSED		
TALENTOSKI	1	5:50
	-------	-------
CV-CLOSED Subtotals:	1	5:50
Service: CV-OPEN		
SU YONG	2	7:55
	-------	-------
CV-OPEN Subtotals:	2	7:55
Service: DENTAL		
TUCKER	1	1:20
	-------	-------
DENTAL Subtotals:	1	1:20
Service: EYE		
GARRETT	2	1:55
	-------	-------
EYE Subtotals:	2	1:55
Service: GEN		
CHAMBERS	3	1:55
DAMON	5	7:15
PUTNAM	1	0:35
SHAPIRO	4	4:40
SIMMS	1	1:20
SPRINGER	2	2:45
VINCENT	4	4:30
	-------	-------
GEN Subtotals:	20	23:00
Service: GU		
ACKER	4	16:09

Exhibit 3-25 Nursing report: operating room (sorted by date/service/surgeon). (Reprinted by permission, ORBIT Software, Enterprise Systems, Inc., 2333 Waukegan Road, Bannockburn, IL 60015-1503.)

COUNTY GENERAL HOSPITAL
O.R. LOG
Sorted by Date/Service/Surgeon

Page 2

Room/ Type	Start/ End	Case Number	Patient	Surgeons	Assistants	Anesth.	Anes. Type	Scrub Nurses	Circ. Nurses

Surgery Date: 05/01/86
Service: NEURO

Room/ Type	Start/ End	Case Number	Patient	Surgeons	Assistants	Anesth.	Anes. Type	Scrub Nurses	Circ. Nurses
08 IP	10:10 11:40	6343193 328744	SCRANTON, MORGAN	BRONSON		PATTERSON STARR	GEN	MAREDA	GAZARRA BARCLAY

Pre-Op Diagnosis
BLOCKAGE OF RVP SHUNT

Procedure
REV OF VP SHUNT RIGHT

Post-op Diagnosis
REPAIR OF R VP SHUNT

Room/ Type	Start/ End	Case Number	Patient	Surgeons	Assistants	Anesth.	Anes. Type	Scrub Nurses	Circ. Nurses
06 IP	10:40 12:25	6344586 365205	VENNER, BRYANNE	BRONSON CURRO		ROTZ STARR	GEN	VALLER	TIETZ DAVIS

Pre-Op Diagnosis
RT CREBERAL EDEMA POSS HEMATOMA

Procedure
INSERTION OF VP SHUNT RIGHT SIDE

Post-op Diagnosis
CEREBRAL EDEMA WITHOUT HEMATOMA

Room/ Type	Start/ End	Case Number	Patient	Surgeons	Assistants	Anesth.	Anes. Type	Scrub Nurses	Circ. Nurses
02 IP	12:35 17:00	6342852 364718	DUNNAN, JENNY	BRONSON CURRO		JONES FOX	GEN	MORRISON MCCULLOM	TURNER GALAY REESE

Pre-Op Diagnosis
POST FPSSA TUMPR POSS CA

Procedure
RE-CRANIOTOMY RESECT POSTERIOR FOSSA TUMOR

Post-op Diagnosis
POST FOSSA TUMOR BENIGN FS

Room/ Type	Start/ End	Case Number	Patient	Surgeons	Assistants	Anesth.	Anes. Type	Scrub Nurses	Circ. Nurses
02 IPAM	07:55 12:25	6331859 363617	WOOLWORTH, SHARYLE	KELLY CURRO		SMITH KARSTEN	GEN	MILLER	MORRISON GALAY

Pre-Op Diagnosis
CONPRESSION CRAN-CER SKULL/NECK -WRECK

Procedure
CRANIO-CERVICAL DECOMPRESSION

Post-op Diagnosis
SAME

Exhibit 3-26 Computerized intraoperative record. (Reprinted by permission, ORBIT Software, Enterprise Systems, Inc., 2333 Waukegan Road, Bannockburn, IL 60015-1503.)

COUNTY GENERAL HOSPITAL 123 Main Street Madison, IL 66666 (312) 555-2000	331-42-6763 RACHEL BONERTZ 42234575 08/06/80 8Y F
INTRAOPERATIVE RECORD	OP

Surgery Date: 01/30/89   Suite: 10
Consent Signed By: MOTHER   Delay Code: Allergies: NONE
Pref. Lists: 10   Delay Time: /   Cancellation Code:

Pre-op Dx: TONSILLITIS AND ADENOIDITIS
Post-op Dx: SAME
Complications: NONE

Procedure 1: TONSILLECTOMY AND ADENOIDECTOMY

Start: 09:00   End: 10:00   Total: 01:00
Procedure 2:

Start: End: Total:

Procedure 1	Procedure 2
Surgeon: BECKER	
Assistant:	
Anes. Staff: BUSCH	
Anes. Asst:	

		Time In	Time Out
Circ RN DOHERTY		08:50	10:05
Scrub Tech./RN KELLEY		08:40	10:05

Case Type: 2   Wound Class: C   Position: SUPINE
Skin Integrity: CLEAR   Skin PrepNONE
Heat Lamp? N   K-Pad? Y   Hypothermia Unit? N   Thermadrape/wrap? N
Patient Temperature: 99.0
EKG Site: YES; PEDIATRIC BACK PAD
Grounding Pad Site: RIGHT THIGH   Size: PEDIATRIC
Equip. Unit Number/Settings: 093456; 30/30
PIV Site/Size: RIGHT HAND; 21 GUAGE ANGIO
Line Site/Size:
IV Pumps: Drain:
Tourniquet On: Off: Location:
Throat Pack In: 09:45   Out: 09:55
Specimen? Y   Frozen Section? N   Culture? N   X-Rays? N
Dressings: NONE

Exhibit 3-27 Recovery room report. (Reprinted by permission, ORBIT Software, Enterprise Systems, Inc., 2333 Waukegan Road, Bannockburn, IL 60015-1503.)

COUNTY GENERAL HOSPITAL

RPT5538 - RECOVERY ROOM REPORT
Sorted By Recovery Room Time
Printed   JUN 01, 1989

Patient Name	Age	Type	Surgeon	Service	Anesth.	Case Type	Procedure Date	Acuity	Arrival	Discharge	Total Time
SCHMIDT, LINDA	44	OP	PIFFINI	GEN	O'DOHERTY	Elective	06/01/89		10:10	11:00	50
GOLD, EVERETT	34	IP	KITTNERS	ENT	PALMER	Elective	06/01/89	1	11:50	12:50	60
JONES, KATHERINE	63	IP	BOWMAN	GEN	ERWIN	Elective	06/01/89	3	09:35	10:45	70
RAGASE, TREY	7	IP	BOND	GEN	ELLIOTT	Emergency	06/01/89	2	14:50	16:30	100
BROWN, MILDRED	69	IP	FITZGERALD	GEN	PALMER	Elective	06/01/89	2	10:50	12:35	105
COOPER, CRIS	30	IP	CIRILLO	GEN	PERUSEK	Elective	06/01/89	1	11:20	13:10	110
SHIELDS, GEORGE	40	IP	ALLAND	GEN	BAILEY	Elective	06/01/89	1	12:25	14:15	110
GOMEZ, JUAN	31	IP	AZIZ	GEN	DAUGHETY	Elective	06/01/89	2	13:30	15:30	120
HENRY, CHARLES	55	IP	BROWN M	GEN	PARSONS	Elective	06/01/89	1	12:05	14:10	125
BYERS, EVA	78	IP	MENG	NEURO	WINDOM	Urgent	06/01/89	1	12:45	14:50	125
HEMSLEY, BLANCHE	66	IP	BECKETTE	GEN	EGAN	Elective	06/01/89	3	12:15	15:45	210

Total Recovery Room Time   1185

This Report Includes All Cases.
This Report Extracted From:

Procedure Dates from 06/01/89 to 06/01/89

Recovery Room Times From 1 to 300 minutes.

Records Printed: 11
Report Complete.

Exhibit 3-28 Computerized discharge planning form. (Reprinted by permission, ORBIT Software, Enterprise Systems, Inc., 2333 Waukegan Road, Bannockburn, IL 60015-1503.)

```
   NURSING: DISCHARGE PLANNING  :   MEDICAL/NURSING NEEDS__

   DX:                                CASE COORDINATOR:
═══════════════════════════════════════════════════════════════

    USE THE LIGHTPEN TO PROBE IDENTIFIED NEEDS:  DATE ADDED    NURSE
                   ! NO MED/NSG/SOCIAL NEEDS        /   /
                   ? DRESSING AND WOUND CARE        /   /
                   ? SPECIAL EQUIPMENT NEEDS        /   /
                   ? REHAB PLANNING/PLACEMENT       /   /
                   ? TERMINAL/PRE-TERMINAL          /   /
                   ? THERAPIES (PT/OT/S&H)          /   /
                   ? TUBES (NG/GT/FOLEY, ETC.)      /   /
                   ? PARENTERAL/IV THERAPY          /   /
                   ? SPECIAL TEACHING NEEDS         /   /
                   ? OSTOMY CARE                    /   /
                   ? NUTRITION (EXCLUDE TUBES)      /   /
                   ? RESPIRATORY                    /   /
                     _____           /   /
═══════════════════════════════════════════════════════════════
                   !*PF18* EDUCATION
    !*PF14* RETURN                     PRESS ENTER TO CONTINUE
```

Part II

Nursing Applications in Ambulatory Surgical Nursing

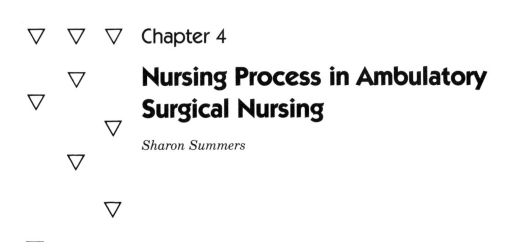

Chapter 4

Nursing Process in Ambulatory Surgical Nursing

Sharon Summers

The five steps of the nursing process have been described in the literature for more than a decade as the foundation for nursing practice, and yet there is still confusion as to how nursing diagnosis fits within the nursing process. Nursing process includes assessment, nursing diagnosis, planning, implementation, and evaluation. Frequently, nursing diagnosis is either omitted from the process or used inappropriately. Thus, the purpose of this chapter is to present strategies for using nursing diagnosis effectively in the ambulatory surgical setting. To accomplish this, nurses must first consider the following questions:

1. How can the nursing process be used with nursing diagnosis as the pivotal point in the process?
2. What are the criteria established by the North American Nursing Diagnosis Association (NANDA) for patterns and taxonomy of nursing diagnosis?
3. Why not adopt the NANDA format to promote standardization of terminology for the development of a body of nursing knowledge?
4. What particular assessment criteria are pertinent in assessing the ambulatory surgical patient, including physiological and psychological stress, and nutritional needs?
5. What guidelines can be utilized for patient assessment and formulation of a nursing diagnosis?
6. What are the similarities and differences that distinguish the standards of care regarding the use of nursing diagnosis established by the Joint Commission on the Accreditation of Hospitals Organization (JCAHO) and those established by professional nursing organizations?
7. Why do nurses need to validate the NANDA format through clinical use and testing?

Exhibits for Chapter 4 are located at the end of the chapter on pages 86–95.

▽

Nursing Process and Nursing Diagnosis

Nursing diagnosis is considered to be the second step in the nursing process, followed by planning, implementation, and evaluation, and yet little agreement exists as to what a nursing diagnosis is, how to write one, or how to use one. Originally, there was agreement as to the meaning of the four-step nursing process outlined in the early literature.[1,2] However, little consensus and few guidelines were found in the literature when nursing diagnosis was added to the nursing process steps.[2,3] Currently, nursing diagnosis is either not included in many nursing texts, or is not used consistently within or among nursing education programs, or both. Consistency in defining and utilizing nursing diagnosis could begin with acceptance of common definitions for nursing process and nursing diagnosis.

Nursing process and nursing diagnosis are defined here for clarity. *Nursing* is defined as "the diagnosis and treatment of human responses to actual or potential health problems."[4] *Process* is defined as "a system of operations in the production of something."[5] Combining the meanings for these two terms, then, *nursing process* can be defined as a systematic process of assessing, formulating nursing diagnoses of actual or potential patient problems, planning, implementing, and evaluating a product— that is, individualized patient care.

Assessment involves the systematic collection of a patient's history and physical/physiological data. Nursing diagnosis is considered to be an outcome of the analysis of these assessment data, and is the basis upon which nursing orders are written and care is planned. The planning component of the nursing process comprises the strategies the nurse will employ to alleviate the patient problems identified through assessment and the derived nursing diagnosis. Implementation is a term that describes the actions the nurse will take to meet a patient's needs based on data derived from the assessment, the nursing diagnosis, and the planning strategies. Evaluation is the analysis of nursing care to determine whether a patient's care was appropriate for the diagnostic statements and whether the nursing orders alleviated the patient problems identified through the assessment and nursing diagnosis steps. Thus, the five steps of the nursing process, as depicted in Figure 4–1, are considered to be cyclical, as evaluation logically links back to assessment.[1,6,7]

Assessment strategies seem to have gained immense popularity, especially when one considers the numerous credit and continuing education courses on physical assessment attended by nurses. For some reason, nurses have become enamored with physical assessment techniques and tools, to the point that many nurses have purchased such items as stethoscopes, otoscopes, ophthalmoscopes, percussion hammers, and the like. Why?

Figure 4-1 Steps in the nursing process.

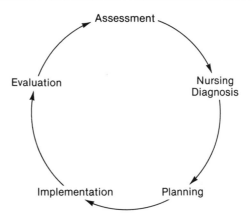

It may be that nurses are more comfortable with the concrete psycho-motor skills required for physical assessment than with the abstract cognitive skills needed to formulate nursing diagnoses. In addition, physical assessment has quickly become valued by many nurses as a necessary basis for patient care, especially in caring for patients with physiological instability. Although nursing diagnosis is an important step in the nursing process, it has not gained the popularity of physical assessment.

Nursing diagnosis may be defined as "a statement that describes the human response (health state or actual/potential altered interaction pattern) of an individual or group that the nurse can legally identify and for which the nurse can order definitive interventions to maintain the health state or to reduce, eliminate, or prevent alterations."[8]

This definition makes three important points: (1) human responses (individual or group) occur according to ordered patterns of behavior, (2) nurses are educated and legally licensed to identify altered human interaction problems, and (3) educated and licensed nurses can legally order interventions to alleviate human interaction problems.

Human response of individuals or groups to health/illness problems has always been a nursing concern. Observations by nurses over time have identified certain patterns of phenomena, such as signs and symptoms of illness. These observations have usually been recorded based on the medical model. When nursing observations and assessments are recorded based on nursing diagnosis, then the NANDA taxonomy can be expanded for current and future patterns.

Altered human responses of individuals or groups have been the main emphasis of nursing education; however, the curriculum traditionally has been organized around the medical model—that is, medical-surgical, pediatric, and obstetrical nursing. As a result, nursing has used the medical model to convey nursing practice to both nurses and physicians. A benefit of this approach has been that nurses and physicians have developed a common, well-defined language with which to communicate. However, the problem with using the medical model is that nursing has failed to develop a separate identity or a precisely defined area of nursing practice. As a result, the cost of nursing services has frequently been included in the room and board charges of hospitalized patients. Thus, adoption and utilization of nursing diagnoses could help to develop a nursing identity and to define the boundaries of nursing practice.

Nurses are both educated and licensed to practice nursing. Many state nursing practice acts have adopted the five-step nursing process, thereby giving nurses the legal right to assess patients and to formulate nursing diagnoses.[9] This license to practice is one of the criteria used to define a profession.

Conway[10] states that the criteria used to define a profession include a body of knowledge, theories about the profession, and control over the practice such that the license to practice establishes the boundaries of the profession. As nursing education frequently is based on the medical model, there is little evidence that nursing has a distinct body of knowledge. Moreover, there is little evidence that nursing has specific theories about the profession of nursing, and may at best have some grand theories, conceptual frameworks, or models.[11] There is little evidence that the license to practice nursing has given rise to clear, well-established boundaries, especially for nurse practitioners, nurse midwives, and home health nurses, as up until the mid 1970s, many nursing practice acts contained regulations requiring nurses to work under the supervision of physicians.[9]

Although nurses are educated and legally licensed to order nursing interventions, few nurses exercise this legal right of the independent practice or role of nursing. Ritter, Crulcich, and McEntegart[12] maintain that nursing practice consists of independent, as well as dependent and interdependent, roles. However, the definition of nursing diagnosis cited earlier refers to the independent practice of nursing, as it specifies that nurses can order specific interventions for a patient.

Therefore, for nursing to be considered a profession, nurses must implement a practice, as outlined by licensing laws, that utilizes the nursing process, including nursing diagnosis, to the full extent of the law. In addition, nurses must develop methods to establish a body of nursing knowledge instead of borrowing from the medical model. A first step toward developing a body of nursing knowledge might be the use of nursing diagnosis patterns and taxonomy as developed by NANDA.[13]

▽

Nursing Diagnosis Patterns and Taxonomy

Nursing diagnosis has not gained the popularity accorded physical assessment. As theorized earlier, it may be that, in a practice profession such as nursing, psychomotor skills are valued more than cognitive skills; this value system, however, ignores the fact that assessment is merely a means of arriving at nursing diagnoses. Moreover, nurses have traditionally conveyed patient assessment data using a medical diagnosis (e.g., inguinal hernia) rather than a nursing diagnosis (e.g., alteration in skin integrity). Why? Medical diagnoses constitute an extensively used, well-defined taxonomy with universal meaning across health care disciplines. By contrast, nursing diagnoses constitute a loosely established taxonomy without universal meaning across health care disciplines, especially when various nursing groups use a variety of diagnostic labels. As Table 4–1 illustrates, medical and nursing diagnoses are also different in form and purpose.[8]

Both the definition of nursing diagnosis and the taxonomy of diagnostic statements have undergone many changes. Although the label *nursing diagnosis* was first used by Fry in 1953,[14] it was not until the early 1970s that formalized activities began to shape and define nursing diagnosis. In 1973, Gebbie and Lavin[3] invited nursing leaders to attend the First National Conference on Classification of Nursing Diagnosis at St. Louis University. It was not until the fifth conference that the group's name was changed to the North American Nursing Diagnosis Association (NANDA).[15] Since then, there have been seven biennial NANDA conferences, and the current membership of the group is approximately 1,450. At the eighth conference in 1988, the membership voted to give NANDA international status, although the name remained unchanged. Currently, several NANDA regional groups and independent regional nursing diagnosis organizations, such as the Mid-America Regional Nursing Diagnosis Conference Group, meet annually to, among other activities, formulate and test nursing diagnoses that are subsequently submitted to NANDA for approval.

An outcome of the work by NANDA members has been the formulation of the nursing diagnosis taxonomy, which is organized around nine functional health patterns. At the 1988 NANDA conference, the 11 health patterns originally proposed by Gordon[16] were reorganized and con-

Table 4-1 A Comparison of Medical and Nursing Diagnosis

Medical Diagnosis	Nursing Diagnosis
Requires physician intervention (e.g., surgery, prescribing of drugs, treatments)	Requires nursing intervention (independent) (e.g., providing comfort, education, emotional support, physical care)
Usually remains constant during illness episode	Diagnoses and interventions may be numerous, and change daily
Defines underlying cause of illness	Care is based on the impact that the illness has on the patient
Care is disease-oriented	Care is patient/family-oriented

Table 4-2 North American Nursing Diagnosis Association 1990 Taxonomy Patterns and Diagnostic Labels

Pattern 1: Exchanging
Nutrition: More than Body Requirements, Altered
Nutrition: Less than Body Requirements, Altered
Nutrition: Potential for more than Body Requirements, Altered
Infection, High Risk for
Body Temperature, High Risk for Altered
Hypothermia
Hyperthermia
Thermoregulation, Ineffective
Dysreflexia
Constipation
Constipation, Perceived
Constipation, Colonic
Diarrhea
Incontinence, Bowel
Urinary Elimination, Altered
Incontinence, Stress
Incontinence, Reflex
Incontinence, Urge
Incontinence, Functional
Incontinence, Total
Urinary Retention
Tissue Perfusion, Altered (specify type) (Renal, cerebral, cardiopulmonary, gastrointestinal, peripheral)
Fluid Volume Excess
Fluid Volume Deficit
Fluid Volume Deficit, High Risk for
Decreased Cardiac Output
Gas Exchange, Impaired
Airway Clearance, Ineffective
Breathing Pattern, Ineffective
Injury, High Risk for
Suffocation, High Risk for
Poisoning, High Risk for
Trauma, High Risk for
Aspiration, High Risk for
Disuse Syndrome, High Risk for
Tissue Integrity, Impaired
Oral Mucous Membrane, Altered
Skin Integrity, Impaired
Skin Integrity, High Risk for Impaired

Pattern 2: Communicating
Communication, Impaired Verbal

Pattern 3: Relating
Social Interaction, Impaired
Social Isolation
Role Performance, Altered
Parenting, Altered
Parenting, High Risk for Altered
Sexual Dysfunction
Family Processes, Altered
Sexuality Patterns, Altered

Pattern 4: Valuing
Spiritual Distress (Distress of the Human Spirit)

Pattern 5: Choosing
Individual Coping, Ineffective
Adjustment, Impaired
Defensive Coping
Denial, Ineffective
Family Coping: Potential for Growth
Noncompliance (Specify)
Decisional Conflict (Specify)
Health Seeking Behaviors (Specify)

Pattern 6: Moving
Physical Mobility, Impaired
Activity Intolerance
Fatigue
Activity Intolerance, High Risk for
Sleep Pattern Disturbance
Diversional Activity Deficit
Home Maintenance Management, Impaired
Health Maintenance, Altered
Self-Care Deficit, Feeding
Breastfeeding, Ineffective
Swallowing, Impaired
Self-Care Deficit, Bathing/Hygiene
Self-Care Deficit, Dressing/Grooming
Self-Care Deficit, Toileting
Growth and Development, Altered

Pattern 7: Perceiving
Body Image Disturbance
Self-Esteem Disturbance

Table 4-2 North American Nursing Diagnosis Association 1990 Taxonomy Patterns and Diagnostic Labels (Continued)

Self-Esteem, Chronic Low	**Pattern 9: Feeling**
Self-Esteem, Situational Low	Pain
Personal Identity Disturbance	Pain, Chronic
Sensory/Perceptual Alterations (specify) (Visual, auditory, kinesthetic, gustatory, tactile, olfactory)	Grieving, Dysfunctional
	Grieving, Anticipatory
	Violence, High Risk for: Self-directed or directed at others
Unilateral Neglect	
Hopelessness	Post-Trauma Response
Powerlessness	Rape-Trauma Syndrome
	Rape-Trauma Syndrome: Compound Reaction
	Rape-Trauma Syndrome: Silent Reaction
Pattern 8: Knowing	Anxiety
Knowledge Deficit (Specify)	Fear
Thought Processes, Altered	

(Used by permission, NANDA, 1990.)

solidated into the currently accepted patterns: Exchanging, Communicating, Relating, Valuing, Choosing, Moving, Perceiving, Knowing, and Feeling.[13]

As illustrated in Table 4–2, the taxonomy of nursing diagnosis involves labels arranged according to nine human response patterns, which conforms to the definition of nursing diagnosis cited earlier.[8] Patterns and taxonomies are easy to understand, as they are used repeatedly in daily living. For example, without a taxonomy, or classification system, it would be difficult to learn all of the medications, or intended uses for those medications, that are currently prescribed for ambulatory surgical patients. Such medications are sorted initially by category or pattern (e.g., oral, inhaled, or parenteral agents); each broad category is then further classified, as in general anesthetic gases or narcotic agonist analgesics. Within each taxonomy are generic chemical names (e.g., nitrous oxide or meperidine hydrochloride), and under each specific generic drug, there are defining characteristics that further delineate each part of the taxonomy and distinguish one drug from another on the basis of chemical composition. Part of the taxonomy then includes the trade names of commercially available products.

The taxonomy of nursing diagnosis is arranged in a manner similar to that of medications. Nine human response patterns are identified, and under each pattern is a pattern-specific taxonomy of nursing diagnosis. Each nursing diagnosis is then further delineated by certain defining characteristics that amplify the diagnostic statement. For example, Table 4–3 presents the nursing diagnosis taxonomy for hypothermia, complete

Table 4-3 Taxonomy of Hypothermia with Defining Characteristics

Pattern	Exchanging
Taxonomy	Hypothermia
Definition	The state in which an individual's body temperature is reduced below normal range
Defining Characteristics	
Major	Reduction in body temperature below normal range; shivering (mild); cool skin; pallor (moderate)
Minor	Slow capillary refill; tachycardia; cyanotic nail beds; hypertension, piloerection
Related Factors	Exposure to cool or cold environment; illness or trauma; damage to hypothalamus; inability to shiver; malnutrition; inadequate clothing; consumption of alcohol; medications causing vasodilatation; evaporation from skin in cool environment; decreased metabolic rate; inactivity; aging

(Used by permission, NANDA, 1990, p. 15.)

with defining characteristics that distinguish this diagnosis from all others. The following list contains suggested perioperative nursing diagnoses that could be used in the ambulatory surgical setting.

Preoperative nursing diagnoses

Individual Coping, Ineffective

Anxiety

Fear

Sleep Pattern Disturbance

Grieving

Knowledge Deficit

Airway Clearance, Ineffective

Thought Processes, Altered

Body Image Disturbance

Nutrition, Altered

Activity Intolerance, High Risk for Self-Esteem Disturbance

Self-Concept Disturbance

Sensory/Perceptual Alterations

Intraoperative nursing diagnoses

Communication, Impaired Verbal

Injury, High Risk for (Nosocomial Infection, Positioning, RX to Prep Solutions)

Skin Integrity, Impaired

Decreased Cardiac Output (Fluid Loss)

Breathing Patterns, Ineffective

Tissue Perfusion, Altered

Hypothermia

Physical Mobility, Impaired

Thermoregulation, Ineffective R/T Medications (Anesthetics, Neuromuscular Blockades)

Fluid Volume Deficit

Anxiety

Sexuality Patterns, Altered (GYN/GU Procedures)

Aspiration, High Risk for

Mucous Membrane, Oral Altered, Dryness)

Sensory/Perceptual Alterations

Swallowing, Impaired

Postoperative nursing diagnoses

Anxiety

Tissue Perfusion, Altered

Breathing Pattern, Ineffective

Airway Clearance, Ineffective

Nutrition, Altered: Less than body requirement

Pain

Skin Integrity, Impaired

Activity Intolerance, High Risk for

Physical Mobility, Impaired

Self-Care Deficit

Fluid Volume Deficit

The taxonomy of nursing diagnosis consists of statements, or prefixes, that have been proposed, discussed, and voted on by the NANDA membership. The first part of the statement consists of these accepted taxonomic prefixes, which are linked to the second part of the nursing diagnosis statement with the phrase *related to* (abbreviated as R/T). It is the second part of the statement that describes the *independent* nursing practice. Remember, nursing diagnosis is a statement, based on the outcome of physical assessment, that is formulated as a problem that nurses are educated and licensed to treat through independent nursing practice. As NANDA members have spent many years working on nursing diagnosis taxonomy and patterns, and since NANDA now consists of international members, why not adopt the NANDA format so that nurses can work together toward a standardized nursing knowledge base?

▽

Standardization of Nursing Knowledge: Forward to Nursing Science

Standardization of nursing knowledge is a prerequisite for the strengthening of the status of nursing, as described in the definition of a profession, and for the establishment of an identity that distinguishes nursing from medicine. Disciplines, such as the biological sciences, have a known body of knowledge that was developed by applying a taxonomy of phenomena. The identified taxonomy was then used to formulate theories, the theories were tested through research, and the body of knowledge that identified the discipline evolved.

For example, preliminary work relating to the germ theory began with Van Leeuwenhoek in 1673 with the development of the first microscope, and then progressed with a classification process developed by Pierre Fidèle Bretonneau (1778–1862).[17] Bretonneau established a doctrine of specific etiologies by advocating that specific diseases were caused by specific organisms found in body secretions; he also speculated that they were contagious. During Bretonneau's time, most diseases were known as fevers. His work classified all diseases that produced a fever, thus building a taxonomy for such diseases as diphtheria, syphilis, scarlet fever, and tuberculosis.[17] Records were carefully kept according to the defining characteristics (i.e., respiratory distress, rash, lesions, or cough) of each disease so that one disease could be distinguished from another. This taxonomy was the forerunner of work by Pasteur, Bassi, Lister, and Koch, thus leading to the germ theory that is the foundation for the discipline of microbiology.[17] Just as the taxonomy of diseases led to the germ theory and the foundation of microbial science, so can the taxonomy of nursing diagnosis lead to nursing theories as the foundation of nursing science.

Nursing science is defined as the dynamic interaction of nursing theory, nursing practice, nursing research, and nursing education.[18] Nursing theory exists for the purpose of describing, explaining, predicting, and controlling nursing phenomena. Nursing practice defines the boundaries of the profession. Nursing research defines activities that validate theory and practice. Nursing education serves to teach others about the theory, the practice, and the research components of nursing. Today, there is little agreement that nursing is a science, as only grand theories, conceptual frameworks, or models have been developed, rather than a well-defined theory.[11] Theories consist of well-defined concepts, and nursing's concepts have yet to be well defined. Moreover, nursing practice is a product of three types of nursing education programs whose graduates take but one licensing examination and then practice nursing according to a particular school's criteria. Nursing research studies are beginning to test nursing practice to document that what nurses do is beneficial to patient health and recovery. A major problem with this cycle of events is that nurses have not defined nursing's concepts. Health, nurse, environment, and client[18] have been described as nursing's concepts; however, they are such complex concepts that they are not useful for guiding day-to-day nursing practice. Before concepts for nursing can be useful, patterns and taxonomies must be developed to define what it is that nurses do. In an attempt to define terms and work toward a conceptual framework, the NANDA patterns and nursing diagnosis taxonomy have been arranged on the basis of a conceptual framework of the Unitary Person; this is a vital first step toward nursing theory and nursing science.[19]

The conceptual framework of the Unitary Person is based on a systems theory and purports that the person is a whole entity interacting with the environment according to the nine functional health patterns adopted by NANDA. Each person consists of a unique organizing pattern.[19] The independent role of nursing is to assess the unitary person according to the nine functional health patterns, and to determine the person's needs with information derived from assessment and nursing diagnosis. This is not intended to negate the dependent or the interdependent roles of nursing, which involves implementing nursing care to meet patient needs based on medical diagnosis.

▽

Assessment of the Ambulatory Surgical Patient

Although it is beyond the scope of this chapter to present indepth assessment strategies, assessment is reviewed and sample assessment forms are presented and discussed. A variety of strategies and forms have been used by nurses to assess patients. Frequently, the forms that nurses have used to record assessment data have been based on the medical model. Although it is important for nurses to have assessment skills, the documentation of the assessment findings does not need to be a replication of what has been recorded by the physician. It is very difficult, if not impossible, to assess patients with forms that were intended to lead to a medical diagnosis and then to miraculously transform the outcome to nursing diagnosis.

Rather, the documentation of assessment findings needs to reflect the nurse's expertise with the nursing process and nursing diagnosis. When the assessment findings are recorded using a form based on the conceptual framework of Unitary Person and the nine functional health patterns, then a frame of reference can be derived as to the meaning of the assessment.

Exhibit 4–1 illustrates a nursing assessment form developed to incorporate the nine NANDA[13] patterns in order to facilitate the utilization of nursing diagnosis. The equipment used for assessment and the methods of systematically examining the patient remain unchanged; however, the structure for assessment is arranged according to the nine functional health patterns, rather than medical systems. When this form is used by a nurse with a knowledge of the nursing diagnosis taxonomy, then it becomes easier to formulate the appropriate nursing diagnosis. This assessment form could benefit from extensive testing and revising by ambulatory surgical nurses to ensure that it is comprehensive enough for a variety of patients. Although this form is lengthy in its present form, it can be shortened with computerization and a copy can be edited for quick, individualized assessment to meet the needs of an individual ambulatory surgical patient.

Assessment Strategies for Ambulatory Surgical Nursing

The long nursing assessment form developed for use in the ambulatory surgical setting can be modified for individualized patient needs. On a busy patient care unit, there is limited time to assess patients, and yet all patients must be assessed thoroughly. With a computerized form, patient assessments can be completed quickly, nursing diagnoses can be formulated, and a care plan can be developed. As depicted in Figure 4–2, there is a sequential flow of reasoning from assessment data through analysis of cues, patterns, and nursing diagnosis.[20] The following case study illustrates the use of the nursing-diagnosis–based assessment form, and compares narrative and nursing-diagnosed–based charting as a hypothetical patient is admitted to the ambulatory surgical unit.

Case Study

Jennifer Simpson is a 30-year-old computer programmer with a medical diagnosis of recurrent cystitis. Her symptoms of frequency and suprapubic pain have interfered with her job performance and social life. Jennifer arrived at the ambulatory surgical unit with preoperative orders from her doctor.

The assessment form was edited to what would be pertinent for Jennifer as a unitary person with a medical problem of recurrent cystitis; the information was then completed on-line, stored as part of her permanent record, and printed as needed. The assessment findings and the nursing diagnoses for Jennifer are shown in Exhibit 4–2. Editing a computerized assessment form to meet Jennifer's individualized needs is more convenient than using the long form which includes several sections not pertinent to her care. When applying the assessment findings and nursing diagnoses to document Jennifer's care, the difference in narrative and nursing diagnosis charting becomes apparent. The narrative charting for Jennifer might resemble that presented in the following list.

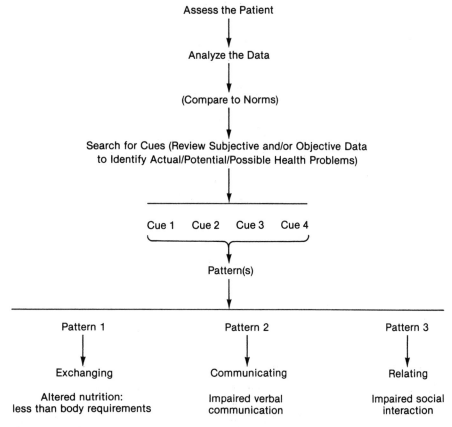

Figure 4-2 Logical flow from assessment to nursing diagnosis.

Admitted for cystoscopy at 1330.

B/P: 120/84, P:84, R:16.

Appears anxious; c/o lower abdominal pain.

Oriented to unit.

It is very difficult to define independent nursing practice using the narrative charting format. When the nursing-diagnosis–based assessment form is used, vital signs and other descriptive information are recorded, but are not focal points of the document. When narrative charting is transformed to the nursing process format (see Exhibit 4–3), preoperative independent nursing practice is easy to define, as care is documented across the five steps of the nursing process and a column is added for ambulatory discharge instruction/evaluation. It is not necessary to rewrite assessment information, but merely to summarize it using the NANDA patterns as a guide.

▽

Standards of Care and Nursing Diagnosis

Standards of care are established by institutions, organizations, or interest groups for the purpose of defining criteria to measure high levels of care. Some standards, such as those established for ambulatory health care by the Joint Commission on Accreditation of Hospital Organization (JACHO), are used to evaluate both institutions and nursing practice.[21] Other standards, such as those established by the American Nurses' Association (ANA),[2] the Association of Operating Room Nurses (AORN),[22] and the American Society of Post Anesthesia Nurses (ASPAN),[23] are considered to be the benchmarks by which nursing care and nursing practice are measured. Both types of standards are reviewed in the following section.

The ambulatory health care standards developed by the JACHO list nurses only under the categories of anesthetist, emergency services, and infirmary and surgical services.[21] The anesthetist section states that policies must exist to define the job description of the nurse anesthetist. The emergency services section specifies that qualified nurses supervise emergency nursing services. The infirmary section specifies that, in units that provide overnight care, qualified registered nurses must be present for each shift the patients are on the unit. The surgical services section specifies that competent nurses assist in providing surgical services and that a competent registered nurse supervises nursing services.[21] These guidelines for nurses are both broad and vague.

The ANA standards for medical-surgical nursing practice[2] present criteria for the professional nurse based on the steps in the nursing process: assessment, nursing diagnosis, formulation of goals, planning of care, and evaluation of care. Steps for the nursing process, especially nursing diagnosis, are broad, and lack specificity for guiding the nurse in the care of a surgical patient.

The standards established by AORN for medical-surgical nursing practice for the professional nurse are formulated around the nursing process model established by the ANA.[22] However, AORN has modified the model, especially for increasing the specificity of outcome criteria (i.e., no infection, patient safety, etc.).[22] In addition, AORN has written specific standards for recovery room care; preoperative patient skin preparation; surgical hand scrubs; sponge, needle, and instrument procedures; in-hospital packaging material; cleaning and processing of anesthesia equipment; and administrative nursing practice.[24]

ASPAN's standards of practice for postanesthesia nursing also follow the steps of the nursing process.[23] Important additions to these standards have been the inclusion of preoperative and postoperative care standards of the ambulatory surgical patient, as well as standards for nursing management.

These standards of practice describe settings and roles for the nurse based on the use of the nursing process. Although the JACHO guidelines for ambulatory health care omit specific reference to the nursing process, they do indicate that the professional nurse must be competent to manage patients in this setting.

The guidelines established by the ANA, AORN, and ASPAN all use the nursing process as the benchmark for judging nursing care. Because nursing diagnosis, as derived from assessment, is the pivotal point of the nursing process, then it can be concluded that nursing diagnosis is the vital step needed to plan and evaluate nursing care. Thus, these standards have several similarities and few differences in that all of them stress the use of the nursing process in judging nursing care. Therefore, it is imperative that nursing diagnosis be validated.

▽

Clinical Validation of Nursing Diagnosis

Although this chapter has described the NANDA taxonomy indepth, what has not been addressed are the methods by which the taxonomy was formulated. Beginning with the first NANDA conference, the taxonomy was formulated by nurses who described patient phenomena based on the experience and observations of these nurses while caring for patients. Subsequent nursing diagnosis conferences added items to the taxonomy that were derived both from experience and from formal research studies. Many of the taxonomic items, however, have not been tested, so there is a need for nurses to validate these diagnostic statements. How can nurses validate nursing diagnoses?

A nursing diagnosis can be validated by nurses in the clinical setting by (1) placing the NANDA criteria for a single diagnosis on a form; (2) using a checklist to record whether patients exhibit the defining criteria; and (3) recording any phenomenon that is not listed but that is frequently observed and that may need to be added to the defining criteria. For example, this process can be used to validate the nursing diagnosis of impaired gas exchange. As Exhibit 4–4 illustrates, impaired gas exchange is first defined, and then both defining characteristics and related factors are listed. Nurses in ambulatory surgical units could test this nursing diagnosis in patients who undergo general anesthesia by checking for the presence or absence of the items on the list. If data were collected on large numbers of patients and if the defining criteria for the nursing diagnosis were present in all of them, then this would be important data to publish or present at conferences. If the data collected did not match that described by NANDA, then this, too, would be very important data to publish or present at conferences. Nurses in ambulatory surgical units are also in a good position to formulate new nursing diagnoses, tested by the same method, and to submit these diagnoses to NANDA for consideration for addition to the taxonomy.

▽

Summary

This chapter has attempted to answer seven questions concerning the use of the nursing process in ambulatory surgical nursing. It can be concluded that the nursing process is an integral part of nursing. Nursing diagnosis can be seen as the pivotal point in the process, as nursing diagnosis is derived from assessment and drives the planning, the implementing, and the evaluation of patient care. Nursing process is intended to guide nurses in caring for patients while communicating in a common language, and consists of nursing activities that include the independent, as well as the dependent and interdependent, roles of nurses. However, the independent role of nurses has been emphasized. Various standards of practice cite the nursing process as the criterion for judging practice. A crucial factor in establishing standards of nursing is the development of a common language, such as that included in the patterns and taxonomy proposed by NANDA. Many will argue that the taxonomy is limited and does not fit all patients; however, it is a starting place for nurses to evaluate practice and to add other taxonomic labels through clinical testing. Therefore, it is recommended that nurses implement and test nursing diagnoses, as defined by NANDA, in order to expedite the building of nursing's knowledge base by defining what nurses do that is unique in the ambulatory surgical setting.

References

1. Yura, H., & Walsh, M. B. (1968). *The nursing process: Assessing, planning, implementing, evaluating.* Washington, D.C.: The Catholic University of America Press, Inc.
2. American Nurses' Association. (1974). *Standards of medical-surgical nursing practice.* Kansas City: American Nurses' Association.
3. Gebbie, K. M., & Lavin, M. A. (1975). *Proceedings of the First National Conference on Classification of Nursing Diagnosis.* St. Louis: C. V. Mosby Co.
4. American Nurses' Association. (1980). *Social policy statement.* Kansas City: American Nurses' Association.
5. *American Heritage Dictionary of the English Language.* (1981, p. 1043). Dallas: Houghton Mifflin, Co.
6. Yura, H., & Walsh, M. B. (1988). *The nursing process: Assessing, planning, implementing, evaluating.* Norwalk, CT: Appleton & Lange.
7. Bulechek, G. M., & McCloskey, J. C. (1985). *Nursing interventions: Treatments for nursing diagnosis.* Philadelphia: W. B. Saunders Co.
8. Carpenito, L. J. (1989–90). *Nursing diagnosis applications to clinical practice.* Philadelphia: J. B. Lippincott Co.
9. Mundinger, M. O. (1970). *Autonomy in nursing.* Germantown, MD: Aspen Systems Corporation.
10. Conway, M. E. (1984). Prescription for professionalization. In N. Chaska (Ed.), *The nursing profession: A time to speak* (pp. 29–37). St. Louis: McGraw-Hill.
11. Walker, L. O., & Avant, K. C. (1989). *Strategies for theory construction in nursing.* Norwalk, CT: Appleton & Lange.

12. Ritter, T., Crulcich, M., & McEntegart, A. (1981). Nursing practice: An amalgam of dependence, independence, and interdependence. In J. C. McCloskey & H. K. Grace (Eds.), *Current issues in nursing* (pp. 5–14). Boston: Blackwell Scientific Publications.
13. North American Nursing Diagnosis Association. (1990). *Taxonomy I Revised 1989 with official diagnostic categories*. St. Louis: North American Nursing Diagnosis Association.
14. Fry, V. (1953). Creative approach to nursing. *American Journal of Nursing, 53*(3), 301–302.
15. Kim, M. J., McFarland, G., & McLane, A. (1984). Classification of nursing diagnoses. *Proceedings of the Fifth National Conference*. New York: McGraw-Hill.
16. Gordon, M. (1982). *Nursing diagnosis process and application*. St. Louis: McGraw-Hill.
17. Dubos, R. (1980). *Man adapting*. New Haven, CT: Yale University Press.
18. Bilitski, C. S. (1981, October). Nursing science and the laws of health: The test of substance as a step in the process of theory development. *Advances in Nursing Science, 4*(1), 15–29.
19. Roy, Sr. C. (1984). Framework for classification system development: Progress and issues. In M. J. Kim, G. McFarland, & A. McLane (Eds.), *Nursing diagnoses: Proceedings of the Fifth National Conference* (p. 40). New York: McGraw-Hill.
20. Carnevali, D. (1983). *Nursing care planning: Diagnosis and management*. Philadelphia: J. B. Lippincott Co.
21. Joint Commission on Accreditation of Hospitals. (1990). *Ambulatory health care standards manual*. Chicago: Joint Commission on Accreditation of Hospitals.
22. The Association of Operating Room Nurses, Inc. (1988). *AORN standards and recommended practice for perioperative nursing*. Denver: The Association of Operating Room Nurses, Inc.
23. The American Society of Post Anesthesia Nurses. (1990). *Standards of nursing practice*. Richmond, VA: The American Society of Post Anesthesia Nurses.
24. The Association of Operating Room Nurses, Inc. (1990). *AORN standards and recommended practices for perioperative nursing*. Denver: Association of Operating Room Nurses, Inc.

Exhibit 4-1 Ambulatory surgical nursing: Nursing diagnosis assessment form based on the nine NANDA patterns.

Name: _____ Date: _____

Address: _____ City _____ State: ___

Phone: (H) _____ (W) _____ SS# _____

Surgical Diagnosis: _____

Medical Diagnosis: _____

Sex: ___ Age: ___ Known Allergies: _____

EXCHANGING

Color oral mucosa: _____ Moist___ Dry ___ Lesions: ___

Teeth _____ Missing _____

Appearance: Well nourished ___ Obese ___ Emaciated ___

Weight: ___ Height: ___ Weight Gain: ___ Weight Loss: ___

Diet Restrictions: _____ Alcohol Intake: ___

Feeding Tubes: ___ Hyperalimentation: ___

Skin: Turgor ___ Intact ___ Lesions ___ Color ___ Temp ___

Fluid Intake: _____

Nursing Diagnosis _____

Exhibit 4-1 (Continued)

Circulation

Temp ___ Pulse ___ BP (Rt arm) ___ (Lt arm) ___

Sitting ___ Standing ___

Apical rate ___ Rhythm: Regular ___ Irregular ___

Heart sounds: S1 ___ S2 ___ S3 ___ S4 ___

Neck veins distended: ___

Peripherial Edema: ___ Location: ___

Pedal Pulse: Rt ___ Lt ___

Calf Tenderness: ___

Extremities: Color: ___ Temp changes: ___

History of: Pacemaker ___ Chest pain ___

Blood Clots: ___ Edema ___

Nursing Diagnosis _____

Respiration

Resp rate ___ Breathsounds ___ Skin Color ___

Cough ___ Productive ___ Sputum Color ___

Smoker ___ Pack years ___

Dyspnea ___ On exertion ___

Nursing Diagnosis _____

Exhibit 4-1 (Continued)

Elimination

Abdomen: Soft___ Firm___ Tender___ Distended___

    Ostomies___ Bowel sounds present___

Stool/day___ Color___ Constipation___ Diarrhea___ Laxative use___

Enema use___ Incontinence of stool___

Urine output/day___ Color___

    Odor___ Urgency___

Frequency___ Nocturia___ Dysuria___ Hematuria___

    Incontinent___ Stress Incontinence___

Nursing Diagnosis___

COMMUNICATING

    Understands spoken language___ Reads___

    Writes___ Reads Lips___ Hearing intact___

    Vision intact___

Nursing Diagnosis___

RELATING

    Marital status: M___ S___ W___ D___ Children___

    Number of Children___ Dependents___

    Occupation___

Exhibit 4-1 (Continued)

Living Arrangements: Home Owner___ Rent___ Others in

    the home___

Support system: Relative___ Friend___

Family concerned about hospitalization___

Gets along with support system___

Personal Behavior: Passive___ Aggressive___ Assertive___

Parent___ Parenting Problems___

Last Menstrual Period___ Menstrual Problems___

Birth Control Methods___ Number of Pregnancies___

Complications of Pregnancies___

Sexual Preference:___

Sexual concerns___ History of STD___

Sexually active:___

Nursing Diagnosis___

VALUING

    Religious Affiliation___ Religious Restrictions___

    Would you like minister: To visit___ To be called___

    Cultural concerns___

    Religious concerns:___

(Continued)

Exhibit 4-1 (Continued)

Nursing Diagnosis ___

CHOOSING

Coping with health problems ___ Verbalizes problems ___

Uses defense mechanisms ___ Can meet role
expectations ___

Family coping: Effective ___ Ineffective ___

Neglectful ___ Self ___ Others ___

Complies with care: ___ Seeks Preventive care: ___

Decision maker: Yes ___ No ___

Nursing Diagnosis ___

MOVING

Ambulates ___ Climbs Stairs ___

Gait: Steady ___ Unsteady ___ Limp ___ Able to walk ___

Prothesis ___ Aids: Cane ___ Walker ___ Wheelchair ___

Fatigue: ___ Tires easily ___

Feels rested after sleep ___ Trouble falling asleep ___

Maintains own home: ___

Able to: Feed Self ___ Bathe Self ___

Needs Help: Feeding ___ Bathing ___ Dressing ___

Exhibit 4-1 (Continued)

Going to bathroom ___
Growth/development problems ___

Nursing Diagnosis ___

PERCEIVING

Body Image Changes ___

Eye contact: Appropriate ___ Downcast ___ Staring ___

Body Posture: Relaxed ___ Stooped ___ Rigid/tense ___

Level of consciousness: Alert ___ Responds to Pain ___

Oriented to: Time ___ Place ___ Person ___

Mood: Calm ___ Sad ___ Angry ___ Withdrawn ___ Other ___

Early a.m. awakening ___

Pupils: Equal ___ Reactive ___

Cognition: Able to follow simple commands: ___

Hearing: Normal ___ Impaired ___ Left Ear ___ Right Ear ___

Vision: Normal ___ Corrected with glasses ___ Prothesis ___

Unilateral Neglect ___

Diversional Activities: ___

Hopelessness ___ Powerlessness ___

Exhibit 4-1 (Continued)

Nursing Diagnosis _____

_____

KNOWING

Cognition Intact___ Recent Memory Change//Deficit___

Difficulty Learning _____

Education level _____

Knowledge deficit:

Regarding Illness:___ Condition:_____

Altered thought process _____

Nursing Diagnosis _____

_____

FEELING

Acute pain:___ Chronic pain___

How pain managed: _____

Anxiety _____

Recent Loss/grief___ Potential Loss/grief___

Potential for violence: Self___ Others___

Fearful___ Post Trauma Experiences___

Post Rape Syndrome: Silent___ Verbalized___

Nursing Diagnosis _____

_____

Exhibit 4-2 Ambulatory surgical nursing case study assessment form based on the nine NANDA patterns.

Legend: X = yes, O = no

Name: ___ Jennifer Simpson ___ Date: 8/19/90

Address: 4576 Oz Lane City Kansas City State: KS

Phone: (H) 864-1234 (W) 556-2363 SS# 654 21-5432

Surgical Diagnosis: Cystoscopy ___

Medical Diagnosis: Recurrent cystitis ___

Sex: F Age: 30 Known Allergies: O

EXCHANGING

Color oral mucosa: pink Moist X Dry O Lesions: O

Teeth X Missing –

Appearance: Well nourished X Obese ___ Emaciated ___

Weight:116 Height: 5'6" Weight Gain: O Weight Loss: O

Diet Restrictions: O ___ Alcohol Intake: O

Feeding Tubes: – Hyperalimentation: –

Skin:Turgor – Intact – Lesions – Color – Temp –

Diaphoresis: –

Fluid Intake: adequate

Exhibit 4-2 (Continued)

Nursing Diagnosis ___

Circulation

Temp 37 C Pulse 84 BP (Rt arm) – (Lt arm) 120/84

Sitting – Standing –

Apical rate 82 Rhythm: Regular X Irregular O

Heart sounds: S1 X S2 X S3 O S4 O

Neck veins distended: No X

Peripherial Edema: No X Location: –

Pedal Pulse: Rt X Lt X

Calf Tenderness: No X

Extremities: Color: pink Temp changes: warm

History of: Pacemaker O Chest pain X

Blood Clots: O Edema ___

Nursing Diagnosis ___

Respiration

Resp rate 16 Breathsounds normal Skin Color pink

Cough O Productive – Sputum Color – Smoker O

Pack years –

Dyspnea O On exertion –

Exhibit 4-2 (Continued)

Nursing Diagnosis_____

Elimination

Abdomen: Soft _X_ Firm___ Tender___ Distended___

Ostomies _O_ Bowel sounds present _X_

Stool/day _–_ Color _–_ Constipation _–_ Diarrhea _–_ Laxative use—

Enema use _–_ Incontinence of stool _–_

Urine output/day _?_ Color **yellow/cloudy**

Odor _X_ Urgency _X_

Frequency _X_ Nocturia _X_ Dysuria _X_ Hematuria _?_

Incontinent _O_ Stress Incontinence _O_

Nursing Diagnosis_____

Understands spoken language _X_ Reads _X_

Writes _X_ Reads Lips _O_ Hearing intact _X_

Vision intact _–_

Nursing Diagnosis_____

RELATING

Marital Status: M___ S _X_ W___ D___ Children _O_

Exhibit 4-2 (Continued)

Number of Children _–_ Dependents _O_

Occupation **Computer programmer**

Living Arrangements: Home Owner___ Rent _X_ Others in

the home _1_

Support system: Relative___ Friend **boyfriend (Jim)**

Family concerned about hospitalization _–_

Gets along with support system _X_

Personal Behavior: Passive_ Aggressive_ Assertive _X_

Parent _–_ Parenting Problems _–_

Last Menstrual Period **8/90** Menstrual Problems _O_

Birth Control Methods **pill** Number of Pregnancies _O_

Complications of Pregnancies_____

Sexual Preference: **heterosexual**

Sexual concerns _O_ History of VD _O_

Sexually active: _X_

Nursing Diagnosis_____

VALUING

Religious Affiliation _–_ Religious Restrictions_____

(Continued)

Exhibit 4-2 (Continued)

Would you like minister: To visit – To be called –

Cultural concerns   O

Religious concerns: O

Nursing Diagnosis

CHOOSING

Coping with health problems X Verbalizes problems

Uses defense mechanisms O   Can meet role

   expectations X

Family coping: Effective –   Ineffective

Neglectful – Self – Others –

Complies with care: Yes X Seeks Preventive care: X

Decision maker: Yes X No

Nursing Diagnosis

MOVING

Ambulates X   Climbs Stairs –

Gait: Steady – Unsteady – Limp – Able to walk –

Prothesis – Aids: Cane – Walker – Wheelchair –

Fatigue: – Tires easily –

Feels rested after sleep – Trouble falling asleep –

Exhibit 4-2 (Continued)

Maintains own home: –

Able to: Feed Self – Bathe Self –

Needs Help: Feeding – Bathing – Dressing –

Going to bathroom –

Growth/development problems –

Nursing Diagnosis

PERCEIVING

Body Image Changes O

Eye contact: Appropriate X Downcast   Staring

Body Posture: Relaxed X Stooped Rigid/tense

Level of consciousness: Alert X Responds to Pain X

Oriented to: Time X Place X Person X

Mood: Calm X Sad Angry Withdrawn Other

Early a.m. awakening –

Pupils: Equal X Reactive X Other –

Cognition: Able to follow simple commands: –

Hearing: Normal – Impaired – Left Ear – Right Ear –

Vision: Normal X Corrected with glasses X Prothesis –

   Farsighted – Nearsighted –

Exhibit 4-2 (Continued)

Unilateral Neglect __–__

Diversional Activities: __–__

Hopelessness __–__ Powerlessness __–__

Nursing Diagnosis _____

KNOWING

Cognition Intact _X_ Recent Memory Change//Deficit _–_

Difficulty Learning _O_

Education level **2 years post high school**

Knowledge deficit:

    Regarding Illness: _O_ Condition: _–_

    Altered thought process _–_

Nursing Diagnosis_____

FEELING

Acute pain: _X_ Chronic pain _X_

How pain managed: **ibuprofin tabs 2, 4 x day**

Anxiety _X_

Recent Loss/grief _–_ Potential Loss/grief _–_

Potential for violence: Self _–_ Others _–_

Fearful _–_ Post Trauma Experiences _–_

    Post Rape Syndrome: Silent _–_ Verbalized _–_

    Nursing Diagnosis_____

Exhibit 4-3 Preoperative care plan derived from the Quick Assessment Form and nursing diagnosis.

PATIENT NAME: Jennifer Simpson   DATE: 9/3/90   TIME: 13:30

MEDICAL DIAGNOSIS: Recurrent cystitis
SURGICAL PROCEDURE: Cystoscopy

Assessment	Nursing Diagnosis	Intervention	Evaluation	Discharge Plan
Exchanging:				
1. Decreased fluid intake	1. Alteration in urinary elimination R/T decreased fluid intake	1. Discuss the importance of adequate fluid intake	1. Discussed the need to increase fluid intake	1. Send home with booklet on fluid/food intake to prevent UTI
Feeling:				
2. Pain	2. Pain R/T infectious processes	2. Position with knees flexed prop with pillows	2. Positioning helped to relieve pain preop hypo also helped decrease pain	2. Verbally reinforce the above booklet on prevention of UTI
3. Anxiety	3. Anxiety R/T impending surgical experience	3. Provide emotional support	3. Anxiety decreased when procedures were explained and by allowing Jennifer to ask questions	

Exhibit 4-4 Checklist for validating nursing diagnosis.

```
                    Impaired Gas Exchange Checklist

Definition: Decreased exchange of oxygen/carbon dioxide between the pulmonary

and cardiovascular system.


Defining Criteria:

Present:

YES        NO
_____

_____|_____Confusion

_____|_____Somnolence

_____|_____Restlessness

_____|_____Irritability

_____|_____Inability to remove secretions

_____|_____Hypercapnia

_____|_____Hypoxia

_____|_____Ventilation perfusion imbalance


Other Characteristics Present:_____

_____

_____

_____
```

▽ ▽ ▽ Chapter 5

▽
▽
New Approaches to Care Planning by
▽
the Ambulatory Surgical Nurse
▽
Utilizing Nursing Diagnosis
▽

Sharon Summers

▽

▽

The previous chapter reviewed the five-step nursing process and de-scribed the process as cyclical or ongoing. As seen in Figure 5–1, it is now proposed that *nursing orders* replace *planning* in the nursing process. When students learn the five steps of the nursing process for the first time, there seems to be confusion as to what belongs in the *planning* column. If the planning phase of the process is perceived as involving only the procedures ordered by the physician, then it is little wonder that prac-ticing nurses do not often receive credit for *nursing*. However, the scope of nursing activities is not limited to merely following medical orders. Thus, this chapter answers the following key questions:

1. Does the nursing practice of the registered nurse consist of three levels (dependent, independent, and interdependent)?
2. What are the differences and similarities of medical diagnosis, care, and orders versus nursing diagnosis, care, and orders?
3. What new approaches to care plan construction, based on nursing diagnosis, could be pertinent for a patient with a surgical problem requiring arthroscopy?
4. How can the logical flow of information from the new care plan format be used to validate quality assurance reports and the standards of practice established by professional organizations?

▽

Levels of Nursing Practice

Nursing practice has been viewed as consisting of three levels: depen-dent, independent, and interdependent.[1] The dependent level of nursing practice is described as that which is determined by others (e.g., giving a preoperative medication as ordered). The independent level of nursing practice refers to that which is not controlled by others (e.g., nursing as-

Exhibits for Chapter 5 are located at the end of the chapter on pages 102–106.

Figure 5-1 Suggested revision of nursing process terminology.

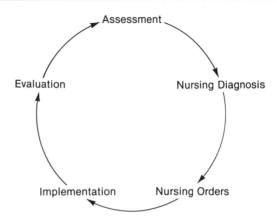

sessment of postoperative nutritional problems and intervention designed to assist the patient/family to promote recovery through proper nutrition). The interdependent level of nursing practice is defined as those nursing activities involving an equal dependence, or mutual responsibility (e.g., adjusting the dosage of pain medication as needed to promote self-care in the ambulatory surgical patient).

Although various nursing practice standards use these three levels of practice as points of reference, the position of the author is that there are only two levels of nursing practice: independent and interdependent. Interdependent nursing practice, or the provision of direct care for patients, is task-oriented (e.g., administering injections), whereas independent or indirect care encompasses all the nontask nursing interventions, such as patient and family emotional support. Indirect patient care is evolving into a more precise definition through the adoption of nursing diagnosis. If nurses work together to validate the North American Nursing Diagnosis Association (NANDA) taxonomy and develop a common standard for practice, then the profession of nursing will be advanced to a higher degree of professionalism.

The criteria distinguishing any profession include a code of ethics, a license to practice, autonomy, and a unique body of knowledge. As a step in the development of a unique body of knowledge, nurses are striving to establish a taxonomy or classification system to define what it is that registered nurses do that is unique. As discussed in Chapter 4, a taxonomy is extremely important, as it is also the first step toward the development of a theory and a science of nursing. Thus, the previously described NANDA nursing diagnosis taxonomy is the first step needed to identify the independent nursing activities. If nurses in an ambulatory surgical setting use the medical taxonomy to document independent surgical nursing care, then it may be difficult to obtain reimbursement or achieve adequate staffing when most acuity scales rate patient problems based on interdependent or direct care. It can be speculated that, when staffing is based on direct care or tasks alone, inadequate staffing may result because professional nursing care consists of more than tasks. Nurses should use NANDA's nursing diagnosis taxonomy, then, to document their assessments according to a standardized format so that nurses can be reimbursed or recognized for giving indirect, as well as direct, nursing care.

▽

Medical versus Nursing Diagnosis, Orders, and Care

Both medical and nursing diagnosis, orders, and care have been compared, contrasted, and described extensively in the literature and are directly related to each profession's definition and state license regulations. Medicine is defined as the science and art for which physicians are licensed to diagnose, prescribe medication for, and otherwise treat disease and cure human ills.[2] Hanft[3] describes physicians as independent practitioners of medicine who work without supervision. Campbell-Heider and Pollock[2] note that physicians have assumed legitimate power based on the historical roles of the educated physician and the role of nurses as physician extenders.

Nursing is defined as "the diagnosis and treatment of human responses to actual or potential health problems" (p. 9).[4] The research of Campbell-Heider and Pollock[2] indicates that nurses have been socialized to work in a team approach, which has resulted in nursing authority being decentralized to a subordinate level. This position is supported by Hanft, who describes the nurse as a "dependent agent who delivers limited services."[2] Historically, the services provided by both physicians and nurses have evolved through and been shaped by licensing regulations and gender issues. Thus, by virtue of each profession's definition and state license regulations, the practice of medicine and the practice of nursing differ. This difference should not, however, imply incompatibilities; rather, it should imply a complementary practice by both professions for one common goal: quality patient care.

▽

Nursing Diagnosis Applications

The case study from Chapter 4 described quick patient assessment and nursing diagnosis strategies for a patient undergoing cystoscopy. A similar case—that of Fred Freeman, a 29-year-old ski instructor admitted to ambulatory surgical services for arthroscopy of the right knee—is presented here to illustrate how medical and nursing diagnoses differ, and how they can complement effective patient care. The strategies proposed in the following discussion are based on the assumption that there are only two levels of nursing practice for registered nurses: interdependent (direct) and independent (indirect).

The nurse completes the admission assessment of Fred, formulates the nursing diagnoses, and writes the nursing orders. This nursing process information is then compared to the physician's history and physical, medical diagnosis, and medical orders. The similarities and differences in the two are noted in Exhibit 5–1.

This case study illustrates the fact that nursing differs from medicine, but the two professions complement each other. It is important to examine the differences and similarities so that nurses can become aware of their levels of nursing practice. All too often, nursing blends so well into medicine that nursing practice is difficult to differentiate, and then it becomes difficult for nurses to be reimbursed for care. Although experienced nurses may not need to define nurse/physician similarities and differences of practice, this complex approach may help inexperienced nurses to clarify the levels of nursing practice. To examine further how the two levels of nursing practice can be used to develop a care plan, data from this case study will now be used to formulate new strategies for care planning in the ambulatory surgical setting.

▽

A New Approach to Care Plan Construction

A new approach to care plan construction is proposed that clearly outlines how nurses can document the two levels of nursing practice. In the past, the traditional format has typically consisted of four columns containing the four steps of the nursing process—assessment, planning, implementation, and evaluation—with the nursing diagnosis listed at the top of the care plan. Confusion among nursing students would usually develop when they were called upon to transform the medical record, as if by magic, into this nursing process format. Since this confusion was the result of trying to "fit" the medical format into the nursing care plan, then it can be assumed that something must be theoretically wrong with how this process is taught. Thus, a new care plan format is proposed, and it is up to the practicing nurse to test the usefulness of this form.

As illustrated in Figure 5–2, the new care plan form consists of five columns: assessment, nursing diagnosis, nursing orders, implementation, and evaluation. Although these categories are not new, what is new are the subcategories included for specifying medical diagnoses and medical orders and for differentiating the two levels of practice (independent and interdependent) as they pertain to implementation. Also, the new care plan offers separate forms for preoperative, intraoperative, and postoperative patient care.

As seen in Exhibits 5–2 through 5–4, the information from the case study presented earlier fits easily into the proposed care plan form for preoperative, intraoperative, and postoperative care. This format not only enhances patient care, but also serves as an easy method for validating quality patient care and for determining whether the nursing care provided meets professional organization standards.

Figure 5-2 New care plan format.

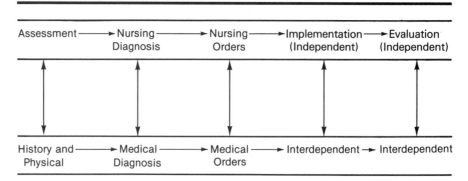

Quality Assurance and Professional Standards of Nursing Practice

The purpose of quality assurance reports is to validate that patients received care that was appropriate for their medical and nursing diagnoses. As described in Chapter 2, the Joint Commission on Accreditation of Health Care Organizations (JCAHO) (1990) mandates that care of the patient in the ambulatory surgical setting be implemented in a safe environment by qualified health care practitioners.[5] Nursing care that is appropriate for an individual ambulatory surgical patient, based on the medical diagnosis and three-part nursing care plans and nursing diagnoses written by the registered nurse, can be well documented using the new care plan strategies that meet the JCAHO criteria.

The purpose of professional organization standards of practice is to validate a level of nursing practice that parallels the purpose and standards of that particular organization. Both the Association of Operating Room nurses (1988) (AORN) and the American Society of Post Anesthesia Nurses (1991) (ASPAN) have established standards of practice. ASPAN, however, also has developed standards for preanesthesia or preprocedural ambulatory care that are based on assessment, nursing diagnosis, care planning, implementation, and evaluation.

In a busy ambulatory surgical setting, the adherence of nurses to quality assurance and standards of practice criteria would be facilitated if the nurse were provided with a form, such as the proposed new care plan, that also paralleled these criteria. Nurses frequently complain about the mountain of paperwork plaguing their practice; most would welcome the use of forms that would eliminate the need for rewriting or searching charts for the standards data. As described in Chapter 3, the use of computers would facilitate the generation of quality assurance reports and care plan formulation/documentation of care. Computerization would also permit prompt retrieval of data, thus avoiding the tedious process of searching for such documentation by hand. With computerization, standard plans of care could be stored, requiring only that the nurse edit these forms appropriately for individualized patient care. It has been stated that nurses effectively use part of the nursing process—that is, assessment and planning—for patient care. However, nursing diagnosis and evaluation of care remain the two weakest areas of documentation for most practicing nurses. If the new care plan were computerized, the computer program could be written so that, in the event that a nurse failed to document any area of the nursing process, an electronic message could be sent, prompting that nurse to enter the omitted information.

▽

Summary

In considering the four basic questions posed in this chapter, one can conclude that it is time for a change in how nursing care plans are written so that nursing care can be distinguished from medical care in the ambulatory surgical setting. It is also time for a change in the way nurses are acknowledged for care provided, with direct care being recognized as task-oriented and indirect care being recognized as the art and science of nursing. Documentation of nursing care could be facilitated by adopting a trilevel approach to care planning in the ambulatory surgical setting, an approach that would differentiate between preoperative, intraoperative, and postoperative care. Although some might interpret this approach as generating additional work, the effort involved in constructing these three-level care plans would be minimized by the use of computers. Once initial care plans were completed and electronically stored, it would be easy to retrieve data and evaluate quality patient care and standards of professional nursing practice. Moreover, such a trilevel approach to care plans could be used to document and acknowledge the activities involved in the professional practice of nursing, thereby advancing the goals of the profession.

References

1. Ritter, T., Crulcich, M., & McEntegart, A. (1981). Nursing practice: An amalgam of dependence, independence and interdependence. In J. M. McCloskey & H. K. Grace (Eds.). *Current Issues in Nursing* (pp. 5–14). Boston: Blackwell Scientific Publications.
2. Campbell-Heider, N., & Pollock, D. (1987). Barriers to physician-nurse collegiality: An anthropological perspective. *Social Science and Medicine, 25*(5), 421–425.
3. Hanft, R. (1981). Health manpower. In S. Jonas (Ed.), *Health Care Delivery in the United States* (pp. 61–64). New York: Springer.
4. American Nurses' Association. (1980). *Nursing: A social policy statement.* Kansas City: American Nurses' Association.
5. *The Joint Commission Accreditation Manual for Hospitals.* (1990). Chicago: Joint Commission on Accreditation of Health Care Organizations.

Exhibit 5-1 Nursing versus medical assessment.

Exhibit 5-1 (Continued)

A

Nursing Assessment

Date: 5/22/92   Time: 07:32
Nursing Assessment

Subjective:
"I'm here to get my knee fixed."

Objective

EENT: Wnl, mouth and lips dry
CV: Apical rate 92, B/P 123/90
      Temp 98

RESP: Breath sounds audible,
Lung fields clear, rate 18
GI/RENAL: Bowel sounds present
in all four quadrants

NEUROMUSC: Alert, nervous,
moving all extremities.

Preoperative Nursing Diagnosis

1. Self-esteem Disturbance:
   R/T job disruption

2. Anxiety R/T operative experience
3. Impaired physical mobility R/T
   recent injury to knee

Intraoperative Nursing Diagnosis

1. Impaired skin integrity R/T
   surgical procedure
2. High risk for injury R/T tissue
   trauma
3. Impaired gas exchange R/T general
   anesthesia use
4. High risk for hypothermia
   R/T cool environment
5. Impaired physical mobility R/T
   unconscious state
6. High risk for infection R/T
   surgical intrusion

B

Medical History & Physical

Date: 5/22/92   Time: 08:20
Medical History & Physical

Subjective:
"Make me like new, Doc."

Objective

H & P dictated.
Chief complaint: Pain in
right knee. Initial
injury occurred in a
skiing accident when a student
fell on him.
C/O instability of the right
knee that prevents him
from working as a ski
instructor
P.E.: Essentially negative
      No visible scars or history of
      previous surgery.

Medical Diagnosis

Instability of right knee
possible rupture of patellar
tendon

C

Postoperative Nursing Diagnosis

1. Pain R/T operative procedure
2. Impaired physical mobility
   R/T immobilizer to knee
3. Impaired skin integrity R/T
   surgically induced wound
4. Alteration in nutrition: less
   than body requirement R/T
   decreased oral intake
5. Knowledge deficit R/T home care
   of wound, crutch walking, and
   nutritional needs

Preoperative Nursing Orders

1. Provide emotional support to
   promote self-esteem
2. Instruct the patient on unit
   routines to decrease anxiety
   I.M. at 08:30

Intraoperative Nursing Orders

1. Carefully monitor surgical prep
2. Monitor surgical procedure
   techniques/equipment use
3. Monitor use of O2 during anesthesia
4. Protect from hypothermia with
   blankets/drapes prn
5. Position patient carefully for
   good body alignment
6. Monitor aseptic techniques of
   the OR team and dressing applications

Postoperative Nursing Orders

1. Monitor pain response
2. Position in proper body alignment
3. Check and maintain DSD - observe
   for drainage
4. Encourage high calorie foods to
   meet energy needs, encourage high
   protein foods to promote wound healing
5. Begin patient teaching for home
   care when awake

D

Preoperative Medical Orders

1. NPO
2. CBC, UA
3. Demerol 100 mg
   Atropine 0.4 mg

4. To OR @ 09.15

Postoperative Medical Orders

1. Tylenol #3 q 3-4
   h for pain
2. Liquid diet prn
3. Instruct patient
   on meaning
   of DSD and knee
   immobilizer
4. Discharge when
   awake with
   crutches
5. Instruct patient to
   avoid driving until
   immobilizer is removed
6. Return to unit on

Exhibit 5-1 (Continued)

Interventions

A Independent Nursing Practice (Indirect Care)	B Interdependent Nursing Practice (Direct Care)
Preoperative 1. Allow patient to verbalize the meaning of his job loss 2. Inform patient of surgical routines to decrease anxiety	1. Give Tylenol #3 prn for pain. Prescription given to wife to be filled in outside pharmacy. 2. Liquids offered and well tolerated. 3. DSD remains intact 4. Discharge home when recovered 5. Inform wife to return patient to unit on 5/29 for suture removal 6. Instruct patient not to drive while wearing knee immobilizer
Intraoperative 1. Monitor surgical procedure and equipment 2. Check temp and cover patient prn 3. Monitor O2 adjunct to anesthesia gases 4. Monitor position on OR table 5. Monitor aseptic technique of OR team members 6. Monitor aseptic technique of dressing application	
Postoperative 1. Monitor pain response 2. Monitor body alignment 3. Check dressing 4. Instruct patient on specific foods that promote wound healing: high protein, high calorie 5. Complete discharge plan by instructing patient on wound care, crutch walking, and when to return for suture removal.	

Exhibit 5-1 (Continued)

Evaluation

C Nursing Ordered Care Provided (Indirect Care)	D Medical Ordered Care Provided (Direct Care)
Preoperative 1. Patient stated he understood that he may be immobile for 4-6 weeks 2. Instruction about OR routine seemed to help patient relax	1. NPO 2. Lab ordered 3. Preop med given
Intraoperative 1. Tissue trauma to be minimized with ice and compression dressing 2. Patient's temp dropped 1.2 and blankets were applied 3. O2 mix to anesthesia appropriate 4. Good body alignment and protection during procedure 5. Aseptic technique maintained during procedure 6. Aseptic technique maintained during dressing applications	
Postoperative 1. Mr. Freeman states he understands why he is not to return to work until the knee has a chance to heal 2. Mr. Freeman states he understands that the dressing over his stitches is to remain dry and intact 3. Mr. Freeman given sample diet forms of high protein-high calorie foods 4. Discharge plan completed and Mr. Freeman and wife were instructed to return to the unit on 5/29 for suture removal. Discharged home to the care of wife at 09:55. 5. Mr. Freeman demonstrated proper use crutches.	1. Patient has not required Tylenol #3 for pain. Prescription given to wife 2. Liquids offered and well tolerated 3. DSD remains intact 4. Discharge home when recovered 5. Wife informed to return the patient to the unit on 5/29 for suture removal. 6. Patient/wife instructed not to drive with knee immobilizer.

Exhibit 5-2 Preoperative care plan.

PATIENT NAME: Fred Freeman

PREOPERATIVE REPORT   DATE: 5/22/90   TIME: 07:32

Assessment	Nursing Diagnosis	Nursing Orders	Implementation	Evaluation
Subjective:				
I'm here to get my knee fixed	1. Self-esteem Disturbance R/T job disruption	1. Provide emotional support to promote self-esteem.	1. Allow patient to verbalize the meaning of his job loss.	1. Patient stated he understood that he may be immobile for 4-6 weeks.
EENT: WNL; mouth and lips dry	2. Anxiety R/T Operative experience	2. Instruct the patient on unit routine to decrease anxiety.	2. Inform patient of surgical routines to decrease anxiety.	2. Instruction about OR routine seemed to help patient relax.
CV: Apical rate B/P 123/90, T 98°F	3. Impaired physical mobility R/T recent injury to knee			
RESP: Breath sounds audible, lung fields clear, rate 18				
GI/RENAL: Bowel sounds present in all four quadrants				
NEUROMUSC: Alert, nervous moving all extremities				

	Medical Diagnosis	Medical Orders	Interdependent	Interdependent
	Instability of rt. knee, possible rupture of patellar tendon	1. NPO	1. NPO Urine to lab	1. NPO
		2. CBC, UA	2. Lab work ordered	2. CBC sample to lab Urine to lab
		3. Demorol, 100 mg Atropine, 0.4mg	3. Preop med given	3. Preop hypo
		4. To OR @ 09:15		

Exhibit 5-3 Intraoperative care plan.

PATIENT NAME: Fred Freeman

INTRAOPERATIVE REPORT   DATE: 5/22/90   TIME: 09:42

Assessment	Nursing Diagnosis	Nursing Orders	Implementation (Independent)	Evaluation (Independent)
1. Surgical prep to rt. knee	1. Impaired skin integrity R/T surgical procedure	1. Carefully monitor surgical prep.	1. Monitor surgical procedures and equipment.	1. Tissue trauma to be minimized with ice & compression dressing.
2. Surgical procedure begun	2. High risk for injury R/T tissue trauma	2. Monitor surgical procedure/techniques and equipment use.	2. Check temp and cover patient prn.	2. Patients temp dropped 1.2° F and blankets applied.
3. Sedated and anesthetized	3. Impaired gas exchange R/T use of general anesthesia	3. Monitor O2 use during anesthesia.	3. Monitor O2 adjunct to anesthesia.	3. O2 mix with anesthesia appropriate.
4. Room temp 62° F	4. Potential for hypothermia R/T cool environment	4. Protect patient from hypothermia with drapes/blankets prn.	4. Monitor position on OR table.	4. Good body alignment and protection during procedure.
5. Placed on narrow table under general anesthesia	5. Impaired physical mobility R/T unconscious state	5. Position patient carefully for good body alignment.	5. Monitor aseptic technique of OR team members.	5. Aseptic technique maintained during procedure.
	6. High risk for infection R/T surgical intrusion	6. Monitor aseptic techniques of OR team and dressing application.	6. Monitor aseptic technique during dressing application.	6. Aseptic technique maintained during dressing application.

Exhibit 5-4 Postoperative care plan.

PATIENT NAME: Fred Freeman

POSTOPERATIVE REPORT   DATE: 5/22/90   TIME: 10:22

Assessment	Nursing Diagnosis	Nursing Orders	Implementation (Independent)	Evaluation (Independent)
1. Recovery from anesthesia begun	1. Pain R/T operative procedure	1. Monitor pain response.	1. Monitor pain response.	1. Patient states he understands why he is not to return to work until the knee has a chance to heal.
2. Immobilizer applied to rt. knee	2. Impaired physical mobility R/T immobilizer	2. Position in proper body alignment.	2. Monitor body alignment.	2. Patient states he understands that the dressing over his stitches is to remain dry and intact.
3. DSD to knee with compression dressing	3. Impaired skin integrity R/T surgical wound	3. Check and maintain DSD, observe for drainage.	3. Check dressing.	3. Patient was given sample diet forms of high-protein, high-calorie foods.
4. Still NPO	4. Alteration in nutrition; less than body requirement R/T decreased oral intake	4. Encourage intake of high-calorie foods to meet energy needs, encourage high-protein foods to promote wound healing.	4. Instruct patient on specific foods that promote wound healing (high-calorie, high-protein foods).	4. Discharge plan completed and the patient was instructed to return to the unit on 5/29 for suture removal. Discharged home to the care of wife @ 10:55.
5. Uninformed as to postop recovery procedures	5. Knowledge deficit R/T home care of wound, crutch walking and nutritional needs	5. Begin patient teaching for home care when awake.	5. Complete discharge plan by instructing patient on wound care, crutch walking, and when to return for suture removal.	

		Medical Orders	Interdependent	
		1. Give Tylenol #3 prn for pain	1. Patient has not required Tylenol for pain. Prescription given to wife to have filled in outside pharmacy.	
		2. Resume liquids prn	2. Liquids offered and well tolerated.	
		3. Instruct patient on meaning of DSD and knee immobilizer	3. DSD remains intact.	
		4. Discharge when recovered	4. Discharge home when recovered.	
		5. Instruct patient to avoid driving until immobilizer is removed.	5. Wife informed to return patient to the unit on 5/29 for suture removal.	
			6. Patient instructed not to drive while wearing immobilizer.	

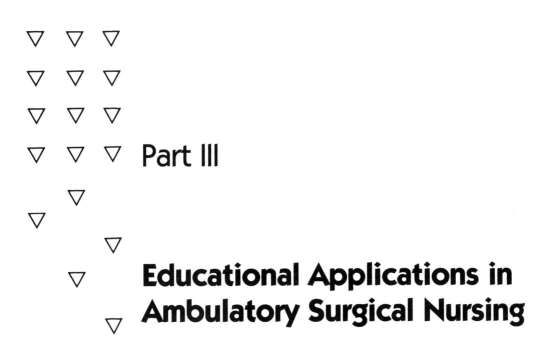

Part III

Educational Applications in Ambulatory Surgical Nursing

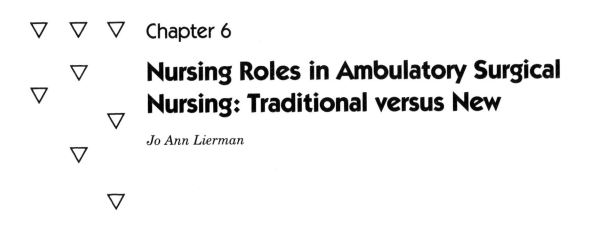

Chapter 6

Nursing Roles in Ambulatory Surgical Nursing: Traditional versus New

Jo Ann Lierman

Ambulatory outpatient care constitutes a large portion of today's health care industry. In 1982, ambulatory surgery procedures represented 20% of all surgical procedures.[1] According to the Health Care Finance Administration, 121, 491 procedures were performed in ambulatory surgery centers in 1986, and it is estimated that by the year 2000, 80% of surgical procedures will be outpatient cases.[2] More surgical procedures are being performed on an outpatient basis because of new developments in anesthesia techniques, fiber optics, and laser technology.[1] Because of advances in technology and our changing social view of health care, the role of the perioperative nurse is changing drastically as well. Several key questions are addressed in this chapter, including:

1. What are the traditional nursing education methods used to prepare the nurse for staff, operating room (OR), and recovery room roles?
2. What are the new educational needs of the nurse for the management of patient admission, patient education, responsibilities in the operating room and recovery room, and discharge planning in the ambulatory surgical setting?
3. What are the inconsistencies between the traditional nursing curriculum and the role expectation of the nurse in the ambulatory surgical setting?
4. What strategies are needed for including educational content in the nursing curriculum to prepare the nurse for a role in the ambulatory surgical setting?

Traditional Role

In the late 1890s, the role of the nurse in the OR was very different from that of today. At that time, the nurse's chief responsibility was to hand sponges to the surgeon. The nurse assisted with dressings and was expected to have a good supply of thread in her dressing basket. Preparation of the OR and care of the patient were not nursing responsibilities.[3] However, with the establishment of training schools in the early 1900s, the OR became a field of practice, and thus the evolution of the OR nurse began.

As scientific knowledge advanced and major discoveries emerged, health care practices and surgery changed, as did the role of the OR nurse. The nurse assumed new responsibilities and the role continually demanded better prepared and more sophisticated nurses. During World War I, nursing practice was primarily limited to caring for the sick and wounded recuperating in hospitals. During World War II, when the personnel shortage was at its height, new roles and responsibilities were created for the nurse. With the development of sulfa drugs and penicillin, wartime surgery became more aggressive, and the nurse was expected to become more specialized. During this period, the OR nurse often was responsible for anesthesia, asepsis, sanitation, instruments, patient preparation, and supervision of other OR personnel, as well as operating room preparation. At the conclusion of the war, nurses returned to civilian hospital duties and wanted to retain these new responsibilities. During the 1940s, nurses managed patient care in the OR and assisted surgeons.[3]

During the 1950s, nurses began to band together to advance the practice of OR nursing. This heralded the formation of the Association of Operating Room Nurses (AORN). During this period, the role of the nurse was centered in the operative suite, and primarily involved patient care during the intraoperative period. During the 1950s and 1960s, the role of the OR nurse was primarily viewed as a technical one because, after all, the patient was asleep. The nurse was considered the "handmaiden" of the surgeon, with responsibility for preparing the operating suite, making sure all supplies were ready, and caring for the patient only during the intraoperative period.[3] Little attention was paid to the other duties the nurse may have been performing, such as patient assessment, psychological and physiological support, and patient teaching. Indeed, it was suggested by some health professionals that the registered nurse was not even needed in the OR since nonnursing personnel, such as operating room technicians, had been trained to perform scrub duties and other duties previously performed by nurses.

As a result of this view of the role of the nurse, delegates at the 1973 AORN Congress approved a statement on the necessity for the registered nurse in the OR. This statement supported the idea that, if surgical patients were to receive optimal care in the OR, a registered nurse was essential because of the nurse's education and background in the nursing process. This statement also implied that nurses have the knowledge base to provide patients with physiological and psychological care, whereas nonprofessional personnel in the OR were trained in the technical aspects of care only, and thus were unable to meet the needs of the surgical patient adequately.[3]

During the 1970s, major events occurred that affected the role of the OR nurse. The *Standards of Nursing Practice: Operating Room,*[4] published in 1975, and the *Operating Room Nursing: Perioperative Role,*[5] developed in 1978, defined clearly the role and scope of practice of the OR nurse. The definition of the perioperative role is based on the following philosophical view:

> Nursing is an independent, autonomous, self-regulating profession with the primary function of helping each person attain his highest possible level of general health. The practice of nursing focuses on assessing people's health status, assets, and deviations from health, and on helping sick people to regain health, and the well or near-well to maintain or attain health through selective application of nursing science and use of available nursing strategies (p. 766).[6]

In 1978, AORN's Project 25 task force defined the role of the perioperative nurse as follows:[5]

> The nurse in the operating room practices in an environment in which basic life-sustaining needs are the highest priority and are predicated upon medical-surgical principles. The role involves the nursing care of patients having known or predicted physiological alterations. The nurse, through collaboration with other members of the health care team, assists in assuring a continuity of care by providing assistance in planning regimens of care in the preoperative, intraoperative, and postoperative periods of the patient's surgical experience. The nurse provides direct care to surgical patients, with primary emphasis on the intraoperative period and responsibility for preoperative assessment and postoperative evaluation. The operating room nurse should possess substantial knowledge, judgment, and skill based on the principles of biological, physiological, behavioral, and social sciences. The nurse makes decisions about the patient's needs and assists and supports the patient in meeting those needs. While the operating nurse works in collaboration with other health professionals to determine and meet patient needs, the nurse has primary responsibility and accountability for nursing care of patients having surgical intervention (pp. 1162–1164).[5]

In 1982, AORN published a statement on the basic competencies of a perioperative nurse that further helped to define the role of the nurse. This statement redefined competency as the "knowledge, skills, and abilities necessary to fulfill the professional role functions of a registered nurse in the operating room" (p. 1).[7] Table 6–1 outlines the expectations of nursing abilities identified by the author.

▽

New Educational Needs

Advances in technology, a changing view of health care, and a more complex patient who needs more information has required concomitant modifications in the role of the perioperative nurse. The perioperative nurse of the 1990s must be knowledgeable in the specialty practice area, utiliz-

Table 6-1 Expectations of Nursing Abilities

To assess the physiological health status of the patient
To assess the psychosocial health status of the patient/family
To formulate nursing diagnoses and goals based on data collected
To plan and implement care
To participate in patient/family teaching
To create and maintain a sterile field
To provide equipment and supplies based on patient needs
To perform specified counts
To administer and monitor the effects of drugs
To monitor the physiological status of the patient intraoperatively
To monitor and control the surgical environment
To respect the patient's rights
To demonstrate accountability in nursing actions
To evaluate patient outcomes
To measure effectiveness of nursing care
To reassess all components of patient care continually, based on new data

ing a holistic patient approach, and possess high levels of skill in business administration, nursing research, and computer science.

Today, ambulatory surgical patients have more complex needs and require more information. The nurse caring for these individuals must be a professional who is highly skilled and well-educated. Minimal credentials should include baccalaureate preparation in nursing, a current nursing license, and at least two years of medical-surgical nursing experience, preferably in critical care. The background of the professional nurse practicing in the ambulatory surgical setting should also include a global perspective derived from the liberal arts and sciences, an emphasis on holistic, family-centered care, and an understanding of the patient's home environment.

The nurse who practices in the ambulatory center of today is an autonomous professional who needs the prerequisite skills to assess and evaluate the patient, the family, and the home environment. In addition, the ambulatory surgical nurse may be called upon to identify or recognize medical problems, develop nursing diagnoses, and follow a set medical protocol. The nurse may be assessing, teaching, and evaluating the patient with regard to the many aspects of the surgical experience, and will be sharing these data with other members of the health care team.

Service, quality care, and compassion constitute the bases for the traditional value system underlying nursing practice. The perioperative nurses of today may experience conflict with their professional value system, however, when the institutions in which they work must adhere to the set fee structure dictated by diagnosis-related groupings (DRGs) and third-party payers. Health care organizations and professionals are now advertising for customers, and the perioperative nurse must be aware of marketing strategies and be very conscious of cost.[8] Perioperative nursing is now faced with many changes and a restructuring of roles. Because the procedure performed determines the patient's length of stay, the nurse must provide quality patient care within this shortened time frame. Indeed, meeting patient care needs during such a shortened length of stay is a good marketing strategy, as satisfied patients will then recommend the ambulatory center to many other people.

The ambulatory surgical unit (ASU) now represents a competitive market that must be both comprehensive and cost-effective. The common goal of most ASUs is to get the patient in and out of the unit with the most efficient use of time and money, while still offering a high standard of care and a low incidence of complications.

The primary force behind the movement from inpatient to outpatient surgery was a change in the health care reimbursement system.[1] This change provided incentives for hospitals to begin to diversify service offerings, especially on the outpatient side. Health industry observers forecasted that by the 1990s, 16% of all inpatient beds would be closed.[9] Current reports estimate that by the year 2000, 25% of the inpatient beds will be closed or 70% of the patients currently treated in hospitals will be treated in alternative settings, such as free standing facilities or physicians' offices.[9]

Because of changing economics, nurses may need to assume additional business management responsibilities in the ASU, thereby adding a new dimsention to the perioperative role. Exposure to the business side of health care may prompt the nurse to become involved in developing innovative nursing care delivery programs, writing business plans for the approval of institutional review boards, and constructing cost-effective staff management programs. Perioperative nurses are now being challenged to learn business principles and management, which may be a new language for them, in order to interact with other health care providers in the health care delivery system. This educational focus is essential for maintaining the integrity of nursing practice within a health care system that utilizes business terminology.

At the current rate of technological advancement, increased knowledge will continue to be at the center of nursing as we progress into the 21st century. New advancements in instruments, equipment, and procedures will allow more complex surgeries to be performed in the ASU. As discussed in Chapter 3, computers, using artificial intelligence, will allow perioperative nurses to access an expert surgical nursing knowledge base. Using robotics, technical tasks, such as cleaning surgical rooms, washing instruments, assembling supplies, and performing repetitive tasks, may become automated. Computers in many institutions are currently performing scheduling, staffing, and other management tasks.[10]

Because we are living in a period of exploding scientific knowledge and the invention of new technology, nursing research is in demand in order to validate new approaches to patient care while maintaining quality. Perioperative nurses are increasingly being asked to participate in research relating to patient care practices, patient care delivery system outcomes, and patients' responses to care. This participation requires the nurse to have a firm knowledge of research principles and methodology.

We are living in a society that has rapidly become health-conscious. This change in health perspective has created a patient who is demanding more information when faced with a surgical experience. Because of this desire for more information and the increased complexity of patients' health problems, the nurse is now required to do more extensive patient teaching, yet with less patient contact and increased time constraints. The main goals of the professional perioperative nurse still remain the same: to ensure patient safety and prevent infection.

With increased utilization of the ASU, patient education has become important to the success of many facilities. The primary goal of patient education is to provide the patient with information to enhance self-care management. Research has shown that patient teaching also reduces anxiety and increases the patient's ability to cope with the surgical experience. This issue is further addressed in Chapter 15. In the ASU, patient teaching is a way to improve patient compliance and nurse–patient interaction. Currently, the role of the perioperative nurse is to provide more comprehensive, complex teaching for patients and their families in a shorter period of time. Time constraints require that nurses be creative and innovative in the delivery of this information.

Another factor that has had an impact on the perioperative role is the changing physiological status of the ambulatory patient. The elderly population continues to grow, with a projected increase to 55 million by the year 2020. Older people, who suffer from more chronic disease and acute illness than their younger counterparts, represent a greater surgical risk.[11] Moreover, the aging process may leave the patient with failing eyesight or hearing, impaired mental ability, impaired mobility, impaired circulation, or other problems associated with aging. These age-related changes may require the nurse to develop special plans for teaching or intraoperative patient care, or these patients may simply warrant more intense nursing care throughout the surgical experience. Thus, the perioperative nurse must be well versed in the aging process and the implications of age-related changes as they relate to the surgical experience.

Perioperative nurses of the future will indeed need to be expert primary nurse practitioners. In the ambulatory surgical setting, perioperative nurses will be practicing in all realms of the surgical experience and functioning autonomously from other health care providers. The nurse will be required to be highly knowledgeable and skillful, as well as have knowledge and ability in business administration, nursing research, and computer science. The nurse will be expected to provide quality nursing care, maintain excellence in practice, and ensure a high level of ethics and values. Perioperative nurses will continually be required to develop new insights into patient care and increasingly effective ways to meet patients' needs. A strong identity will be essential for the nurse in this expanded role, as will continuing education and a commitment to life-long learning in order for the nurse to survive in a world of rapid technological advancement and changing health care practices.

▽

Traditional Nursing Education and Ambulatory Surgical Nursing Practice

The first known instance of OR training occurred in 1876 when Professor Henry Jacob Bigelow took nursing pupils into the OR at Harvard Medical School for instruction. This was perhaps the beginning of OR nursing education.[12] In an article on early OR nursing, Metzger quotes Walsh, who in 1880 stated, "The development of modern surgery made it absolutely necessary that nurses should be trained, educated women, so as to be able to be proper auxiliaries for the surgeons" (p. 80).[12] When training schools first started, curriculum guides or standards were unknown. Excellence was derived from whoever was in charge of the school. At the turn of the century, hospitals were primarily intended for care of surgical patients.[3] Because of this, surgery probably played a major role in the development of nursing education.

Metzger further indicated that, in the early 1900s, nurses received instruction in business ethics of the OR as their responsibilities included material management.[12] The OR nurse's responsibilities were increasing, but it was not until 1917 that the first national curriculum was established by the National League of Nursing Education. This first curriculum included instruction in surgical disease, OR technique, and bacteriology.[12]

Throughout nursing history, education and practice have been closely related. In the area of perioperative nursing, academic curriculum and instruction has become increasingly devoid of OR content, and has seriously lagged behind the times in meeting the educational needs associated with a rapidly evolving and expanding perioperative role. In our health care system, emphasis is no longer placed on traditional hospital-based nursing practice, but rather on a practice requiring highly skilled and qualified nurses functioning in an autonomous expanded role. Today, perioperative nurses are actively involved in ambulatory surgical care.

Traditional baccalaureate curricula divide content into conventional subject areas, such as medical-surgical nursing, pediatric nursing, psychiatric-mental health nursing. The major goal of this type of curriculum is to produce a generalist nurse who has a scientific knowledge base of nursing and who can analyze and synthesize nursing information. To some degree, this goal has met the needs of hospital-based nursing services that are interested in graduates who are technically competent and who can be assimilated immediately into the work environment. Currently, though, throughout the United States, the emphasis is on baccalaureate education as a prerequisite for entry into practice. The catalyst for more education has been derived from a variety of sources, such as state nursing boards requiring the baccalaureate degree for entry into practice, health care organizations' promotion requirements, satisfaction of personal needs on the part of individual nurses, and recognition by various professional organizations that more indepth knowledge is required for modern nursing practice. Perioperative nursing is currently viewed as a specialty area; consequently, specific perioperative nursing content has been eliminated from traditional, generalist nursing curricula.

A recent descriptive study of 230 students enrolled in associate and baccalaureate degree programs in the Denver area looked at some basic questions about perioperative nursing education.[13] The questions were:

1. How much time do students actually spend in the OR?
2. What activities are the students involved in while in the OR?
3. What activities are most interesting to the students?
4. Is the OR experience a planned activity for students?

The results showed that students received little exposure to the OR; 76.9% of the respondents spent less than five days in the OR throughout their entire nursing education program, and half of those students did so for observation experiences only, with no required written or oral assignment to complete. The students were most interested in the role of the nurse in the OR. Most of the students did not have a preplanned experience.

Results of this study are typical of most traditional nursing curricula. Whereas students are usually well versed in the preoperative and postoperative care of a patient on a typical hospital unit, the medical-surgical component of their educational program typically offers little, if any, exposure to intraoperative nursing care. A one- or two-day observational experience limits the student's ability to gain a comprehensive understanding of the perioperative role. Students tend to see the OR nurse as someone who merely performs technical work, and they frequently miss altogether the concept of nursing process as it applies to the intraoperative role. Exposure to the new expanded role of the perioperative nurse in an ambulatory surgery center is all but nonexistent.

Some schools of nursing do offer elective courses in perioperative nursing, which provide a more global view of perioperative nursing and allow students to experience many aspects of the role. However, these elective courses tend to focus on the intraoperative period of patient care, often to the exclusion of the preoperative and postoperative phases. The student thus does not gain a full, comprehensive view of the perioperative role.

Present curriculum designs tend to focus the student's attention on other areas of nursing practice. Because of the limited exposure of traditional nursing students to perioperative nursing, it is difficult, if not impossible, for new graduates to enter this specialty area of nursing practice. For economic reasons, most hospitals are unwilling to provide inservice education in the OR for new graduates because of the time and expense involved before they are competent to function independently in this setting. Staffing shortages in many hospitals further aggravate the problem by eliminating the availability of staff members to serve as a preceptor to new graduates.

Experienced nurses who wish to change practice settings find it difficult to move into the perioperative role. Orienting registered nurses with little, if any, OR experience is time-consuming and expensive; consequently, job vacancies are usually filled by experienced OR nurses. Some specialty courses designed for registered nurses offer OR training and experience, but these courses are usually lengthy and quite costly, and the nurse is often unable to continue employment while attending the specialty course.

As hospitals seek ways to improve business, ORs have gained popularity as large revenue-generators. According to the latest American Hospital Association figures, more than 50% of hospital admissions are surgery-related.[14] Alternative health care delivery systems, such as ambulatory surgery centers, are growing in numbers. These facts, coupled with increasingly autonomous and informed patients, the growing number of elderly patients, explosive technological advances, and changing societal health views, lend support to the movement to make perioperative nursing a recognized specialty area. If this goal is to be realized, educational methods will need to change to meet the challenge of providing qualified nurses in this practice area.

▽

Strategies for Educational Change

One of the first steps in making education congruent with perioperative practice is to achieve agreement between educators and nurses in practice on the nursing roles being performed and the optimal preparation for the perioperative nurse. This is increasingly important in light of the new role of the perioperative nurse in the ambulatory outpatient area and the possible change and expansion of this role in the near future. Once this has been accomplished, effective means can be devised for educating a high-quality nurse who is prepared to deal with the expectations and demands of this practice area.

Baccalaureate programs need to consider ways to integrate perioperative content into their curricula. At a recent nurse education conference, Rothrock stated that some of the competencies in perioperative nursing, as defined by AORN, could be integrated into a traditional generalist curriculum. Schools of nursing might want to integrate such content into a leadership course, into the medical-surgical nursing component, or perhaps within the maternal/child course. These basic competencies can be applied to all areas of nursing. Students thus would gain the advantages of an introduction to the basic principles of perioperative nursing care, a chance for experience in this nursing area, enhancement of their development and growth as students, and encouragement from practicing perioperative nurses to consider this specialized area of nursing practice after graduation.[14]

At the 1989 Nurse Education Conference, Murphy has expanded on how perioperative nursing content could be taught to meet the objectives of existing courses in basic nursing programs.[14] Basic content areas, such as change theory; leadership strategies; research findings and their application to practice; collaborative roles of the health care team; moral, legal, and ethical principles in nursing practice; and certain psychomotor skills, can be incorporated into a clinical experience in perioperative nursing.[11]

Because of increasing technology, the use of noninvasive techniques is increasing in ambulatory surgery settings. Students need additional experience in meeting the emotional needs of patients. Clinical experience in an ambulatory surgery setting could allow students an opportunity to expand their experience in psychosocial care and in the use of nonpharmacologic pain management strategies, such as relaxation techniques and guided imagery. The nursing procedures listed in Table 6–2 could also be incorporated into this type of clinical experience. If the ambulatory surgery center is performing preoperative assessment and teaching visits with patients prior to the day of surgery, the student experiences all aspects of the nursing process, as well as patient teaching. Students could be paired with preceptors for clinical monitoring. Clinical competencies could be matched with course objectives just as easily in this type of clinical setting as in an inpatient hospital surgical setting. During a semester-long medical-surgical rotation offered by a traditional baccalaureate program, students could spend at least one fourth of the rotation in a perioperative clinical setting.

Elective course offerings may also be an option (see Chapter 17). This type of course could be taught as a regular course or as independent study. Elective courses can vary in length from several weeks during a mid-term period, to a summer-long course offering. Perioperative nurses could be used as preceptors or guest instructors. With these types of courses, exposure to the perioperative role and scope of practice experience is limited only by the instructor's creativity.

Registered nurses frequently request accessible educational programs. Offering specialization courses within the framework of a school of nursing, perhaps as a continuing education offering, could be a good marketing strategy for attracting practicing nurses back to an educational program. Successful completion of this kind of a course within an academic setting might encourage practicing nurses to continue their ed-

Table 6-2 Suggested Experiences for Students in the
Perioperative Area

Assessment of physiological health status
Assessment of psychological health status
Development of nursing diagnoses
Development of care plans
Patient teaching
Development of outcome statements
Development of criteria for goal measurement
Documentation and accountability for patient care
Evaluation and revision of care of plans
Professional behavior
Organization of work and setting of priorities
Patient positioning and preparation
Surgical hand scrub
Methods of gowning and gloving
Creation and maintenance of a sterile field
Performance of sponge, sharps, and instrument counts
Containment/isolation procedures
Monitoring of intake and output
Administration of medications
Catheterization

ucation, perhaps completing a baccalaureate or higher degree in nursing. This type of course could prepare beginning level perioperative nurses for immediate employment in local health care facilities, and it would also enhance the relationship between education and the practice areas. A course of this nature needs to be offered at times that are convenient for most practicing nurses. Flexibility in schedules and extended learning environments that are not locked into a college campus routine will also enhance the popularity of the course for nurses wishing to change practice careers.

The registered nurse could independently master the knowledge necessary for the professional practice of perioperative nursing through the use of well-constructed resource materials and self-directed educational programs. Methods of delivery might include computer-assisted instruction, assigned readings, audiotapes and videotapes with written learner guides, or interactive video instruction. Free access to an instructor via telephone would facilitate the answering of questions, as would the presentation of lectures via teleconference. Lectures and demonstrations could be presented across the country by telecommunication methods. This type of independent study would allow nurses to learn content while off-campus. For some adults, this is a viable way of learning and allows flexibility in their schedules. Clinical experience could follow the course work through cooperation with preceptors in local hospitals close to the learner's home. Again, creativity is the only limitation.

Continuing education programs for practicing perioperative nurses is vital. Considering the fast pace with which changes occur in OR practice, nurses must keep their competencies up to date in order to assimilate these changes in their practice and continue to provide quality patient care. Continuing education offerings are also a way for health care facilities to attract and retain nurses. In 1988, a study involving 416 hospital nurses showed that continuing education offerings were one of seven items that nurses considered when looking for a job, and they were also appreciated highly by nurses already employed by a health facility.[15] One study, designed to assess the impact of continuing education on nursing practice, showed that continuing education programs significantly improved the quality of nursing practice and patient care.[16] The study documented an 18% rise in the quality of care and found that continuing education programs increased participants' awareness, created more positive attitudes, increased interest in quality patient care, and improved the health facility climate. Nursing needs for the study were determined from nursing audits.[16] Nursing audits, as well as surveys of patient expectations, responses, and evaluations regarding care, can be used to provide information concerning the types of course offerings needed to keep nurses abreast of advances in the perioperative practice area.

▽
Summary

The scope of perioperative nursing practice is continually changing and expanding. Changing health views, economics, technologic advances, and increased responsibilities and expectations are all factors contributing to this change in practice. Perioperative nursing is a segment of the health care system and, as is true for any professional segment of nursing, the continuity, growth, and well-being of the professional area is contingent upon education and research. It is imperative that attention be given to the educational needs of the practicing nurse, as well as to the preparation of future nurses in this specialty area. It is only through education and research that the profession will remain viable and continue to provide quality patient care. Through a futuristic vision, an understanding of the current dynamics of the health care system, and creative educational strategies, the educational challenge currently facing perioperative nursing can be met.

References

1. Olson, L. L. (1984). Providers preparing for major battle over market for outpatient surgery. *Modern Health Care, 84,* 82–88.
2. Lehr, P.S. (1988). Ambulatory Surgery Conference Highlights Gains, Problems Facing Industry. *Journal of the Association of Operating Room Nurses, 48,* 194–199.

3. Lee, R. M. (1976). Early operating room nursing. *Journal of the Association of Operating Room Nurses, 24,* 124–138.
4. Association of Operating Room Nurses—American Nurses' Association Division on Medical-Surgical Practice. (1975). *Standards of Nursing Practice: Operating Room.* Kansas City: American Nurses' Association.
5. Operating room nursing: Perioperative role. (1978). *Journal of the Association of Operating Room Nurses, 27,* 1156–1175.
6. Schlotfeldt, M. (1973). Planning for progress. *Nursing Outlook, 21,* 766–769.
7. Association of Operating Room Nurses. (1986). Competency statements in perioperative nursing. *Journal of the Association of Operating Room Nurses, 43,* 244–261.
8. Beyers, M. (1987). Future of nursing care delivery. *Nursing Administration Quarterly, 11,* 71–80.
9. Michel, L. L. and Myrick, C. (1990). Current and future trends in ambulatory surgery and their impact on nursing practice. *Journal of Post Anesthesia Nursing, 5,* 347–349.
10. Harvey, C. K. (1987). Future trends in perioperative nursing and technology. *Nursing Administration Quarterly, 12,* 38–41.
11. Bailes, B. K. (1988). Changes in perioperative nursing require higher education. *Journal of the Association of Operating Room Nurses, 48,* 124–126.
12. Metzger, R. S. (1976). Early operating room nursing. *Journal of the Association of Operating Room Nurses, 24,* 73–90.
13. Gutierrez, K., McCormack, C., & Villaverde, M. (1989). Perioperative nursing in the college curriculum. *Journal of the Association of Operating Room Nurses, 49,* 1052–1064.
14. Nurse educator conference focuses on "how." (1989). *Journal of the Association of Operating Room Nurses, 49,* 312–321.
15. Neathawk, R. D., Dubuque, S. E., & Kronk, C. A. (1988). Nurses' evaluation and retention. *Nursing Management, 19,* 38–45.
16. Meservy, D., & Monson, M. A. (1987). Impact of continuing education on nursing practice and quality of patient care. *The Journal of Continuing Education in Nursing, 18,* 214–220.

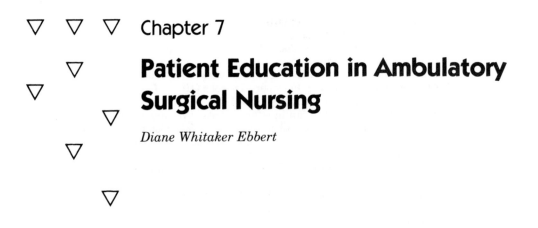

Chapter 7

Patient Education in Ambulatory Surgical Nursing

Diane Whitaker Ebbert

The concept of ambulatory surgery is not new. In fact, as early as 1909, Nicholl[1] reported performing over 7,000 operations on ambulatory patients. However, there has been a dramatic increase in the utilization of ambulatory surgery in the last 15 years. It is estimated that today, more than 20 million procedures are performed annually on an ambulatory basis.[2] Within this expanding arena for health care, a group of patients with unique learning needs has arisen.

A broad research base has been established to verify the effectiveness of preoperative patient teaching in reducing postoperative anxiety, pain, nausea, and length of stay in the hospitalized, elective surgical patient.[3] Likewise, it would be reasonable to assume that an ambulatory surgery patient who receives quality patient education preoperatively would experience similar results.[4] An extensive search of the literature yielded very few research studies that focused on ambulatory surgery, and no studies were found in which outcomes of patient education interventions with ambulatory surgery patients were examined.

Nurses are no longer afforded the luxury of spending several hours the evening before surgery preparing patients for the impending event. Moreover, patients no longer remain in the hospital several days postoperatively to learn how to change their bandages, walk with crutches, or learn other self-care activities. Typically, ambulatory surgery patients enter the hospital or facility in the morning, undergo surgery, and return home in the afternoon. Within this limited time frame, the nurse must establish rapport with patients, admit them, perform an assessment, establish a plan of care, initiate the plan of care, and discharge patients to their homes to recover from the surgery. Thus, the time available for the nurse to teach the patient in the ambulatory surgery setting is extremely limited. This time limitation makes it imperative for perioperative nurses to identify the specific learning needs of ambulatory surgery patients and to implement an individualized teaching plan to meet those needs.

This chapter discusses patient education in the ambulatory surgery setting. The following questions will serve as the framework for the discussion:

1. What are the basic principles of adult education as they relate to ambulatory surgery patients?
2. What are the learning needs of the patient undergoing ambulatory surgery?
3. Do inconsistencies exist between patients' recognized learning needs and what nurses perceive as the learning needs of ambulatory surgery patients?
4. How can patient education be implemented in the ambulatory surgery setting?

▽

Principles of Adult Education

The role of patient educator is one that nurses have embraced and incorporated into the practice of nursing for many years. Like other components of nursing practice, effective patient education occurs as a result of utilization of nursing's strong knowledge base. Providing patient education requires nurses to draw on that knowledge base, which incorporates scientific principles and theories of learning. Theories help to organize and guide a nurse's plan of action for patient education, thereby enhancing the process of learning. Without a definite plan, patient education lacks direction, making evaluation difficult, if not possible.

It is beyond the scope of this chapter to present the magnitude of learning theories that exist; however, many have been cited that apply to adults.[5–9] Within the ambulatory surgery setting, where many patients are adults, utilization of the basic principles of adult education can be extremely helpful in directing the educational component of patient care.

Hoffman[10] identified 12 generally recognized principles of learning that were gleaned from a variety of sources and can no longer be identified with a particular author. Ten of the principles deemed to be appropriate for use with ambulatory surgery patients are listed below. The descriptions following each principle have been added by the author, together with examples of how they might be applied directly to the ambulatory surgery learner. Although these principles have not been tested specifically in ambulatory surgery patients, the assumption can be made that, as with other nurse–patient teaching situations, these principles should increase the likelihood that patients will learn what to expect and that their ability to care for themselves will ultimately increase.

1. *Perception is necessary for learning.* Perception requires that the patient be able to respond to verbal and written information. If adult ambulatory surgery patients are being instructed through the use of written materials, those materials must be designed to facilitate the learner's perceptual abilities

(e.g., the use of large print on nonglare pages for patients with visual impairments).

2. *Learning, because it is considered a change in behavior, is threatening. Therefore, learning takes place more readily when threats are kept to a minimum.* Providing a quiet, private environment for teaching will help to decrease the level of anxiety or potential threat perceived by patients.

3. *Learning is more effective when it is in response to a felt need of the learner.* By thoroughly assessing the learning needs of the ambulatory surgery patient, the nurse is then able to structure her teaching plan to include those needs perceived to be important by the patient. For example, the nurse, when trying to instruct a patient who is totally consumed with the worry of how their blood sugar will be maintained when they will not be allowed to eat until after surgery, will have the greatest success if instruction begins with preoperative teaching about the rationale for NPO (nothing by mouth) status.

4. *Learning is made easier when the material to be learned is related to what the learner already knows.* Adult patients present with various life experiences. By carefully assessing the patient, these previous experiences can be incorporated into the teaching plan. For instance, in teaching a patient to assess the amount of vaginal bleeding they experience after undergoing a laparoscopic tubal ligation, the patient may not understand what would be considered "excessive" bleeding. However, most patients would be able to understand if "normal bleeding" were placed in the context of their normal menstrual period.

5. *Learning is facilitated when the material to be learned is meaningful to the learner.* Nurses have a tendency to teach patients the same way they were taught in nursing school. By accurately assessing the ambulatory surgery patient, it will be quite obvious to the nurse which patients have a need to know how the medial nerve became entrapped, thus necessitating a carpal tunnel release, and which patients simply want to know how they are to care for themselves at home with their hand splinted.

6. *Active participation on the part of the learner is essential if learning is to take place.* An environment conducive to learning is an integral component of this principle. Patients cannot be expected to learn when they are concentrating on a television program. Learning is also facilitated when patients are allowed to demonstrate the skills they are taught. The probability of patients performing postoperative knee exercises is much greater if the nurse has discussed the exercises and has allowed the patient to demonstrate them, than if the patient is simply sent home with an instruction sheet.

7. *Learning is retained longer when it is put into immediate use than when its application is delayed.* If there is a delay between the time a patient is instructed how to perform a skill and when they actual perform the skill, it may be difficult for them to remember the process. For ambulatory surgery patients undergoing septoplasty, for instance, learning is enhanced if these patients are allowed to change their own mustache dressing, as needed, while at the facility, giving them the opportunity to become familiar with the technique prior to discharge.

8. *Learning must be reinforced.* This principle is similar to the previous one. Reviewing what has previously been taught, as well as any new information, reinforces its importance for the patient and increases the likelihood of its retention.

9. *Organization promotes retention and application of learning.* A well-organized teaching plan that flows logically helps the patient remember and use the information presented. Ambulatory surgery patients who receive information organized according to the logical order of preoperative, intraoperative, and postoperative time frames have a frame of reference for what should happen when, which in turn enhances learning.

10. *Accountability for learning rests with the learner.* Nurses, as nurturing and caring individuals, often assume responsibilities that are not theirs to bear. Although nurses assume responsibility for teaching patients how to care for themselves within their limitations so that they may function at their highest level of ability, nurses cannot assume the responsibility of learning for the patient. That responsibility rests with the patient alone. Not every patient is interested in learning, and not every patient will learn, through no fault of the nurse.

A logical framework for educating the ambulatory surgery patient, utilizing the above principles, closely parallels the nursing process. The perioperative nurse assesses the patient's learning needs, focusing on what the patient perceives as important. Together, the patient and nurse then establish short- and long-term objectives, and develop an individualized teaching plan. This plan is then implemented and the plan is evaluated for patient outcomes. The following section will help the perioperative nurse to begin the process of determining the learning needs of the ambulatory surgery patient.

▽

Learning Needs of Patients

Although studies have been conducted to determine the learning needs of surgery patients,[11–13] the specific learning needs of ambulatory surgery patients have not been addressed. Typically, the patient teaching performed preoperatively has involved information nurses wanted patients to know in order to expedite the surgical procedure. Ambulatory surgery patients present unique learning needs. Not only do these patients need to know what to expect and how to react to happenings the day of surgery, they also must learn how to care for themselves and handle situations that may arise after their discharge home. Although many of the learning needs of ambulatory surgery patients may be generalized, each patient, as an individual, may present specific needs. The majority of studies conducted about preoperative teaching has involved evaluation of patient outcomes based on skills taught or the format in which the information was presented. Few studies have approached the issue of patients' preoperative learning needs by actually asking patients what it is they want to know in order to enhance their surgical experience. This author designed and conducted a small pilot study to begin identifying what patients perceive as their learning needs before undergoing ambulatory surgery.[14]

Pilot Study

The study was conducted to identify categories of learning needs for ambulatory surgical patients undergoing arthroscopic knee surgery. Data were collected from two groups of subjects using a qualitative, descriptive research design. The first group consisted of patients selected from a Midwest, suburban, orthopaedic surgery practice. The second group was composed of perioperative nurses practicing in a hospital-based ASU in a Midwest, suburban, community hospital. Participants were asked to complete two questionnaires, one of which was designed to collect demographic data and the other to identify learning needs.

Subjects

The group of patients completing questionnaires included an equal number of males and females. The mean age of the participants was 28 years, with a range of 18 to 41 years of age. The average number of years of education completed was 13, with a range of 11 to 14. All participants had previously had an experience in surgery.

The group of perioperative nurses completing questionnaires consisted of females who worked an average of 40+ hours per week. The average number of years the subjects had been employed in perioperative nursing was 15.8, with the extent of individual experience ranging from 4 to 26 years. All participants routinely provided patient education as part of their employment responsibilities and all had experience providing patient education to ambulatory surgery patients.

Instrument

The instrument utilized to identify learning needs was the Object Content Test (OCT). The OCT was developed from Kuhn's[15] Twenty Statement Test and was extended by Hartley.[16] The OCT is an unstructured, single page, paper and pencil test. The test consisted of the question, "What do I need to know as a patient scheduled for outpatient knee surgery?" which was followed by 20 numbered blanks for subjects to record their responses. The question perioperative nurses were asked to answer was, "What are the learning needs of the patient scheduled for outpatient arthroscopic knee surgery?"

Subjects were informed that they were not limited to 20 responses and were also free to use the back of the test. The OCT was self-administered, and subjects were encouraged to record their responses without regard to grammar or complete sentences. Reliability of the OCT has been established.[17] The instrument is considered public domain.

Data Analysis

Content analysis was used to categorize the subject's responses. Responses to the OCT were transcribed verbatim onto 3×5 index cards. Individual responses were then sorted into categories by two perioperative nursing experts. The categories were validated by a qualitative nursing research expert experienced with the OCT.

The categories identified by patients are listed as follows, and definitions of needs are included within each category.

1. *Preadmission learning needs*—Needs with content that would best lend itself to presentation during the preadmission period, from the time the decision for surgery was made until presentation of the patient to the ambulatory surgery facility.
2. *Preoperative learning needs*—Learning needs with content involving the preoperative time period, from arrival at the ambulatory surgery facility until transfer to the operating room bed.
3. *Intraoperative learning needs*—Needs involving information pertaining to the time period from transfer to the operating room bed to transfer to the recovery room.
4. *Postoperative learning needs*—Those needs involving information regarding the time period from transfer to the recovery room to discharge home.
5. *Postdischarge learning needs*—Needs involving information related to the time period after discharge from the facility.
6. *Other learning needs*—Those needs that did not readily fit into the categories previously listed. Needs classified in this category involved issues of accountability on the part of the health care profession.
7. *Psychosocial needs*—Needs which, to be met most effectively, would require specific interventions throughout the perioperative experience, rather than at specific time periods.

▽

Comparison of the Perceived Learning Needs of Patients and Nurses

For the purpose of simplifying this comparison of the perceived learning needs of patients and nurses, the reader may want to refer to Tables 7–1 through 7–11, which contain the information obtained from both groups in the study. The items in each table are listed in the order of the most frequent response to the least frequent.

Table 7–1 presents the categories of learning needs identified by both patients and nurses. Those categories identified by both subject groups were: (1) preadmission learning needs, (2) preoperative learning needs, (3) intraoperative learning needs, (4) postoperative learning needs, and (5) postdischarge learning needs. In addition, the patient subject group identified two other categories of learning needs: (1) other learning needs, and (2) psychosocial needs.

Four of the six preadmission learning needs identified by patients (Table 7–2) were also identified by nurses (Table 7–3). Those needs identified by both groups were (1) NPO, (2) location, (3) personal items, and (4) arrival time. Other learning needs perceived by the nurses and listed in Table 7–3 were: (1) transportation, (2) waiting area for family, (3) medications/allergies, (4) need for operative consent, (5) scheduled OR time, and (6) the admission procedure.

In the category of preoperative learning needs, nurses identified all of the learning needs listed by patients (Table 7–4). The needs jointly identified were: (1) anesthesia, (2) length of stay, (3) length of procedure, and (4) recovery room time. The learning needs that were perceived exclusively by nurses are listed in Table 7–5. These needs included: (1) shave/scrub preparation, (2) blood test(s), (3) intravenous (IV) line, (4) preoperative antibiotics, (5) preoperative care, (6) sequence of events, and (7) waiting time for the family.

Nurses perceived the same intraoperative learning needs that the patients identified: the need for information regarding what will be done

Table 7-1 Categories of Learning Needs Identified by Patients and Nurses

1. Preadmission learning needs
2. Preoperative learning needs
3. Intraoperative learning needs
4. Postoperative learning needs
5. Postdischarge learning needs
6. Other learning needs*
7. Psychosocial needs*

*Indicates a category identified only by patients

Table 7-2 Categories of Preadmission Learning
Needs Identified by Patients

NPO*	Nail polish
Location*	Privacy
Personal items*	Arrival time*

*Indicates a need also identified by nurses

Table 7-3 Categories of Preadmission Learning
Needs Identified by Nurses

NPO*	Waiting area for family
Arrival time*	Medications/allergies
Location*	Operative consent
Transportation	Scheduled OR time
Personal items*	Admission procedure

*Indicates a need also identified by patients

Table 7-4 Categories of Preoperative Learning
Needs Identified by Patients

Anesthesia*
Length of stay*
Length of procedure*
RR time*

*Indicates a need also identified by nurses

Table 7-5 Categories of Preoperative Learning
Needs Identified by Nurses

Shave/scrub preparation	Preoperative care
Length of stay*	Sequence of events
Blood test	Length of procedure*
Intravenous (IV) line	Waiting time for family
Anesthesia*	Recovery room time*
Antibiotics	

*Indicates a need also identified by patients

Table 7-6 Categories of Intraoperative Learning Needs Identified by Nurses

Skin preparation	Monitoring of equipment
Incisions	Explanation of procedure*
Tourniquet placement	Placement of patient on operating room bed

*Indicates a need also identified by patients

during the operative procedure. Other intraoperative learning needs identified by nurses were: (1) skin preparation, (2) incisions, (3) placement of the tourniquet, (4) monitoring of equipment, and (5) placement of the patient on the operating room bed (Table 7–6).

Three of the four postoperative learning needs identified by patients (Table 7–7), were also identified by nurses (Table 7–8). The needs identified by both groups were: (1) amount/type of pain, (2) postoperative care, and (3) discussion of findings with the physician after surgery. Table 7–8 lists other learning needs identified only by nurses, including: (1) type of dressings, (2) diet, (3) what to expect in the recovery room, (4) removal of the IV, and (5) dismissal criteria.

Nurses identified four of the seven learning needs that patients had relating to the postdischarge period (Tables 7–9 and 7–10). The needs identified by both groups were: (1) notifying the physician of problems, (2) sensations to expect the first days at home, (3) possible physical reactions, and (4) the need for crutches. Other learning needs perceived only by nurses were: (1) use of pain medications, (2) postoperative activity level, (3) postoperative ambulation/exercise, (4) elevation of the leg, (5) care of dressings, (6) return visit to physician, (7) other comfort measures, (8) normal postoperative occurrences, (9) postoperative instructions, (10) self-care at home, (11) postoperative phone call from the nurse, and (12) return to work (Table 7–10).

Nurses were most successful in matching patients' responses in the category of preoperative learning needs. There were no learning needs perceived by nurses that could be categorized into patient-identified categories of "other learning needs" or "psychosocial needs" (Table 7–11).

Table 7-7 Categories of Postoperative Learning Needs Identified by Patients

Amount/type of pain*
Postoperative care*
Discussion with physician after surgery*
Possibility of a drainage tube

*Indicates a need also identified by nurses

Table 7-8 Categories of Postoperative Learning Needs Identified by Nurses

Type of dressings	Discussion with physician after surgery*
Diet	Removal of IV line
What to expect in the recovery room	Dismissal criteria
Postoperative discomfort*	Immediate postoperative care*

*Indicates a need also identified by patients

Table 7-9 Categories of Postdischarge Learning Needs Identified by Patients

Rehabilitation	Possible physical reactions*
How to reach the physician if problems developed*	Resuming sports activity
Degree of drowsiness after discharge	Need for crutches*
Sensations during first days at home*	

*Indicates a need also identified by nurses

Table 7-10 Categories of Postdischarge Learning Needs Identified by Nurses

Postoperative activity level	Normal postoperative occurrences
Postoperative complications*	Postoperative instructions
Postoperative ambulation/exercise	Self-care at home
Elevation of leg	Notifying the physician of problems*
Sensations during first days at home*	
Care of dressings	Postoperative phone call from nurse
Return visit to physician	
Crutches*	Return to work
Other comfort measures	

*Indicates a need also identified by patients

Table 7-11 Other Learning Needs Identified by Patients

General Needs	Psychosocial Needs
Reputation of surgeon	Reassurance
Hospital reputation	Support of family/friends
Risks of operation	
Total cost	
Cause of problem	
Probability of recurrence	

Overall, the nurses identified 76% of the learning needs that patients themselves had listed. However, patients only identified 31% of the learning needs that nurses perceived for patients. Admittedly, the sample size used in this study was small, so one cannot generalize the results. However, the results do indicate that nurses identify more learning needs for patients than patients identify for themselves. A possible explanation for this incongruence might be that ambulatory surgical patients are basically in an unfamiliar environment and may be unable to identify all of their learning needs. Because responses to the OCT were written and the investigator did not discuss the answers with the subjects, some of the differences in identified needs may be purely a matter of semantics. Also, patients in the study were tested prior to surgery. It is possible that preoperative anxiety may have prohibited their recognition of learning needs.

A large percentage of the learning needs identified by nurses were procedural in nature. Knowledge of these procedures may or may not have an impact on patient outcomes. Most nurses are very methodical and procedure-oriented; therefore, these identified needs might more accurately reflect what nurses would want to know if they were patients, rather than what patients actually are interested in knowing.

Based on the findings of this pilot study, further study is needed to define the specific learning needs of the ambulatory surgery patient. This study, despite its small size, clearly demonstrated that, although many needs of the patient are being met with preoperative teaching, some, and perhaps the most important needs of the patient, are not being met. The ability of ambulatory surgery patients to return to the home environment and manage their own care may depend on meeting some of these currently unmet learning needs. Once ambulatory surgery patients' learning needs are clearly identified, legitimate research regarding the impact of perioperative teaching on patient outcomes can be undertaken.

▽

Implementing Patient Education Programs

Before embarking on a project as involved as perioperative patient education, nurses must first define their goals. The most common goal would be to provide patients with information that would meet their learning needs, as well as promote their safety and well-being, so as to make the ambulatory perioperative experience as positive as possible. This involves a comprehensive process that cannot be left to chance and that depends on many factors.

Successful implementation of a patient education program within the ambulatory surgery setting depends on the existence of supportive links between administration, perioperative nurses, surgeons, and willing patients. A break in any one of these links seriously weakens the program.

Once the mechanics of a new patient education program have been decided upon, the program should be shared with the surgeons. Program information is not presented for their approval, but rather for communication purposes and pertinent input. With the current atmosphere of competition for patients, an effective education program is a wonderful marketing tool for nurses, surgeons, and health care facilities alike. Moreover, because surgeons do assume responsibility for the patient's care following discharge, it is essential that they know what instructions and teaching their patients are receiving. Patients who have been well prepared and had their learning needs met tend to be satisfied patients who will tell others of their favorable experience.

The actual teaching plan for ambulatory surgery patients will differ with each facility and with each patient. Although each patient is an individual and has specific learning needs, many of those needs will be the same as those of other patients. Therefore, a facility may want to consider the use of standardized teaching plans that can be modified to incorporate individual needs. If standardized care plans are not available, the teaching plan like other nursing care, becomes part of the patient's nursing care plan.

The plan is initiated as the result of a careful and accurate assessment of the patient's learning needs. Once the assessment is completed, a nursing diagnosis is made. For example, during a preoperative interview with Mr. K., a 76-year-old widower, it is learned that he will be returning home after ambulatory knee surgery to care for himself. He relates that he has always maintained his independence and has rarely been ill. He thinks of the surgery as a mere inconvenience, and is looking forward to being "as good as new" afterward. An accurate nursing diagnosis based on the assessment of Mr. K. might be "Knowledge deficit related to self-care activities following discharge." This diagnosis basically deals with the need for procedural information. Other diagnoses may involve psychosocial or sensory information needs.

After pertinent nursing diagnoses are formulated, the next step is for the patient and nurse to identify mutual learning objectives. An objective in Mr. K.'s situation might be "Mr. K. will demonstrate the ability to change his dressing, utilizing sterile techniques, prior to discharge." This process of identifying goals does not have to be a formal one, and in the reality of a fast-paced ambulatory surgery setting, it may be the result of a conversation with the patient. For example, the nurse may state: "Mr. K., when you go home, you will need to change the dressing on your knee in two days. Have you ever changed a surgical bandage before?" To which Mr. K. might reply, "No, I don't believe I have. Will you show me exactly how I should do that?" Thus, a learning objective is mutually identified.

The intervention component of the teaching plan is the one many nurses deal with so frequently that they often forget to individualize this portion of the plan. Not only do nurses need to recall and utilize the principles of adult education discussed earlier, but they must also consider that not all patients learn in the same way, and most do not learn at the same speed. On a busy day, when it takes four demonstrations before Mr. K. learns how to open a package of 4×4 gauze bandages correctly, without contaminating it, the teaching process becomes a frustrating experience. It is also frustrating for the patient, who feels rushed and who may never have seen a package of 4 × 4's before! Remember that one of the principles of adult education is that learning is enhanced by an environment conducive to learning.

The next phase of the teaching plan is evaluation. If outcomes are not evaluated, then it is impossible to determine the impact of the teaching. Evaluation also provides an opportunity for teaching plans to be modified in an attempt to attain different outcomes. If Mr. K. is unable to demonstrate the correct method for changing his dressing after being shown several times, the nurse can rethink the intervention and try another teaching approach. Perhaps if he had written instructions that complemented the demonstration, he would be able to synthesize the process successfully.

The process of educating the ambulatory surgery patient spans the entire perioperative period, as it begins prior to the patient's admission to the facility and ends post discharge. Many facilities complete this process through the use of preadmission phone calls and postoperative follow-up calls. Others have instituted a policy that brings patients to the facility a day or two ahead of surgery for laboratory work, at which time a few minutes are spent assessing and educating the patient.

As many homes are equipped with videocassette recorders, an alternative for some institutions is to produce a videotape of the institution's standard preoperative instructions which patients can view at their convenience, in their own home. Including a telephone number and the name of a resource person will help to clarify any questions the patient might have.

The surgeon's office is often an untapped source for initiating the educational process. Tastefully prepared brochures presenting basic preoperative information can be supplied by the ambulatory surgery unit and distributed via the office. The instructions contained in the brochure would be an adjunct to the information provided by office staff, and would prompt patients to identify their own needs prior to receiving the call from the perioperative nurse before surgery.

With the expanding use of home health agencies, surgeons may want to consider having a home health nurse (preferably one with perioperative experience) visit patients preoperatively to begin the teaching process. This approach can be extremely helpful when it is speculated that a patient will require help with care after returning home from ambulatory surgery.

▽

Summary

This chapter has answered four questions that are imperative to successful education of the ambulatory surgery patient. One of the roles of a perioperative nurse is that of teacher, and so the nurse must, at the very least, be familiar with the basic principles underlying adult learning. The nurse must also be able to assess a patient's learning needs as promptly and as accurately as a patient's physical needs. By utilizing the nursing process and nursing diagnoses, the nurse is then able to incorporate the meeting of those needs into the patient's overall plan of care. Many mechanisms are available to nurses today to aid in implementing the educational process with patients. Nurses should be guided by the basic principles of adult education, as well as their own creativity and experience. Regardless of the mechanism used, the essential component for ensuring success is the involvement of committed individuals with a common goal of providing quality patient care, of which education is an integral component.

References

1. Nicholl, J. H. (1909). The surgery of infancy. *British Medical Journal, 2*, 253–254.
2. Wolcott, M. W. (Ed.). (1988). *Ambulatory surgery and the basics of emergency surgical care.* Philadelphia: J. B. Lippincott.
3. King, I., & Tarsitano, B. (1982). The effect of a structured and unstructured preoperative teaching: A replication. *Nursing Research, 31*(6), 324–329.
4. Stewart, S. M. (1987). Who is your same day surgery learner? *Perioperative Nursing Quarterly, 3*(2), 14–18.
5. Gagne, R. (1970). *The conditions of learning* (2nd ed.). New York: Holt, Rinehart, and Winston.
6. Knowles, M. D. (1970). *The modern process of adult education: Andragogy versus pedagogy.* New York: Associated Press.
7. Redman, B. K. (1981). *Issues and concepts in patient education.* New York: Appleton-Century-Crofts.
8. Skinner, B. F. (1950). Are theories of learning necessary? *Psychological Review, 57*(4), 193–216.
9. Snelbecker, G. (1974). *Learning theory, instructional theory, and psychoeducational design.* New York: McGraw-Hill.
10. Hoffman, S. E. (1987). Planning for patient teaching based on learning theory. In C. Smith (ed.), *Patient education: Nurses in partnership with other health professionals.* Orlando, FL: Grune & Stratton.
11. Miller, Sr. P., & Strada, E. A. (1978). Preoperative information and recovery of open-heart surgery patients. *Heart & Lung, 7*, 486–493.
12. Markin, D. A. (1986). Preoperative concerns of the patient undergoing craniotomy. *Journal of Neuroscience Nursing, 18* 275–278.
13. Miler, R., & Drake, M. (1980). Standards of nursing performance: Tools for assuring quality care. *ORB, 5*, 16–19.
14. Ebbert, D. (1989). *Learning needs of ambulatory surgery patients as perceived by patients and nurses.* Unpublished manuscript.
15. Kuhn, M. H., & McPortland, T. S. (1954). An empirical investigation of self attitudes. *American Sociological Review, 19*, 68–78.
16. Hartley, W. S. (1970). *Manual for the twenty statements problem (Who am I?)* (rev.) Unpublished manuscript, Department of Human Ecology and Community Health, University of Kansas Medical Center, Kansas City, KS.
17. Jauernig, P. R. (1984). *Jauernig's framework for the concept of forced fluids.* Unpublished master's thesis, University of Kansas Medical Center, School of Nursing, Kansas City, KS.

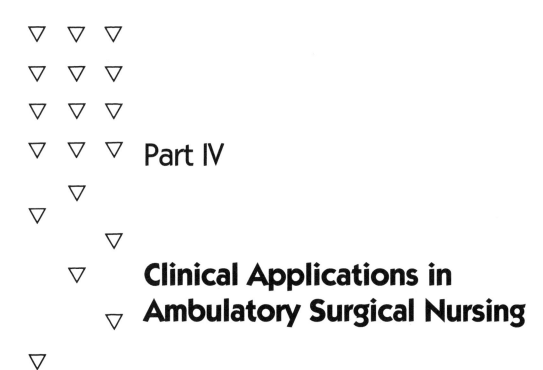

Part IV

Clinical Applications in Ambulatory Surgical Nursing

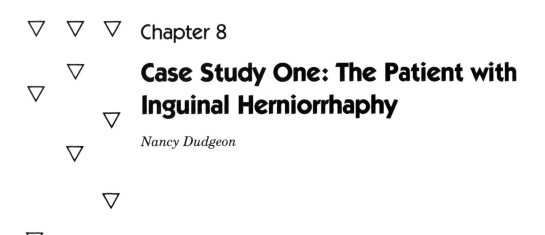

Chapter 8

Case Study One: The Patient with Inguinal Herniorrhaphy

Nancy Dudgeon

Nurses are charged with giving quality care to patients. In this time of limited financial resources for medical care, limited numbers of hospital/facility-based nurses, and greater demand for health care, nurses are mandated to use nursing resources as efficiently as possible. To deliver quality care, nurses must gather data and analyze that data to establish nursing diagnoses and to plan, implement, and evaluate patient care. Today's rapid movement toward ambulatory surgery as a cost-containment effort now requires that nurses deliver quality care in the most efficient manner within the shortest period of time. The purpose of this chapter is to discuss the care of a patient admitted to the ambulatory surgical unit (ASU) for an inguinal herniorrhaphy, addressing the following questions:

1. What are the nursing assessment techniques needed to assess the patient, including specific institutional forms?
2. What information from the patient assessment data can be used to formulate nursing diagnoses?
3. How can a perioperative care plan be developed for this ambulatory surgical patient?
4. What methods can be used to evaluate patient outcome on the basis of patient education, discharge planning, and follow-up care?

Nursing Assessment Techniques

Ambulatory surgical nursing is a relative new concept for patient management. As a result, there have been few guidelines as to methods and forms for patient assessment. One solution has been to take existing assessment forms and adapt them to the ambulatory patient setting. A problem exists, however, when multiple health care providers repeatedly

Exhibits for Chapter 8 are located at the end of the chapter on pages 145–160.

collect the same information with lengthy forms. Patients frequently complain that there is little evidence that the information provided is shared among health care professionals. There is a need for an organized, easy-to-use form that is convenient for the nurse to record information and convenient for health professionals to retrieve that information at a later time.

The nursing assessment form discussed in Chapter 4 will be used for initial patient assessment. In addition, a form will be used to demonstrate a consistent, continual flow of information using a single form. As seen in Exhibit 8–1, this assessment form is applicable for any adult patient as it allows for total body assessment and the formulation of nursing diagnoses according to the nine NANDA patterns.[1]

Case Study

Tom Smith, a 25-year-old construction worker, presented to the ambulatory surgery department with a one-week history of sudden pain and bulging in his right groin upon lifting a 75-pound barrel. Since that time, he has been unable to bear down or lift without discomfort. In an upright position, he has a mild aching in his right groin that is relieved by lying down. Tom saw Dr. McClurg in the surgery clinic and was scheduled for a right inguinal hernia repair today.

Upon Tom's admission to the ASU, the nurse completed a preoperative assessment form. As can be determined from the data in Exhibit 8–2, Tom is relatively healthy, and the only physical problem noted is an occasional cough associated with his 10-pack year (1 pack per day × 10 years) smoking history. It can be concluded that the assessment form was adequate for assessing Tom on admission. The next logical step, then, is to use this assessment data to establish nursing diagnoses for Tom.

▽

Formulating Nursing Diagnosis

As described in the American Society of Post Anesthesia Nurses' (AS-PAN's) standards of practice, several nursing diagnoses are appropriate for the patient admitted for inguinal herniorrhaphy, including pain, anxiety, fear, knowledge deficit, fluid volume deficit, and alterations in skin integrity.[2] As noted in Exhibit 8–2, the nursing diagnoses for Tom include: fear related to (R/T) a perceived threat to job stability/security, knowledge deficit R/T a lack of familiarity with the surgical experience, and anxiety R/T loss of control.

Nursing diagnoses formulated from the admission assessment are then used to develop the perioperative care plan. The care plan format used to plan Tom's nursing care is based on the plan outlined in Chapter 5, and is described in this chapter for the preoperative, intraoperative, and postoperative phases of Tom's care.

▽

Perioperative Care Plan

In a busy ASU, it is a time-saving practice to use a care plan to facilitate patient care. As seen in Exhibits 8–3 through 8–5, the care plan for Tom personalizes his care while providing continuity. During Tom's postanesthesia recovery, the intraoperative care plan can be used as baseline information as the nurse records Tom's recovery (Exhibits 8–6 and 8–7).

▽

Evaluation of Patient Outcome

Evaluation of patient outcomes is comprised of effectiveness of patient education, discharge planning, and follow-up care. An inguinal hernia repair is one of the most commonly performed surgical procedures, and is one that is predominately performed on an ambulatory surgery basis. Given the shortened time frame of this setting, one preadmission teaching method might be the development and production of a videotape that would demonstrate care pertinent to these patients. This film could be viewed in a variety of places and at a number of times, the doctor's office or the ASU, during the patient's preoperative visit for pertinent laboratory studies or at the time of the preoperative visit with the anesthesiologist on the day of surgery. Moreover, with so many people owning videocassette recorders, the film could also be checked out or mailed to the patient to be viewed preoperatively in the comfort of his home. In this case, the phone number of a resource person could be provided for answering any questions that might arise prior to the day of surgery. Learning could be measured by a one-page questionnaire completed at the time of videotape viewing, and returned upon admission.

There are many methods that can be used to evaluate the outcomes of the care that all team members have provided for patients. ASPAN requires that written instructions be part of the minimum standards of nursing practice.[2] The standards established by the Joint Commission for Accreditation of Hospital Organizations (JCAHO)[3] also require written instructions for follow-up care, including information on how to obtain assistance in the event of postoperative problems. These standards further mandate a predischarge review of the instructions with the patient or with a person responsible for the patient. These standards ensure that patients and their family members will be provided written reinforcement of the verbal instructions. Reviewing the written instructions with the patient prior to discharge may also prompt further questions from the patient. A sample form that can be used for patients' postoperative instructions can be found in Exhibit 8–8.[4] This form might be revised to include an area for identification of the patient and date; a checklist to identify potential problems that should prompt the patient to call the physician; an area for the patient's signature to verify that the instructions have been reviewed with them; and a statement advising the patient to avoid alcoholic beverages, operation of any motor vehicle, important decision making, or signing of any important documents for 24 hours. This instruction sheet provides flexibility for individualization of the instructions, and encompasses the areas that should be addressed with the ambulatory surgery patient.

For Tom, as an example of a typical patient who undergoes an inguinal herniorrhaphy, it is important that he be taught how to lift properly to prevent damage to his surgical site and to prevent recurrence of the hernia. The immediate postoperative period may not be the ideal time to teach patients new lifting skills. Problems, such as sedation from the anesthetic agents, postoperative pain medications, the potential distraction of postoperative pain, and possible nausea or vomiting, may interfere with such learning. However, for the ambulatory surgical patient, this may be the only opportunity for patient teaching. Patient education materials must address the prevention of hernia recurrence, and a printed copy of the information should be given to the patient to review both during instruction and after discharge at a less stressful time. The content should include how to lift, how to transport heavy objects, and how to practice good body mechanics.

To evaluate the resolution of the nursing diagnoses, the nurse would refer to the care plan forms that were begun preoperatively and carried out postoperatively. The care plan documentation indicates the care provided the patient from the time of admission through discharge. The forms document which nursing diagnoses were formulated and how they were resolved. Evaluation of care depends on both verbal statements and any nonverbal feedback offered by the patient and family members. The evaluation process can also provide feedback, as with a return demonstration of the proper technique for dressing changes.

One method of evaluation is to call the patient the evening of surgery or the next day. During this phone call, the nurse can inquire how the patient is feeling and whether there are any problems or questions to be answered. The nurse may also ask specific questions as to the appearance of the wound or the degree of the patient's postoperative pain.

Another method of evaluation involves the use of a questionnaire that is completed by the patient at home and mailed back to the unit, preferably as an adjunct to the postoperative phone call. A questionnaire is most likely to be returned if it is simple and quick to complete, and if postage is prepaid. This questionnaire could invite suggestions from the patient as to what might be done to enhance the surgical experience, and would aid in identifying which aspects of care were helpful to the patient.

One additional method of evaluation involves the use of a retrospective or concurrent audit of the chart. This can be accomplished with a simple questionnaire and checklist answer form designed to analyze the five steps of the nursing process. Problem areas can be identified and a method for resolution of problems can be instituted to improve patient care.

▽

Summary

In answering the four questions posed earlier in this chapter, it has been demonstrated that quality care can be delivered and documented in the ambulatory surgical setting effectively and efficiently. Duplication of effort can be avoided in assessment and nursing diagnosis documentation by the development of standardized perioperative care plans designed for the most common surgical procedures. These care plans could be inserted in a patient's record, with space provided for information relating specifically to an individual patient. With the advent of advanced technology, like laser surgery, more procedures will be performed on an ambulatory surgery basis. The nursing care approaches discussed in this chapter can be applied to any patient problem managed in the ASU.

References

1. North American Nursing Diagnosis Association. (1989). *Taxonomy I Revised—1989*. St. Louis: North American Nursing Diagnosis Association.
2. The American Society of Post Anesthesia Nurses. (1986). *Standards of practice*. Richmond, VA: The American Society of Post Anesthesia Nurses.
3. *The Joint Commission Accreditation Manual for Hospitals*. (1990). Chicago: The Joint Commission on Accreditation of Hospitals.
4. University of Kansas Medical Center. (1989). *Post-surgical instructions to the patient*. Kansas City, KS.

Bibliography

American Society of Post Anesthesia Nurses. (1985). *The post anesthesia nursing review for certification*. Richmond, VA: American Society of Post Anesthesia Nurses.

American Society of Post Anesthesia Nurses. (1991). *Standards of nursing practice*. Richmond, VA: American Society of Post Anesthesia Nurses.

Carpenito, L. J. *Handbook of nursing diagnosis 1989–1990*. (1989). Philadelphia: J. B. Lippincott.

Doenges, M. E., Moorhouse, M. F., & Geissler, A. C. (1989). *Nursing care plans: Guidelines for planning patient care* (2nd ed.). Philadelphia: F. A. Davis.

Drain, C., & Christoph, S. (1987). *The recovery room: A critical care approach to postanesthesia nursing* (2nd ed.). Philadelphia: W. B. Saunders.

Fraulini, K. E. (1987). *After anesthesia: A guide for PACU, ICU, and medical-surgical nurses*. Norwalk, CT: Appleton & Lange.

Gulanick, M., Klopp, A., & Glanes, S. (eds.). (1986). *Nursing care plans: Nursing diagnosis and intervention*. St. Louis: C.V. Mosby.

Guzzetta, C. E., Bunton, S. D., Prinkey, L. A., Sherer, A. P., & Seifert, P. C. (1989). *Clinical assessment tools for use with nursing diagnoses*. St. Louis: C. V. Mosby.

Liechty, R. D., & Soper, R. T. (1989). *Fundamentals of surgery* (6th ed.). St. Louis: C. V. Mosby.

North American Nursing Diagnosis Association: *Taxonomy I Revised—1989.* (1989). St. Louis: North American Nursing Diagnosis Association.

Smith, S., & Duell, D. (1989). *Clinical nursing skills* (2nd ed.). Norwalk, CT: Appleton & Lange.

Ulrich, S. P., Canale, S. W., & Wendell, S. A. (1986). *Nursing care planning guides: A nursing diagnosis approach.* Philadelphia: W. B. Saunders.

Exhibit 8-1 Ambulatory surgical nursing diagnosis assessment form (based on the nine NANDA patterns).

Name _____ Date: _____
Address _____ City _____ State _____
Phone:(H) _____ (W) _____ SS# _____
Surgical Diagnosis: _____ Medical Diagnosis: _____
Sex _____ Age _____ Known Allergies _____

EXCHANGING

NUTRITION

Oral mucosa: Color _____ Moist _____ Dry _____ Lesions _____
Teeth _____ Missing _____
Dentures _____ Upper _____ Lower _____ Partial _____
Appearance: Well nourished _____ Obese _____ Emaciated _____
Weight: _____ Height: _____ Weight Gain: _____ Weight Loss: _____
Diet Restrictions: _____ Alcohol Intake: _____
Feeding Tubes: _____ Hyperalimentation: _____
Skin: Turgor _____ Intact _____ Lesions _____ Color _____
Temp _____ Diaphoresis _____
Fluid Intake _____
Nursing Diagnosis _____

Circulation

Temp: _____ Pulse: _____ BP: (Rt arm) _____ (Lt arm) _____
Sitting _____ Standing _____

Exhibit 8-1 (Continued)

Apical rate _____ Rhythm: Regular _____ Irregular _____
Heart sounds: S1 _____ S2 _____ S3 _____ S4 _____
Neck veins distended: _____
Nailbed color _____ Cap refill _____ Radial pulses _____
Peripheral Edema: _____ Location: _____
Pedal Pulse: Rt _____ Lt _____ Capillary refill _____
Calf Tenderness: _____
Extremities: Color _____ Temp changes _____
History of: Pacemaker _____ Chest pain _____
Blood Clots _____ Edema _____
Nursing Diagnosis _____

Respiration

Resp rate _____ Breath sounds _____ Skin Color _____
Cough _____ Productive _____ Sputum color _____
Smoker _____ Pack years _____
Dyspnea _____ On exertion _____
Nursing Diagnosis _____

Elimination

Abdomen: Soft _____ Firm _____ Tender _____ Distended _____
Ostomies _____ Bowel sounds present _____
Stool/day _____ Color _____ Constipation _____ Diarrhea _____
Last BM _____ Character _____
Laxative use _____ Enema use _____ Incontinence of stool] _____

(Continued)

Exhibit 8-1 (Continued)

Complications of Pregnancies_____ Sexual Preference_____
Sexual concerns_____ History of STD_____
Nursing Diagnosis_____

VALUING

Religious Affiliation_____ Religious Restrictions_____

Would you like minister: To visit_____ To be called_____
Cultural concerns_____
Nursing Diagnosis_____

CHOOSING

Coping with health problems_____
Verbalizes problems_____
Uses defense mechanisms_____ Can meet role expectations_____
Family coping: Effective_____ Ineffective_____
Neglectful_____ Self_____ Others_____
Complies with care:_____ Seeks Preventive care_____
Decision maker:_____
Nursing Diagnosis_____

MOVING

Ambulates_____ Climbs Stairs_____
Gait: Steady_____ Unsteady_____ Limp_____ Able to walk_____

Exhibit 8-1 (Continued)

Urine output/day_____ Color_____ Odor_____ Urgency_____
Frequency_____ Nocturia_____ Dysuria_____ Hematuria_____
Incontinent_____ Stress Incontinence_____
Nursing Diagnosis_____

COMMUNICATING

Understands spoken language_____ Reads_____
Writes_____ Reads Lips_____ Hearing intact_____
Vision intact_____
Verbal/Non Verbal:_____

Nursing Diagnosis_____

RELATING

Marital Status: M__ S__ W__ D__ Children_____
Number of Children_____ Dependents_____
Occupation_____
Living Arrangements: Home owner_____ Rent_____ Others in the Home_____
Support system: Relative_____ Friend_____ wife_____
Family concerned about hospitalization_____
Gets along with support system_____
Personal Behavior: Passive_____ Aggressive_____ Assertive_____
Parent_____ Parenting problems_____
Last Menstrual Period_____ Menstrual Problems_____
Birth Control Methods_____ Number of Pregnancies_____

Exhibit 8-1 (Continued)

Prosthesis_____ Aids: Cane_____ Walker_____ Wheelchair_____

Fatigue:_____ Tires easily_____

Feels rested after sleep_____ Trouble falling asleep_____

Insomnia_____/Sleeping aids_____

Maintains own home:_____

Able to: Feed Self_____ Bathe Self_____

Needs Help: Feeding_____ Bathing_____ Dressing_____

Going to bathroom_____

Growth/development problems_____

Nursing Diagnosis_____

PERCEIVING

Body Image Changes_____

Eye contact: Appropriate_____ Downcast_____ Staring_____

Body Posture: Relaxed_____ Stooped_____ Rigid/tense_____

Level of consciousness_____ Alert_____ Responds to_____

Oriented to: Time_____ Place_____ Person_____

Mood: Calm_____ Sad_____ Angry_____ Withdrawn_____ Other_____

Early a.m. awakening_____

Pupils: Equal_____ Reactive_____ Other_____

Cognition: Able to follow simple commands:_____

Hearing: Normal_____ Impaired_____ Left Ear_____ Right Ear_____

Vision: Normal_____ Corrected with glasses_____ Prosthesis_____ Farsighted_____

Nearsighted_____

Exhibit 8-1 (Continued)

Unilateral Neglect_____

Diversional Activities:_____

Hopelessness_____ Powerlessness_____

Nursing Diagnosis_____

KNOWING

Cognition intact_____ Recent Memory Change/Deficit_____

Difficulty Learning_____

Education level_____

Knowledge deficit:_____

Regarding Illness:_____ Condition:_____

Altered thought process_____

Nursing Diagnosis_____

FEELING

Acute pain:_____ Chronic pain_____

How pain managed:_____

Recent Loss/grief_____ Potential Loss/grief_____

Potential for violence:Self_____ Others_____

Fearful_____ Post Trauma Experiences_____

Post Rape Syndrome: Silent_____ Verbalized_____

Nursing Diagnosis_____

Exhibit 8-2 Ambulatory surgical nursing diagnosis assessment form (based on the nine NANDA patterns).

Name Tom Smith _____ Date: 8/21/91 _____

Address 6032 Fenway Rd _____ City Middleton _____ State NE _____

Phone:(H) 432-6428 _____ (W) 431-9564 _____ SS# 594-71-4238 _____

Surgical Diagnosis: Right inguinal hernia Medical Diagnosis: Right inguinal hernia

Sex M _ Age 25 _ Known Allergies: NONE _____

Current medications: Occasional tylenol. Denies use of recreational drugs

Previous surgeries/anesthetics: T & A at age 5 years under general anesthesia without

complications. Informant: self DOB: 8/13/64 _____

Hx of current c/o "Sudden onset of pain 1 wk. ago upon lifting 75# barrel off truck.

Noted to have bulge in groin (L). Not able to bear down/lift without pain/discomfort.

Chronic Illnesses: None

Patient Explanation of Procedure: "I am here to have this hernia fixed."

Patient Expectations of outcome of procedure: "I'll be able to return to my work."

EXCHANGING

NUTRITION

Oral mucosa: Color Pink Moist 0 Dry X Lesions 0

Teeth 1 Missing 0 Multiple fillings, no caps or loose teeth

    Dentures 0 Upper 0 Lower 0 Partial 0

Appearance: Well nourished Lean/muscular Obese 0 Emaciated 0

Weight: 80kg Height: 6ft. Weight Gain: 0 Weight Loss: 0

Diet Restrictions: None Alcohol Intake: Social 6 pk/wk

No. of Meals Daily: 3 Last Meal: Dinner/Yesterday

Exhibit 8-2 (Continued)

Feeding Tubes: 0 _____ Hyperalimentation: 0 _____

Skin: Turgor Good Leathery Intact X Lesions 0 Color Deeply Tanned

Conjunctiva/Sclera White _____

Temp warm Diaphoresis X _____

Fluid Intake 6-8 glasses/day- H₂O/Coffee/milk/soda

    Calluses: both hands, rough, dry

Nursing Diagnosis _____

Circulation

Temp: 37⁵ °C Pulse: 80ap. BP: (Rt arm) 130/70 (Lt arm) 124/74

    Sitting X Standing 0

Apical rate 80 Rhythm: Regular X strong Irregular 0

Heart sounds: S1 X S2 X S3 0 S4 0

Neck veins distended: 0

Nailbed color Pink Cap refill 2 sec Radial pulses 2+

Peripheral Edema: 0 Location: ankles/feet bilat

Pedal Pulse: Rt 2+DP/2+PT Lt 2+DP/+2+PT Capillary refill 2 sec

Calf Tenderness: 0

Extremities: Color Pink Temp changes equally warm

History of: Pacemaker 0 Chest pain 0

Blood Clots 0 Edema 0

Nursing Diagnosis _____

Respiration

Resp rate 24 Breath sounds clear Skin Color deeply tanned

Exhibit 8-2 (Continued)

(Continued)

RELATING

Marital Status: M X S ___ O ___ W ___ D ___ D ___ Children _none_ (Married; 1 year;

wife pregnant)

Number of Children _none_ Dependents _1_

Occupation _Construction Worker_

Living Arrangements: Home owner _0_ Rent _X_ Others in the Home _–_

Support system: Relative _0_ Friend _0_ spouse/significant other _X_

Family concerned about hospitalization _X_

Gets along with support system _____

Personal Behavior: Passive _0_ Aggressive _0_ Assertive _X_

Parent _0_ Parenting problems _0_

Concerns: "I want to get this fixed for good. My wife is pregnant. Mine is the

only income! I get laid off if business slacks off. Sometimes 1-2 weeks at a time.

I need to go to work when the work is there.

Last Menstrual Period _n/a_ Menstrual Problems _n/a_

Birth Control Methods _n/a_ Number of Pregnancies _n/a_

Complications of Pregnancies _n/a_ Sexual Preference _____

Sexual concerns _0_ History of STD _0_

Nursing Diagnosis _____

VALUING

Religious Affiliation _no pref._ Religious Restrictions _____

Cultural concerns _____

Exhibit 8-2 (Continued)

Cough X _occ am_ Productive _X_ Sputum color _white_

Smoker _1_ ppd Pack years _10_

Dyspnea _0_ On exertion _0_

Nursing Diagnosis _____

Elimination

Abdomen: Soft _X_ Firm _X_ right inguinal mass Tender _X right inguinal_

Distended _X right inguinal_

Ostomies _0_ Bowel sounds present _X all 4 quadrants_

Stool/day _q am_ Color _Brown_ Constipation _0_ Diarrhea _0_

Last BM _yesterday_ Character _Firm_

Laxative use _0_ Enema use _0_ Incontinence of stool _0_

Urine output/day _____ Color _med. yellow_ Odor _0_ Urgency _0_

Frequency _6x_ Nocturia _0_ Dysuria _0_ Hematuria _0_

Incontinent _0_ Stress Incontinence _0_

Nursing Diagnosis _____

COMMUNICATING

Understands spoken language _X_ Reads _X_

Writes _X_ Reads Lips _0_ Hearing intact _0_

Vision intact _X_

Verbal/Non Verbal: _Glances at wife frequently. Wife at side holding husband's_

jacket. Brief short m-m. Clasping and unclasping hands. cracks knuckles.

Nursing Diagnosis _____

Exhibit 8-2 (Continued)

Growth/development problems _____

Limitations imposed by illness: **Most comfortable reclining. Duration: 1 wk.**

Guards affected area. Sits leaned to the left and slouched.

Nursing Diagnosis _____

PERCEIVING

Body Image Changes _____

Eye contact: Appropriate X Downcast ___ Staring ___

Body Posture: Relaxed ___ Stooped ___ Rigid/tense X

Level of consciousness ___ Alert X Responds to ___

Oriented to: Time X Place X Person X

Mood: Calm ___ Sad ___ Angry ___ Withdrawn ___ Other X

Early a.m. awakening 5 am

Pupils: Equal X Reactive X Other ___

Cognition: Able to follow simple commands: X

Hearing: Normal X Impaired ___ Left Ear ___ Right Ear ___

Vision: Normal X Corrected with glasses 0 Prosthesis 0 Farsighted 0

Nearsighted 0

Unilateral Neglect 0

Diversional Activities: lifts weights/socializes with friends

Hopelessness 0 Powerlessness 0

Stress factors: "Long hours., boring job." Relieves stress by staying busy and an occasional "boys' niteout. "NOTE: FIDGETY, CONSTANT MOTION, IMPATIENT

Nursing Diagnosis (1) Anxiety R/T lack of familiarity with surgical experience, loss of control. (2) Fear R/T perceived threat to job stability/security.

Exhibit 8-2 (Continued)

Nursing Diagnosis _____

CHOOSING

Coping with health problems X **"Get this taken care of"**

Verbalizes problems X

Uses defense mechanisms ___ Can meet role expectations X

Family coping: Effective X Ineffective ___

Neglectful 0 Self 0 Others 0

Complies with care: X Seeks Preventive care 0 **"never had any problems"**

Decision maker: X

Nursing Diagnosis _____

MOVING

Ambulates X Climbs Stairs ___

Gait: Steady X Unsteady 0 Limp __ **favors R side** Able to walk ___

Prosthesis 0 Aids: Cane 0 Walker 0 Wheelchair 0

Fatigue: 0 Tires easily ___

Feels rested after sleep **6 hrs.** Trouble falling asleep ___

Insomnia ___ /Sleeping aids ___

Maintains own home:

Able to: Feed Self X Bathe Self __ **pm: usually on arrival home. shower**

Needs Help: Feeding 0 Bathing 0 Dressing 0

Going to bathroom 0

Exhibit 8-2 (Continued)

KNOWING

Cognition intact _X_ Recent Memory Change/Deficit _0_

Difficulty Learning _0_

Education level _High school completed_

Information deficit:

    Regarding Illness: _X_ Condition: _X_

    Altered thought process_

Nursing Diagnosis _Information deficit R/T lack of familiarity with surgical experience_

FEELING

Acute pain: _X_ Chronic pain_

How pain managed: _laying down_

Recent Loss/grief _0_ Potential Loss/grief _0_

Potential for violence:Self _0_ Others _0_

Fearful _X_ Post Trauma Experiences_

Post Rape Syndrome: Silent_ Verbalized_

Nursing Diagnosis _Pain R/T injury_

Exhibit 8-3 Preoperative care.

Assessment	Nursing Diagnosis	Nursing Orders	Implementation (Independent)	Evaluation (Independent)
Subjective "I want to get this hernia fixed for good. I can't afford to be off work during the busy season."	1. Fear R/T perceived threat to job stability	1a. Provide emotional support for job concerns. 1b. Provide information about occurrence/ prognosis.	1a. Allow patient to verbalize concerns. 1b. Inform the patient re cause, repair, and prevention of hernias. Provide printed information on good body mechanics for lifting.	1b. The patient stated he understands how hernias occur and how to prevent recurrence. Patient began to leaf through handout.
Objective C/V: BP = Right arm 130/70 Left arm 126/74 Apical pulse = 80, regular Neuro: Alert, oriented, appropriate verbal interaction. Fidgeting, impatient. Resp:Breath sounds clear to ausculation. Respir. easy and nonlabored. Rate = 24. GI: Bowel sounds present in all four quadrants. Abdomen soft.	2. Knowledge deficit R/T unfamiliarity with surgical experience	2. Provide information re surgical experience pertinent to : a. the patient b. the family member or surrogate.	2a. Describe events that will occur inter-operatively and postoperatively. 2b. Instruct the patient and family members where/ when the surgeon will communicate with them and what must be accomplished prior to discharge, opportunities to ask questions.	2a. The patient verbalized understanding of peri-operative events. Asked appropriate questions. Anticipated next step in experience. 2b. The patient's wife indicated understanding of peri-operative events.
HEENT: Mucous membranes pink, dry. GU: Voided last at 06:30	3. Anxiety R/T loss of control.	3. Allow patient to verbalize concerns.	3. Ask patient if they have any questions/concerns re information or issues which you may not have addressed.	3. Patient appeared relaxed. Admitted to feeling more comfortable.

	Medical Diagnosis	Medical Orders	Implementation (Interdependent)	Evaluation (Interdependent)
	Right inquinal hernia	1. NPO after midnight	1. NPO status maintained	1. Patient verifies NPO status since midnight.
		2. HBG/Hct and electrolytes	2. Lab work ordered, specimen obtained/ delivered to lab.	2. Lab results in chart.
		3. Surgeon's history/ physical present in chart.	3. History/physical placed in chart.	3. History/physical available in chart.
		4. Surgical permit signed and in chart.	4. Signed permit placed in chart.	4. Signed permit present in chart.
		5. Patient must be in the company of a family member or surrogate overnight.	5. Verify wife will be driving patient home and remain at home tonight in event of problems and to offer assistance/care.	5. Patient and wife understand instructions.

Exhibit 8-4 Intraoperative care.

Assessment	Nursing Diagnosis	Nursing Orders	Implementation (Independent)	Evaluation (Independent)
1. Patient is sedated. Patient requires an advocate.	1. Potential for injury R/T surgical environment and anesthetized state	1. Provide for patient safety.	1a. Remove dentures, partials, contacts, glasses, jewelry, hearing aids, any prosthesis.	1a. N/A to this patient
			1b. Verbally verify patient's name/ procedure. Compare patient chart, name band, and surgical schedule.	1b. All information correlates.
			1c. Transfer patient to OR table with all brakes intact and with patient's assistance.	1c. Transfer occurred without incident.
			1d. Secure patient to OR table in good body alignment with extremities supported.	1d. Peripheral pulses present. Patient offers no complaints of circulatory impairment prior to discharge.
			1e. Place cautery pad.	1e. There is no evidence of electrical burns.
			1f. Avoid pooling of prep. solutions.	1f. There is no evidence of chemical burns.
			1g. Verify sponge, needle, instrument, and blade counts.	1g. All counts are correct.
2a. Surgical scrub to right groin	2. Impaired skin integrity R/T surgical incision	2a. Prepare operative site.	2a. Scrub/shave surgical site according to specific procedure.	2a. Patient was prepped as described in procedure.
2b,c. Open surgical wound		2b. Monitor surgical team's aseptic technique.	2b. Identify breaks in technique and resolve immediately.	2b. No breaks in technique were identified.
		2c. Monitor aseptic technique for application of surgical dressing.	2c. Identify breaks in technique and resolve immediately.	2c. No breaks in technique were identified. Dry, sterile dressing in place and intact.

		Medical Orders	Interventions (Interdependent)	Evaluation (Interdependent)
		1. Prevent hypo/ hyperthermia	1a. Maintain average OR temperature at 37° C.	1. Patient's temperature was monitored per anesthesia and ranged 36-37° C without adjunctive treatment.
			1b. Maintain communication with anesthesia re patient's temperature.	
			1c. Have warming blanket placed on OR table for standby use.	

(Continued)

Exhibit 8-4 (Continued)

3. Patient anesthetized	3. Impaired physical mobility R/T anesthetized state	3. Protect patient during emergence and during transfer to cart.	3a. Maintain restraints until time for transfer. 3b. When ready to transfer explain to patient quietly, briefly, simply that he will be moved, he needs to lie quietly and his operation is over. 3c. Coordinate surgical team to provide smooth transition to cart.	3c. Patient was moved to cart without incident or injury.

Exhibit 8-5 Postoperative care.

Assessment	Nursing Diagnosis	Nursing Orders	Implementation (Independent)	Evaluation (Independent)
1. Patient groaning, grimacing, calling out. C/V: BP = 150/80 Apical pulse = 104 regular Resp.: rate = 36	1. Pain R/T surgical intervention	1a. Monitor c/o pain — verbal or behavioral cues.	1a. Review anesthesia record for medications given pre-operatively or in the OR; check for localized reaction. Evaluate pain based on patient's description as to location and intensity (describe on scale of 1-10).	1a. Patient reports pain is decreased and level is tolerable.
		1b. Monitor vital signs every 15 min., or more frequently as needed.	1b. Evaluate vital signs.	1b. Patient's vital signs are WNL of pre-op baseline and stabilized.
		1c. Monitor response to interventions.	1c. Reposition, once patient is reactive, with head of bed elevated and knee slightly flexed. Ambulate with minimal assistance prior to discharge.	1c. Patient is in good body alignment. Patient ambulated independently without complaints of faintness and with steady gait.
		1d. Provide information and emotional support.	1d. Acknowledge patient's c/o pain. Explain how he will be assisted. Explain what he can do to help his pain (e.g. deep breathing, pleasant thoughts, relaxation).	1d. Patient is able to relax and rest when undisturbed. Patient is able to assist in pain control.
		1e. Educate patient re breathing, splinting, coughing.	1e. Patient instructed on frequent deep breathing. Splinting demonstrated to patient.	1e. Patient provided a return demonstration of splinting upon deep breathing.
		1f. Educate patient re constipating effects of alteration in diet, fluid intake, and codeine in pain medication.	1f. Explain return to normal diet. Discuss foods/fluids which promote bowel function for him. Discuss effect of straining in relation to comfort/stress on surgical incision.	1f. Patient states he understands why constipation is undesirable and how it may be avoided.

(Continued)

Exhibit 8-5 (Continued)

Assessment	Nursing Diagnosis	Nursing Orders	Implementation (Interdependent)	Evaluation (Interdependent)
	1. Right inquinal herniorrhaphy	1a. Fentanyl 50 mcg; may repeat x 1 for c/o severe pain while in PACU. 1b. Tylenol #3 tabs, 1-2 po q 3-4 hrs PRN pain.	1a,b. Medicated with Fentanyl; 30 min later, Fentanyl repeated and Tylenol #3 tabs two given concomitantly. Instruct patient in appropriate use of medications for pain and action to take if pain is not relieved.	1a,b. Patient now rates pain as a 3 on a scale of 1–10. Patient verbalized understanding if safe use of pain medication and importance of notifying his doctor if prescribed dosing does not relieve pain.
		1c. Apply ice bag to surgical site for first 24 hrs. 1d. Scrotal support	1c,d. Ice bag and scrotal support obtained and placed on patient.	1c,d. Patient understands use of ice and scrotal support to minimize edema/swelling and prevent swelling/pain.
2. "When can I go home?" C/V:BP = 134/72 right arm Apical pulse = 88, regular Neuro: Alert, oriented. Dozes off when undisturbed. Resp.: Breath sounds coarse, clear with coughing, respers easy and nonlabored. Rate = 20 GI: Abdomen soft. HEENT: Mucous membranes pink, dry GU: No void since 6:30 A.M.	2. Information deficit R/T behaviors to be demonstrated prior to discharge to home.	2. Provide instruction in and rationale for: 2a. Ability to tolerate oral fluids prior to dismissal	2a. Offer ice chips and sips of fluid (preferably water). Offer soda crackers if patient c/o nausea or has been treated for emesis.	2. Patient stated he understands criteria for dismissal to home.
		2b. Ability to ambulate with minimal assistance prior to dismissal	2b. Gradually change position throughout PACU stay to head of bed elevated 90°, dangle feet, stand, sit up in chair, ambulate with minimal assistance.	
		2c. Maintenance of stable vital signs within normal limits of pre-op range without adverse affects from position changes prior to dismissal	2c. Evaluate vital signs in relation to pre-operative baseline/position and any c/o nausea or color change in skin and diaphoresis.	
3. "When can I go back to work?"	3. Information deficit R/T postoperative care/ concerns.	3a. Review with patient good body mechanics. Provide information.	3a. Instruct patient re restrictions on lifting/ strenuous activities. Discuss required activities of his job. Provide printed material on safe lifting.	3a. Patient understands he may have activity restrictions for up to six weeks. Expresses need to learn new ways of lifting heavy materials.
		3b. Review with patient the signs which require communication with his doctor.	3b. Instruct patient that he should call his doctor if he has drainage from his wound (especially foul smelling), inordinate swelling accompanied by pain and/or unre-lieved by pain medi-cation as ordered; an elevated temperature; separation of edges of wound.	3b. Patient verbalized that his wound will be bruised/reddened, will have no drainage, will be soft around incision, edges will be closed, discomfort will be relieved with pain medi-cation and that he should not have a temperature. Patient's dressing is dry and intact. IV line was discontinued.

Exhibit 8-5 (Continued)

Assessment	Medical Diagnosis	Medical Orders	Interventions (Interdependent)	Evaluation (Interdependent)
	Discharge when stable	1. Void prior to discharge to home	1. Offer fluids. Ambulate to bathroom with assistance.	1. Patient voided 250 cc of urine. Patient states he feels he emptied his bladder. Patient states he feels less pressure near his wound.
		2. Discharge to home when recovered from anesthesia; send home a copy of the postoperative instructions.	2a. Review postoperative instructions re: diet, activity, scheduled postoperative appointment, care of incision (dressing changes and bathing instructions), phone numbers and who to call if problems or concerns develop, prescriptions. Review dressing change.	2a. Patient nodded head to instructions. Denies any questions. Prescription available for pick up in pharmacy. Verbally demonstrated how to change dressing. Understands he may not drive for one week.
			2b. Review with patient avoidance of alcoholic beverages, operating any motor vehicle, making any important decisions, signing any important documents for 24 hours due to the effects of anesthetic agents.	2b. Patient stated he understood the precautions.
				2c. Patient dismissed to ambulatory surgery area via wheelchair with copy of instructions, supplies. Instructions reviewed with wife. Discharged home in company of wife.

Exhibit 8-6 Perioperative record.

```
                    PERIOPERATIVE RECORD        Name    Tom Smith
                                                Number  70000178

Anesthesia Report by:    J. Simmons, M.D.
Medications/Agents
  N/A  Pre-op
  N/A  General
  N/A  Muscle Relaxant Agent(s)
                         Reversal
  N/A  Regional: Type _____ Agent _____
  N/A  Local Agent(s):
   X   Other intra-op meds: Versed 5mg; Fentanyl 200mcg
       (MAC) Reglan 10mg

Fluids:
  Loss: EBL  50cc   V/O  0    Other   N/A
  Replacement: Crystalloid=Type   LR   Amount   1100
               Colloid   0  ; Other   0

Allergies    None Known
Vital Signs:Intra BP 100-120/70-80P  80-120 R  16-20T 36 - 37 core

PACU Admission Information:
  Time   0915   Admitted by   N. Dudgeon, RN
  Operation Performed
  Airway Support:   None  x  Airway(type) _____
                    Endotracheal _____ Trach _____
  Oxygen Support:   None  x  ; Nasal Cannula _____ LPM _____
                    Blow by  /Mask  /Shield ____ LPM ____ %
                    Bagged _____
  Breath Sounds:    Clear  x   Other _____
  EKG:  NSR _____ Other _____
  Skin Condition: Warm/Dry  x  Color  Pink  Other _____
  Dressings: Site _____ Type _____ None  x
  IV: SiteLeft Hand Condition0 Redness, 0 Swelling None
  IV Fluids: Type Hanging  LR  Amount Remaining900ccNone
  Position of Patient  OOB up 45 degrees, holes gatched

Discharge Information:
  Time   10:30   Dismissed by   N. Dudgeon, RN
  Breath Sounds: Clear  x   Other  Respir easy/nonlabored
  Extubated N/A;TV N/A NIF N/A Grips/Head lift/Swallow N/A
  Airway Dc'd    N/A    ; 02 Dc'd    N/A
  EKG: NSR  X   Other  0 ectopy noted
  Skin Condition: Warm, dry  x   Color  Pink  Other _____
  Dressings: Dry, intact  x   Other _____
```

Exhibit 8-6 (Continued)

```
Drains (output): Color _____ Amount _____ None
  IV Dc'd   1015   Condition of Site  0 redness, 0 swelling
  Pain Level  Minimal 3 on a 1-10 scale
Post-op Instructions:
  Copy sent with patient   x   Signed by patient   x
  Reviewed with patient   x   /significant other    x wife
  Indicates understanding  x Demonstrates skills   x dressing
                                                    change
  Prescriptions provided for  Tylenol #3
Ambulatory: Without assist  N/A  With assist  N/A  Type  N/A
            Other  N/A    Transported via  Wheelchair
Tolerating Fluids: Yes  x  No
Special Instructions  Dressing changes; lifting precautions
Supplies Provided  1-10 pack 4 x 4's: paper tape
Designated/Responsible accompanying adult  Wife - Sue Smith
```

Exhibit 8-7 Perioperative charting.

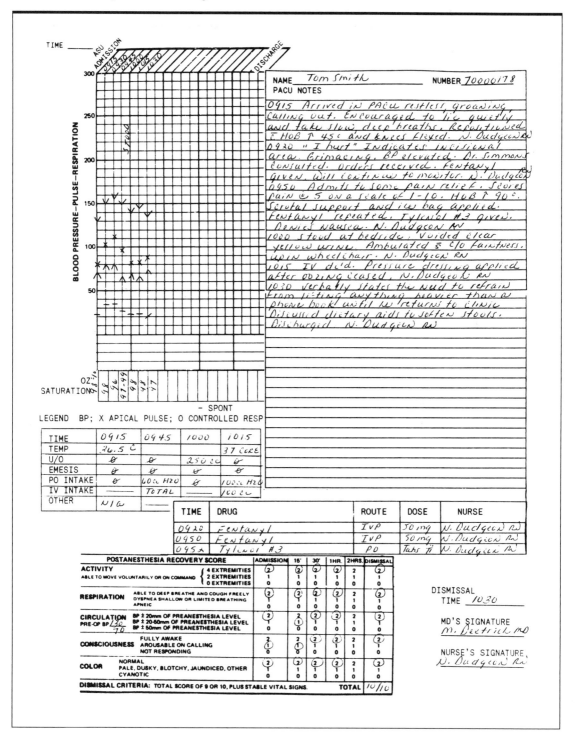

TIME _____

NAME *Tom Smith*   NUMBER *70000178*

PACU NOTES

0915 Arrived in PACU restless, groaning, calling out. Encouraged to lie quietly and take slow, deep breaths. Repositioned c̄ HOB ↑ 45° and knees flexed. N. Dudgeon RN
0920 "I hurt" Indicates incisional area. Grimacing. BP elevated. Dr. Simmons consulted. Orders received. Fentanyl given. Will continue to monitor. N. Dudgeon RN
0950 Admits to some pain relief. Scores pain @ 5 on a scale of 1-10. HOB ↑ 90°. Scrotal support and ice bag applied. Fentanyl repeated. Tylenol #3 given. Denies nausea. N. Dudgeon RN
1000 Stood at bedside. Voided clear yellow urine. Ambulated c̄ c/o faintness. Upon wheelchair. N. Dudgeon RN
1015 IV dc'd. Pressure dressing applied after oozing ceased. N. Dudgeon RN
1030 Verbally states the need to refrain from lifting anything heavier than a phone book until he returns to clinic. Discussed dietary aids to soften stools. Discharged. N. Dudgeon RN

LEGEND BP; X APICAL PULSE; O CONTROLLED RESP   - SPONT

TIME	0915	0945	1000	1015
TEMP	26.5 C			37 core
U/O	∅	∅	250 cc	∅
EMESIS	∅	∅	∅	∅
PO INTAKE	∅	60 cc H2O	∅	100 cc H2O
IV INTAKE	—	TOTAL	—	100 cc
OTHER	N/G			

TIME	DRUG	ROUTE	DOSE	NURSE
0920	Fentanyl	IVP	50 mg	N. Dudgeon RN
0950	Fentanyl	IVP	50 mg	N. Dudgeon RN
0950	Tylenol #3	PO	Tabs ii	N. Dudgeon RN

POSTANESTHESIA RECOVERY SCORE		ADMISSION	15'	30'	1HR.	2HRS.	DISMISSAL
ACTIVITY ABLE TO MOVE VOLUNTARILY OR ON COMMAND	4 EXTREMITIES	2	2	2	2	2	2
	2 EXTREMITIES	1	1	1	1	1	1
	0 EXTREMITIES	0	0	0	0	0	0
RESPIRATION	ABLE TO DEEP BREATHE AND COUGH FREELY	2	2	2	2	2	2
	DYSPNEA SHALLOW OR LIMITED BREATHING	1	1	1	1	1	1
	APNEIC	0	0	0	0	0	0
CIRCULATION PRE-OP BP 130/70	BP ±20mm OF PREANESTHESIA LEVEL	2	2	2	2	2	2
	BP ±20-50mm OF PREANESTHESIA LEVEL	1	1	1	1	1	1
	BP ±50mm OF PREANESTHESIA LEVEL	0	0	0	0	0	0
CONSCIOUSNESS	FULLY AWAKE	2	2	2	2	2	2
	AROUSABLE ON CALLING	1	1	1	1	1	1
	NOT RESPONDING	0	0	0	0	0	0
COLOR	NORMAL	2	2	2	2	2	2
	PALE, DUSKY, BLOTCHY, JAUNDICED, OTHER	1	1	1	1	1	1
	CYANOTIC	0	0	0	0	0	0
DISMISSAL CRITERIA: TOTAL SCORE OF 9 OR 10, PLUS STABLE VITAL SIGNS.						TOTAL	10/10

DISMISSAL TIME *1030*

MD'S SIGNATURE
M. Beetrick MD

NURSE'S SIGNATURE
N. Dudgeon RN

Exhibit 8-8 Postsurgical instructions for patients (day surgery center). (Reprinted with permission, University of Kansas Medical Center, Kansas City, KS.)

SURGEON'S INSTRUCTIONS:

1. Diet Instruction:_____
    _____

2. Activity:_____
    _____

    Restrictions:_____
    _____

3. Call Clinic (phone number)_____and schedule a return appointment for

    (date)_____.

4. Instructions for care of incision:

    a. Dressing changes:_____
        _____

    b. Bathing instructions:_____
        _____

5. Prescriptions written for:_____
    _____

6. If you should have problems, call_____, after clinic hours call

    _____and ask for_____

7. You will need these special supplies:_____
    _____
    _____

8. Special instructions:_____
    _____

    _____

                    Physician's Signature:_____

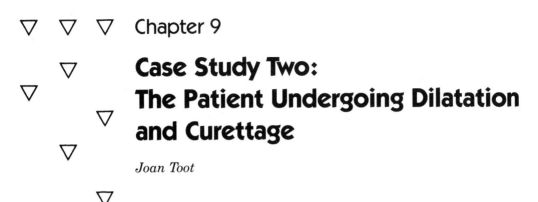

Chapter 9

Case Study Two:
The Patient Undergoing Dilatation
and Curettage

Joan Toot

Women who are admitted to an ambulatory surgery unit (ASU) for dilatation and curettage (D & C) frequently have both physical and psychological needs. As nurses are aware, the D & C procedure is performed for diagnostic purposes, such as uterine bleeding or incomplete abortion. By the very nature of this procedure, then, it is important to assess patient needs and to plan nursing interventions to minimize patient stressors in the ASU.

The purpose of this chapter is to present the care of a patient admitted to the ASU for a D & C by answering the following questions:

1. What are the nursing assessment techniques needed to assess the patient, including interviewing techniques and specific institutional forms?
2. What information from the patient assessment data can be used to formulate nursing diagnoses?
3. How can a perioperative care plan be developed for this type of ambulatory surgical patient?
4. What methods can be used to evaluate patient outcomes, including patient education, discharge planning, and follow-up care?

Nursing Assessment Techniques

The perioperative nurse working in the ASU functions in a unique environment. The nurse-patient relationship is limited to a short but intense time frame. Good interpersonal communication and physical assessment skills, combined with a knowledge of surgical procedures, are essential requirements for a perioperative nurse in the ambulatory surgery setting. Within the abbreviated time frame that is typical of this setting, the nurse must establish a therapeutic relationship, assess the psychosocial

Exhibits for Chapter 9 are located at the end of the chapter on pages 174–185.

and physical status of the patient, and meet the needs of patients during the three phases of care in the ASU.

Perioperative Phases

The perioperative surgical experience is divided into three time periods: the preoperative phase, the intraoperative phase, and the postoperative phase. The *preoperative phase* may begin when the patient elects to have surgery. The ASU often provides information booklets to be distributed to the patient at the physician's office. The initial verbal contact may begin with a preoperative phone call to the patient the evening before surgery.

This initial contact allows the nurse to inquire about special needs or concerns that the patient or family may have. A phone call documentation record, such as the one shown in Exhibit 9-1, can be used as an information guide; it includes specific guidelines for instructing patients on preparing themselves for the surgical procedure.

The nurse may initiate the nursing process when the patient is admitted to the ASU. (An in-depth discussion of the nursing process is provided in Chapter 4.) Nursing assessment requires interpersonal communication and technical skills. During assessment, the nurse obtains patient data by interviewing and examining the patient. The preoperative phase terminates with the admission of the patient into the operating room.

The *intraoperative phase* includes all nursing activities undertaken while the patient remains in the operating room (OR). The *postoperative phase* is initiated with admission of the patient into the recovery room and can extend to postoperative follow-up in the patient's home. The perioperative nurse utilizes the postoperative phase to evaluate patient outcomes.

Interview Process

The interview process, an integral part of nursing assessment, requires the nurse to be skillful in interviewing techniques. By developing and practicing good interviewing techniques, the ambulatory nurse can effectively collect data within a restricted time frame.

Bullock and Bamford describe three phases of the interviewing process:[1] the introductive phase, the working phase, and the termination phase. The nurse establishes trust and rapport with the patient and family in the *introductive phase*. This is done by identifying one's self as the nurse assisting with and planning the patient's care. Once rapport is established with the patient and family, the nurse can progress into the working phase of the interview.

In the *working phase,* the nurse strives to obtain data systematically through a structured interview and physical examination of the patient.

Informing patients that the purpose of the interview is to collect clinical information regarding their health status and to plan nursing care frequently elicits their cooperation. A comfortable, private environment also helps to facilitate a successful patient interview.

The interview or therapeutic relationship ends in the *termination phase*. At that time, the nurse informs the patient and family that the interview is completed. Often in the nurse-patient relationship, the primary responsibility for care shifts to the family during the termination phase. The nurse informs the patient and family that the relationship will be terminating. The termination phase involves dismissal of the patient from the ASU.

The nurse incorporates various forms and skills into the interviewing process. The use of an assessment form guides the nurse through a systematic assessment of the patient. The assessment form provides a directed, structure approach. Utilizing such a written assessment form (Exhibit 9-2) as a guide, the nurse uses directive and indirective questions for gathering information.

Directive interview questions are usually close-ended. Directive interviewing techniques allow the nurse to control the purpose and pace of the interview. Factual historical data are obtained as a result of well-structured questions. The *nondirective approach,* which uses open-ended questions, is less structured, and allows patients to set the pace and direction of the interview. This approach encourages patients to verbalize needs, and is an effective means of eliciting their perception of the current situation at their level of readiness. Verbal and nonverbal therapeutic communication techniques are also essential skills required of the professional nurse when implementing the directive and nondirective approaches. A combination of directive and nondirective approaches assists the nurse in gathering comprehensive data within a limited time frame.

Physical Assessment

Upon completion of the nursing interview, the nurse conducts the preoperative physical assessment of the patient. The technical skills needed for physical assessment may include observation, auscultation, inspection, palpation, percussion, and consultation. Past and present medical records, if available, also provide valuable medical and nursing history. Unusual concerns or abnormal findings are reported to the surgeon, anesthesiologist, and perioperative nursing staff.

Assessment of all body systems completes the preparation of the patient for surgery. Laboratory tests include hemoglobin and hematocrit levels, as well as other tests that may be indicated based on the patient's current medical history. Regardless of the patient's age, the nurse must inquire about potential problems relating to the hip joints or lumbar back region. This information assists the perioperative nurse in safely positioning the patient in the OR. The lithotomy position is utilized in performing a D & C. This position places the patient at risk for potential injury to the joints, muscles, and nerves of the pelvic and lumbar regions. After the nurse assesses the patient and records the data, the nursing diagnoses can be formulated.

▽

Nursing Diagnosis

Formulation of nursing diagnoses is the weakest link in the nursing process; however, the Association of Operating Room Nurses (AORN) Standard II, which states that nursing diagnoses are derived from health assessment data, challenges the perioperative nurse to formulate nursing diagnoses.[2] Gordon defines nursing diagnosis as a statement that describes actual or potential health problems for which nurses, by virtue of their education and experience, may independently prescribe primary intervention.[3] The perioperative nurse organizes, interprets, analyzes, and prioritizes the information needed to formulate a nursing diagnosis.

Frequently, the perioperative nurse tends to neglect the formulation of nursing diagnoses. The nurse does not purposely neglect this stage of the assessment phase. Rather, the omission results from health assessment forms that do not lend themselves to the clinical use of nursing diagnosis, thereby failing to incorporate nursing theory into the clinical practice of nursing. Nurse educators, nursing managers, and clinical practicing nurses have neglected to develop nursing assessment forms that encourage formulation of nursing diagnoses. At the present time, most nursing assessment records are based on body systems and medical terminology. A review of the literature reveals a severe shortcoming in ASUs in instituting assessment forms that encourage the nurse to formulate nursing diagnoses.

The North America Nursing Diagnosis Association (NANDA) created a Unitary Person Framework as a conceptual model for formulation of nursing diagnosis.[4] This conceptual framework theorizes that each person's health is manifested by the nine human response patterns (Table 9-1). These human response patterns represent categories that form the basis for development of a holistic assessment that is derived from nursing data. NANDA published *Taxonomy I* in an attempt to standardize the use of nursing diagnosis according to the nine human response patterns.[4] Previously, nursing diagnoses had been arranged alphabetically.

Taxonomy I lists a definition of and describes the defining characteristics for each diagnosis. The use of *Taxonomy I* could standardize the formulation of nursing diagnoses for the nursing profession. The preoperative assessment form (see Exhibit 9-2), which is based on the nine functional patterns of unitary man, directs the nurse in an assessment of the patient's sociocultural, psychological, and physical status. This form, which was recently developed, requires in-depth clinical testing.

Table 9-1 Nine Human Response Patterns in the
Conceptual Framework of the Unitary Person

Pattern	Definition
Exchanging	A human response pattern involving mutual giving and receiving
Communicating	A human response pattern involving sending messages
Relating	A human response pattern involving establishing bonds
Valuing	A human response pattern involving the assigning of relative worth
Choosing	A human response pattern involving the selection of alternatives
Moving	A human response pattern involving activity
Perceiving	A human response pattern involving the reception of information
Knowing	A human response pattern involving the meaning associated with information
Feeling	A human response pattern involving the subjective awareness of information

(From the North American Nursing Diagnosis Association, St. Louis, 1989.)

To facilitate adaptation of *Taxonomy I* to clinical practice, nursing assessment forms need to be revised to reflect the nine human response patterns. With development of nursing assessment forms based on these nine human response patterns, nursing diagnoses can readily be identified from the data base. Reconciling the nursing diagnosis to the categories presented in *Taxonomy I* promotes standardization of terminology in the nursing profession.

By combining individual patient assessments based on NANDA's nine human response patterns with the nurse's knowledge of the potential problems inherent to a specific surgical procedure, nursing diagnoses will become apparent from the data. A concise, well-structured nursing assessment form that requires documentation of nursing diagnoses promotes usage of nursing diagnoses by perioperative nurses in the ASU.

The following case study is used to demonstrate the formulation of nursing diagnoses from the patient assessment data. Each nursing diagnosis will be listed under the appropriate human response pattern. There may not be a nursing diagnosis identified for each human response pattern. The initial assessment and formulation of nursing diagnoses are usually accomplished during the preoperative phase. The perioperative nurse is responsible for continually reassessing the patient through each perioperative phase to identify new problems and related nursing diagnoses.

Case Study

Mrs. B., a 35-year-old white female, presents to the ASU for a D & C. Mrs. B.'s diagnosis is incomplete abortion at nine weeks' gestation. Mrs. B. is observed to be tearful and anxious. She complains of uterine cramping and vaginal bleeding of 12-hour duration. Mr. B. and their minister have accompanied Mrs. B. to the ASU. Mrs. B. verbalizes her concerns about her inability to carry a pregnancy to term. She states that this is her second first-trimester miscarriage in 18 months. Mrs. B., a lawyer, now questions her decision to delay pregnancy until after her professional career was established.

Mrs. B.'s history includes a D & C performed 12 months ago, also for an incomplete, spontaneous abortion, and a fractured pelvis 10 years ago, which resulted in limited range of motion of the left hip. She walks with a slight limp and complains of chronic left hip pain. She was diagnosed as having Raynaud's disease 5 years ago.

Mrs. B.'s present medications include prenatal vitamins. She also takes ibuprofen for chronic hip pain when not pregnant. She denies any allergies to medications.

Mrs. B.'s physical assessment reveals an alert, crying, but cooperative adult female. Her skin is warm and dry with evidence of adequate hydration and nutrition. She ambulates with a slight limp and limited range of motion of the left hip and leg. Assessment of her vital signs reveals that her blood pressure is 100/60, her pulse is 90, and her respirations are regular, with a rate of 18. She is complaining of pelvic discomfort and vaginal bleeding. She describes the amount of vaginal bleeding as being similar to a heavy menstrual period. She denies the ingestion of food or liquids during the previous 10 hours. Mrs. B. asks that her husband and minister be allowed to remain with her preoperatively and postoperatively. Using these assessment data and derived nursing diagnoses (Table 9-2), the nurse can then develop the nursing care plan.

▽

Perioperative Care Plan

The AORN *standards of practice* recommend the use of care plans in the practice of perioperative nursing.[2] In addition, the Joint Commission on Accreditation of Health Care Organizations' (JCAHO's) Standard H01.5 mandates that "hospital-sponsored ambulatory care meet[s] the same standards of quality that apply to inpatient care provided by the hospital (p. 54)."[5] However, care plans are noticeably absent in many ASUs. Most nursing care plan formats developed for intermediate or long-term hospital stays are not applicable to short-term patients. The task of developing ambulatory surgical care plans becomes the responsibility of the nurse specializing in this clinical area. Using the diagnostic categories

Table 9-2 Suggested Nursing Diagnosis Formulated for Mrs. B.

Pattern	Related Nursing Diagnosis
Communciating	No problem identified preoperatively
Valuing	No problem identified preoperatively
Relating	Altered sexual patterns R/T postoperative restriction of sexual intercourse
Knowing	Potential knowledge deficit R/T surgical procedure
	Potential knowledge deficit R/T pattern of habitual spontaneous abortion
Feeling	Pain R/T uterine cramping
	Grieving R/T loss of pregnancy
Moving	Impaired physical mobility R/T decrease range of motion in left hip
	High risk for injury (left hip) R/T lithotomy position for surgical procedure
Perceiving	Situational low self-esteem R/T inability to maintain viable pregnancy
Exchanging	Potential altered peripheral tissue perfusion R/T history of Reynaud's disease
	High risk for fluid volume deficit R/T decreased fluid intake (NPO status)
	High risk for fluid volume deficit R/T blood loss
	High risk for infection R/T surgical procedure
	High risk for infection R/T impaired uterine tissue
Choosing	Decisional conflict R/T career goals versus delayed pregnancy

from NANDA's *Taxonomy I* and Mrs. B's assessment data, an individualized nursing care plan (Exhibit 9-3) has been written.

Realistically, developing an individualized nursing care plan from a blank piece of paper is not an efficient use of nurses' time in the ASU. Thus, a care plan format that is practical for ambulatory surgery is a standardized one. The development and use of standardized care plans have reduced the amount of time required to develop a care plan for each patient. Alfaro and Hanson-Smith support the use of standardized care plans, but recommend that the nurse incorporate individual needs of patients into the standard care plan.[6,7]

A review of the literature revealed few published standardized care plans for ASUs. Jan Branham, R.N., B.S., Ellie Godfrey, R.N., B.S.N., and

Barbara Moore, R.N., M.S.N. of Seton Medical Center, Austin, Texas published a care plan they developed (Exhibit 9-4).[8] This care plan represents a practical variation of a standardized care plan. The care plan incorporates the capacity to individualize patient care within a standard care plan format.

Ideally, the nurse who develops the patient care plan provides patient care preoperatively and postoperatively. It becomes the responsibility of the intraoperative nurse, then, to review the care plan and to become familiar with the patient's needs. The intraoperative nurse then plans the care provided in the OR accordingly, taking into consideration the needs of the individual patient and the proposed surgical procedure. To illustrate the practical application of a nursing care plan, a discussion of nursing care actions implemented for Mrs. B. during each operative phase is presented.

Preoperative Care Plan

Mrs. B. presents herself to the ASU accompanied by her husband and their minister. The nurse introduces herself to Mr. and Mrs. B. To provide privacy for Mrs. B. during her assessment, the nurse instructs the minister to remain in the waiting room. The minister and Mrs. B. are informed that he may join Mr. and Mrs. B. after she is admitted.

The nurse quickly observes that Mrs. B is tearful. The nurse assesses the reason for Mrs. B.'s tearfulness. Through questioning and encouraging Mrs. B. to verbalize her feelings, the nurse ascertains that Mrs. B. must be given time to verbalize her emotional distress related to her miscarriage. Empathizing with Mrs. B. enhances the development of a therapeutic relationship. The nurse completes Mrs. B.'s physical assessment and health history. The nurse then escorts the minister into Mrs. B.'s room. Completion of the initial assessment provides data for the nurse to identify nursing diagnoses and to develop the nursing care plan.

Effective preoperative and postoperative teaching depends on quickly decreasing Mrs. B.'s emotional distress. Mrs. B.'s primary concerns related to the surgical procedure are prevention of increased hip pain and decreased perfusion to her fingers. The nurse explains to Mrs. B. the intended nursing actions related to her physical concerns. A careful preoperative assessment of Mrs. B.'s gait and present circulatory status of her fingers provides information for postoperative comparison.

Preoperatively, the nurse determines that Mrs. B. is at high risk for fluid volume deficit. The laboratory results of the preoperative hemoglobin and hematocrit tests are documented. The intravenous intracatheter to be inserted by the nurse should be a minimum of 18 French to accommodate the potential need for rapid infusion of fluid or blood products. In Mrs. B.'s individual case, postoperative teaching is not instituted preoperatively, as her main concern is to have a sufficient amount of private time with her husband and minister. Detailing the technical aspects of her surgical procedure was not considered an important aspect of patient teaching for Mrs. B due to her familiarity with the D & C procedure and her present state of emotional stress.

Intraoperative Care Plan

The OR nurse assumes the responsibility for planning Mrs. B.'s nursing care while in the OR. The nurse prepares the OR with the standard supplies used for a D & C. Consultation with the preoperative nurse and a review of the care plan provide the intraoperative nurse with the information needed to plan for individualized care of Mrs. B. In Mrs. B.'s situation, the nurse plans for a warmer physical environment in the OR and a warm covering for Mrs. B.'s hands and forearms to prevent altered tissue perfusion of the fingers. Mrs. B.'s limited range of motion in her left hip requires careful attention while positioning her in the lithotomy position. During the intraoperative phase, the nurse documents any resolution of identified nursing diagnoses included in the care plan.

Postoperative Care Plan

The intraoperative nurse accompanies Mrs. B. to the recovery room and terminates the intraoperative care phase by giving a verbal report to the recovery room nurse. The initial assessment of Mrs. B.'s cardiovascular and respiratory status is a priority nursing action, as is the assessment and documentation of vaginal bleeding. The intravenous intracatheter is examined for patency. As Mrs. B. arouses from the general anesthesia, the nurse orients her to the surroundings. Emotional support continues as an important aspect of Mrs. B.'s care. If pain medication is required, small doses of short-acting intravenous analgesia are preferred. In the absence of nausea, oral fluids are then encouraged. Ice chips are the first choice, and if these are tolerated, Mrs. B. is advanced to clear liquids.

Upon dismissal from the recovery room, Mrs. B. is reunited with her husband and minister, at her request, in a private patient room. Allowing her to spend time with her support system in private encourages Mrs. B. to verbalize the emotional aspects of her spontaneous abortion.

Utilizing the nursing care plan as a guide, the nurse continues to monitor Mrs. B. for discomfort, vaginal bleeding, oral fluid intake, and urinary output. The peripheral perfusion in Mrs. B.'s fingers requires assessment to determine whether the nursing actions were adequate. As Mrs. B. begins to ambulate, the nurse observes her for any change in gait or verbalization of increased left hip pain.

When the nurse determines that Mrs. B. is ready for postoperative teaching, a dismissal instruction sheet (see Exhibit 9-5) is reviewed with her and her husband, and any questions regarding these instructions are answered by the nurse. A copy of the written dismissal instruction sheet is sent home with Mrs. B. Mrs. B. is prepared for discharge when the nurse determines that the dismissal criteria have been met. The surgeon is notified of Mrs. B.'s readiness for dismissal and Mrs. B. is discharged home with her husband. Mr. and Mrs. B. are instructed that a nurse from the ASU will be calling them later in the evening to check on Mrs. B.'s recovery.

▽

Methods for Evaluating Patient Outcomes

The nursing profession requires nurses to evaluate patient outcomes continually. Quality assurance is the process by which patient outcomes are evaluated. Craighead states that quality assurance addresses the gaps between the caregiver's intention and the care given.[9] Quality assurance examines both the assets of and the discrepancies in nursing care. The goal of quality assurance is to improve patient care. Regardless of the positive intent of quality assurance studies, nurses view them as time-consuming and problematic in that they create additional paperwork. However, nurses are concerned about outcomes of patient care, patient education, and discharge planning, and quality assurance studies are essential for ensuring high standards of nursing care in these areas.

Ambulatory surgery has brought many changes in the patient care delivery system. When hospitalization for a D & C was the norm, patients usually remained in the hospital several days postoperatively. This meant that patient education and discharge planning evolved over an extended period of time. The nurse had a reasonable amount of time to evaluate the patient's response to nursing care and postoperative teaching. Moreover, the nurse was actively involved in assisting the patient and family to achieve the desired outcomes. However, ambulatory surgery has altered this nurse-patient relationship drastically. The perioperative nurse now has limited time for patient teaching and discharge planning. The patient returns home before the nurse can evaluate the outcomes of patient education and discharge planning. The short-term stay of ambulatory surgical patients requires creative approaches to assess patient outcomes. Quality assurance studies are needed to evaluate these new methods to ensure optimal patient care standards. Commonly used methods include concurrent and retrospective chart audits, telephone interviews, and questionnaires.

A well-constructed nursing care plan provides a format for conducting concurrent and retrospective chart audits. The content of a nursing care plan is based on standardized language and measurable criteria. The nursing diagnosis documents the focus of patient care, the goal statement defines the intended outcome, implementation involves the methods used to achieve the patient goals, and the evaluation of patient outcomes verifies the results of the nursing actions. Thus, a nursing care plan lends itself to quality assurance audits. Peer review of the content of a nursing care plan can identify the areas responsible for failed patient outcomes. On a positive note, nursing care plan audits may also identify innovative nursing actions that can be shared with other nurses to enhance nursing care.

Successful patient education and discharge planning are critical factors influencing the outcome of the patient's surgical experience. The nurse instructs the patient regarding postoperative instructions and co-ordinates discharge planning. The teaching process involves the patient and other persons participating in postoperative care. Discharge instructions are written in a concise format using simple language. The nurse then reviews the written instruction sheet with the patient and family. A copy of the written instruction sheet is sent home with the patient. The patient is encouraged to schedule a postoperative follow-up visit with the surgeon before dismissal. The time of the follow-up appointment is then written on the instruction sheet.

Auditing a patient's questions regarding the home care that is based on the discharge instructions is also a means of evaluating the outcome of patient teaching. Additionally, the peer review audit determines the accuracy of the nursing responses to the patient's questions. An excessive number of questions regarding home care instructions may reveal a possible deficiency in postoperative discharge teaching either on the part of the nursing staff or the attending physician. Alternatively, a lack of correct or appropriate responses by the nurse to a patient's questions indicates a need for staff education. A continuous, systematic audit of postoperative patient outcomes provides quality assurance data and perpetuates a high standard of patient care. Telephone interviews are helpful in the audit process.

Telephone interviews provide immediate and personal contact with the patient. Ideally, the postoperative follow-up telephone contact occurs within 24 hours after dismissal. A form (Exhibit 9-1) may assist the interviewer in standardizing the content of the telephone interview, as well as in covering all pertinent areas of inquiry. The questions refer to the patient's physical well-being and understanding of the discharge instructions. An astute and intuitive perioperative nurse can listen to the patient or caregiver responses and detect potential problems. Referral or follow-up telephone contact may be necessary if a potential problem is suspected by the nurse. Thus, the form becomes a legal document that states the outcome of the telephone interview and the recommendations made by the nurse.

Standardized postoperative telephone interview records (Exhibit 9-1) can be audited on a regular basis. The audit summary sheet (Exhibit 9-6) evaluates the outcomes of patient teaching and the patient's physical status after dismissal. Questions one through four of the audit summary sheet evaluate the patient's physical status after dismissal. A patient compliance level that is less than the assigned desired outcome standards alerts the nursing staff of a potential problem with the ASU dismissal criteria or the nursing staff's judgment of the patient's readiness for dismissal.

Another means of outcome evaluation involves the use of written questionnaires (Exhibit 9-7), which may be sent to patients one week after their ambulatory surgical experience. If a patient has a negative comment about their ASU experience, they may hesitate to express an opinion during a personal telephone interview. Thus, the use of a less personal method, such as a questionnaire, allows patients to express their opinions in a nonthreatening, anonymous way. The questionnaire addresses the environmental setting of the ASU, and also evaluates the success of the interdisciplinary team approach involving surgeons, perioperative nurses, and anesthesia personnel.

A successful patient surgical outcome requires an interdependent team effort by the surgeons, the anesthesia team, and the perioperative nurses. A positive professional relationship between the surgeons and the perioperative nursing staff encourages sharing of patient information. After dismissal of the patient, the perioperative nurse maintains a limited contact with the patient. After follow-up visits with the patient the surgeon can provide information to the nursing staff about patient outcomes. The surgical patient benefits from informative communication from all members involved in caring for the patient.

▽

Summary

This chapter has presented some approaches to the role of the nurse in caring for a patient admitted for a D & C. By answering the four questions listed at the beginning of the chapter, the intent has been to guide the nurse through the five steps of the nursing process: assessment, nursing diagnosis, planning, implementing, and evaluating patient care. Emphasis has been placed on interviewing techniques, perioperative care plan development, and methods for evaluating patient outcomes.

References

1. Bullock, J., and Bamford, P. (1984). *Nursing assessment: A multidimensional approach*. Montery, CA: Wadsworth Health Science Division.
2. Association of Operating Room Nurses, Inc. (1988). *AORN practices for perioperative nursing*. Denver, CO: Association of Operating Room Nurses, Inc.
3. Gordon, M. (1982). *Nursing diagnosis: Process and application*. New York: McGraw-Hill.
4. North American Nursing Diagnosis Association. (1989). *Taxonomy I with official diagnostic categories* (rev. ed.). St. Louis: North American Nursing Diagnosis Association.
5. Joint Commission on Accreditation of Hospital Organizations. (1990). *An ambulatory health care standards manual*. Chicago: Joint Commission on Accreditation of Hospital Organizations.

6. Alfaro, R. (1989). *Applying nursing diagnosis and nursing process: A step-by-step guide. (2nd ed.)* Philadelphia: J. B. Lippincott.
7. Hanson-Smith, B. (1989). *Nursing care planning guides for childbearing families*. Baltimore: Williams & Wilkins.
8. Staff (1989, July). Texas center initiating outpatient care plan during preadmission visit. *Same-Day Surgery* 13 (7); 97–100.
9. Craighead, J. (1987). Accountability in clinical judgment and decision making: How can we assure quality? In K. J. Hannah, M. Reiner, W. Mills, and S. Lelourneau (Eds.), *Clinical judgment and decision making: The future with nursing diagnosis* (pp. 449–452). New York: Wiley Medical Publications.

Exhibit 9-1 Out-patient surgery pre- and post-op visit checklist. (Reprinted by permission, Lawrence Memorial Hospital, Lawrence, KS.)

OUT-PATIENT SURGERY
PRE- AND POST-OP VISIT CHECKLIST

NAME _____ AGE _____ PROCEDURE _____

SURGEON _____ DATE OF SURGERY _____ ARRIVAL TIME _____

PHONE # _____

PRE-OP   VISIT _____ PHONE CALL _____

	YES	NO
1. Patient or family contacted.	_____	_____
2. If general or regional, remind patient to have nothing by mouth after midnight.	_____	_____
3. Does patient have a responsible adult to drive him home?	_____	_____
4. Do you wear glasses _____ contact lenses ____ (check one if applies) (Remind to bring contact case if needed.)	_____	_____
5. Remind patient to leave jewelry and money at home.	_____	_____
6. Suggest patient bring slippers to wear while at hospital.	_____	_____
7. Suggest apparel appropriate for surgery.	_____	_____
8. Has patient completed required lab work?	_____	_____
9. Instruct patient what time to arrive.	_____	_____
10. Location of outpatient check in /parking	_____	_____
11. Medication	_____	_____
12. Recently ill, cold, fever.	_____	_____
13. Waiting area for visitors.	_____	_____
14. Expected length of stay.	_____	_____
15. Bring papers from Doctor's office (Insurance Form, Health Care Plus).	_____	_____

COMMENTS: _____

_____

_____
Signature

POST-OP

	YES	NO
1. Patient or family contacted.	_____	_____
2. Did patient experience any nausea/vomiting?	_____	_____
3. Was patient able to eat or drink fluids?	_____	_____
4. Was pain medication taken?	_____	
5. Was pain medication adequate?	_____	_____
6. Was any drainage observed from surgical site?	_____	_____
7. Further questions regarding home care.	_____	_____
8. Questions regarding discharge instructions.	_____	_____
9. Reminder to schedule post-op appointment.	_____	_____

COMMENTS: _____

_____

_____

_____
Signature

Exhibit 9-2 Preoperative assessment form.

Surgeon _____ Proposed Procedure _____ Date _____

Anesthesia _____ Proposed anesthesia _____ Allergies _____

Exchanging: A pattern involving mutual giving and receiving.

Ht. _____ Wt. _____ B/P _____ P. _____ regular/irregular R. _____ SAO₂% _____

Breath sounds _____ Dyspnea _____ on exertion _____ Smoke/Chewing tobacco _____

Cough _____ Dry/Productive Dentures: upper/lower plate Partial: upper/lower

Crowns: _____ Loose teeth: _____ Appearance: well nourished obese emaciated

Skin: Turgor _____ Lesions _____ Bruises _____ Abrasions _____

Extremities: Peripheral edema: _____ Location _____ Pedal pulse R _____ L _____

Capillary refill: adequate slow absence(specify) _____

Elimination: Ostomies _____ Urinary:frequency urgency dysuria hematuria retention

Review of systems: Health problems past and present

	Yes	No		Yes	No		Yes	No
Thyroid			Steroid therapy			Cardiac/vascular disease		
Diabetes			Hypertension			Renal		
Arthritis			CVA			Hematologic		
Gastrointestinal			Cancer			Seizures		
Hepatic/Hepatitis			Respiratory			Alcohol intake		
Caffiene intake			Neuro/muscular					

Exhibit 9-2 (Continued)

Nursing Diagnosis; Actual or potential

Fluid volume: deficit/excess Impaired tissue perfusion Injury(specify) _____

Impaired gas exchange Impaired skin integrity Nutrition: more/less than body

Urinary: retention urgency hematuria frequency dysuria requirement _____

Knowing: A pattern involving the meaning associated with information

Current medication (including O.T.C.) _____

Drug _____ Dosage _____ Last Dose _____

Previous illness/hospitalizations/surgeries (specify dates)

_____

History of nausea or vomiting with previous anesthesia Yes No Date _____

Learning difficulties: Yes(specify) _____ No _____

Knowledge deficit: regarding illness _____ sugical routine _____ home care _____

Memory intact: yes _____ no _____ recent _____ remote _____

Nursing Diagnosis: actual or potential

Knowledge deficit(specify) _____ Level of orientation _____

(Continued)

Exhibit 9-2 (Continued)

Marital status: M S W D   Children: Adult____ dependent minors____

Support system: relatives friends availability for assistance:____

Family and patient concerns R/T surgery:____

Nursing Diagnosis: actual or potential

Impaired support system__ Impaired family process__ Other____

Valuing: A pattern involving the assigning of relative worth

Religious affiliation:_____ Religious restrictions:____

Minister present: yes no   Cultural practices:____

Nursing Diagnosis: actual or potential

Spiritual state: despair distress Other____

Perceiving: A pattern involving the reception of information

Eye contact: appropriate downcast staring avoidance

Body posture: relaxed rigid tense   Mood: calm tearful withdrawn anxious

Affect: normal flat   Cognitive: ability to follow simple commands yes no

Hearing: normal impaired left ear right ear   Hearing aide: Left Right

Vision:normal impaired glasses contacts:Right Left Removed preoperatively yes no

Concern about body image changes R/T surgical procedure:____

Nursing Diagnosis: actual or potential

Body image changes self esteem visual auditory powerlessness

Exhibit 9-2 (Continued)

Confusion_____   Memory_____   Others_____

Moving: A pattern involving activity

Ambulates: by self___ with assistance____   Prosthesis(specify)____

Aids: cane walker wheelchair___ Gait: Steady unsteady limp

Range of Motion: normal____ abnormal(specify extremity and limitation)____

Self care: Self care deficit yes__ no__ (specify)____

Discharge planning needs:____

Nursing Diagnosis: actual or potential

activity intolerance impaired physical mobility self care deficit

Communicating: A pattern involving sending messages

understands English language yes no other____ reads yes no writes yes no

Reads lips yes no   sign language yes no

Hearing intact R L deficit R L Vision intact R L Deficit R L

Assistive devices used for communication:____

Physical limitation of speech (specify):____

Nursing Diagnosis: actual or potential

Impaired communication: verbal visual auditory

Relating: A pattern involving establishing bonds

Exhibit 9-2 (Continued)

Feeling: A pattern involving the subjective awareness of information

Physical pain: acute   chronic

location _____   Duration _____

Emotional intregity: recent loss/grief   yes   no   fearful   yes   no

Specify: _____

Nursing Diagnosis: actual or potential

Pain: acute chronic grieving anxiety fear

Choosing: A pattern involving the selection of alternatives

Coping with health problems   yes   no

Verbalizes problem: _____

Family coping: effective ineffective

Compliance:

Compliance with past/present health care regimens: yes   no

Willingness to comply with future health care regimens: yes   no

Nursing Diagnosis: actual or potential

Ineffective individual family coping Noncompliance past present future

Exhibit 9-3 Perioperative care plan.

Assessment	Nursing Diagnosis	Patient Goal	Nursing Intervention	Outcome
Subjective "I have been bleeding for 10 to 12 hours." **Objective** Documented active vaginal bleeding	**Exchanging:** High risk for uterine infection R/T impaired tissue of uterine cavity **Exchanging:** High risk for infection R/T surgical procedure	Patient will be free of infection with no evidence of fever, increased uterine or abdominal pain, or foul vaginal discharge 72 hours after surgery.	1. Adhere to strict surgical aseptic technique. 2. Instruct patient regarding reportable signs and symptoms of infection. 3. Acquaint patient and husband with dismissal instructions related to prevention of infection (refer to dismissal instruction sheet). 4. Send copy of dismissal instruction sheet home with patient.	Resolved: Time _____ Initial _____ Reassessed: _____ Initial _____
Subjective "Please keep my hands warm. If they get cold it is very painful." **Objective** Documented history of Reynaud's disease.	**Exchanging:** Potential altered peripheral tissue perfusion R/T history of Reynaud's disease	Patient will not experience pain or decreased perfusion to hands during confinement in ambulatory surgical unit.	1. Provide warm coverings for hands. 2. Provide warm environment when possible. 3. Provide restful environment to decrease anxiety.	Resolved: Time _____ Initial _____ Reassessed: _____ Initial _____
Subjective "My lower stomach hurts. Feels like cramps." **Objective** Documented incomplete abortion. Holding lower abdomen.	**Feeling:** Pain R/T uterine cramping	Patient will verbalize adequate pain relief within 30-45 minutes after administration of post-operative analgesias.	1. Encourage patient to evaluate pain on scale of 1-10 and reevaluate 30-45 minutes after administration of oral pain medication. 2. Provide a quiet restful environment.	Resolved: Time _____ Initial _____ Reassessed: _____ Initial _____

Subjective
 	
"I have been bleeding and cramping since last night."
 	
Objective
 	
Active vaginal bleeding of slight amount of bright blood
	Exchanging:
	
	High risk for fluid volume deficit R/T blood loss (active vaginal bleeding)
		Patient will exhibit vaginal bleeding that is within normal limits.	1. Monitor vaginal bleeding by:
			  a. Noting the amount and number perineal pads used.
			  b. Observing for blood clot formation.
			2. Administer postoperative IV Pitocin as ordered by physician.
			3. Complete preoperative testing of hemoglobin and hematocrit to assess patient's preoperative status.
				Resolved:
				Time _____
				Initial _____
				
				Reassessed: _____
				Initial _____

Exhibit 9-3 (Continued)

Assessment	Nursing Diagnosis	Patient Goal	Nursing Intervention	Outcome
Subjective "I have not had anything to eat or drink since, for 10 hours." **Objective** Confirmed NPO status	**Exchanging:** High risk for fluid volume deficit R/T decreased fluid intake	Patient will maintain normal fluid volume as evidenced by stable blood pressure, pulse, respiration, adequate urine output, and no evidence of vomiting.	1. Monitor vital signs as required by status of patient. 2. Monitor oral and IV fluid intake. 3. Monitor urine output. 4. Monitor status of any nausea and vomiting. 5. Administer antiemetic medications as ordered by physician.	Resolved: Time _____ Initial _____ Reassessed: _____ Initial _____

Subjective
 	
"I injured my left hip 10 years ago. There are some activities I cannot do. My hip does not move right."
 	
Objective
 	
Ambulates with limp, left leg limited R.O.M. on abduction and flexion
	Moving:
	
	High risk for injury (left hip) R/T lithotomy positioning for surgical procedure
		Patient will not experience increased left hip pain or disability in gait.	1. Position patient according to proper protocol once patient is relaxed.
			  a. Position legs in stirrups by elevating simultaneously.
			  b. Avoid excessive abduction of hip joints.
			  c. Lower legs slowly while being well supported at termination of procedure.
			  d. Return patient to proper body alignment.
				Resolved:
				Time _____
				Initial _____
				
				Reassessed: _____
				Initial _____

Subjective "We want this baby so much. I just don't know why I lost the baby. Can my husband and minister stay with me?" **Objective** Tearful; downcast eyes	**Feeling:** Grieving R/T loss of pregnancy	Patient will complete therapeutic grieving process as evidenced by maintaining normal functional activities.	1. Allow husband and minister to remain with patient. 2. Provide privacy for family and minister. 3. Respond to patient or husband with therapeutic communication techniques encouraging verbalization of their loss.	Resolved: Time _____ Initial _____ Reassessed: _____ Initial _____
Subjective ""I wonder if I waited too late to have a family." **Objective** 35-year old professional with history of repeated spontaneous incomplete abortions. Relates information about deciding to delay pregnancy until professional career was established.	**Choosing:** Decisional conflict R/T delaying pregnancy versus career goals	Patient and husband will be able to discuss Mrs. B's decision to delay pregnancy in order to establish her career. Mrs. B will be able to accept her decision without feelings of guilt.	1. Encourage patient to discuss feeling of doubt about her decision. Explore possibility of counseling to explore feelings of guilt regarding career goals versus parenthood.	Resolved: Time _____ Initial _____ Reassessed: _____ Initial _____

(Continued)

Exhibit 9-3 (Continued)

Assessment	Nursing Diagnosis	Patient Goal	Nursing Intervention	Outcome

Subjective
 	
None
 	
Objective
 	
Postoperative patho-physiology of uterus makes patient at risk for uterine infection
	Relating:
	
	Altered sexuality patterns R/T restricted sexual intercourse
		Patient and husband will verbalize an understanding of restricted intercourse after receiving post-operative instructions.	1. Educate patient and husband regarding reasons for abstaining from sexual inter-course until vaginal bleeding stops or until instructed otherwise by physician.	Resolved:
				   Time _____
				   Initial _____
				
				Reassessed: _____
				   Initial _____

Subjective
 	
"I had a fractured pelvis and left hip 10 years ago. My left hip does not move properly. I have to be careful."
 	
Objective
 	
Limited R.O.M. with decreased abduction and flexion; ambulates with limp of left leg.
	Moving:
	
	Impaired physical mobility R/T decreased R.O.M. in left hip
		Patient will not exper-ience increased pain or disability of left hip. Patient's altered gait will not be compromised upon dismissal from ambulatory surgical unit.	1. Assist the patient in ambulating post-operatively to prevent injury to left hip.
			
			2. Provide support until patient can ambulate with steady gait and no evidence of dizziness.
				Resolved:
				   Time _____
				   Initial _____
				
				Reassessed: _____
				   Initial _____

Subjective
 	
"What is wrong with me. Why can't I have a baby like everyone else? Maybe I waited too long. I am 35-years old.
 	
Objective
 	
35-year old female who intentionally prevented conception until establishment of career. Repeated first trimester incomplete abortions.
	Perceiving :
	
	Situational low self-esteem R/T inability to maintain viable pregnancy
		The patient will ver-balize the need to seek counseling if unable to resolve feeling of low self esteem.	1. Encourage the patient to discuss feelings of failure with her hus-band, minister, and physician.
			
			2. Discuss possibility of counseling to explore situational conflicts R/T repeated abortions.
			
			3. Encourage patient to discuss physiological factors with physician to increase knowledge of physiological factors regarding spontaneous abortions.
				Resolved:
				   Time _____
				   Initial _____
				
				Reassessed: _____
				   Initial _____

Exhibit 9-4 Day surgery/P.A.T. nursing care plan. (Reprinted with permission of the Seton Medical Center, Austin, TX.)

(Continued)

Seton Medical Center
Day Surgery/P.A.T. Care Plan

Page 1

DATE TIME INIT	NURSING DIAGNOSIS/ ETIOLOGY	NURSING INTERVENTION	DATE TIME INIT	COMMENTS (Date, time and initial each comment)	OUTCOME
	Anxiety Potential 1) Fear of unknown 2) Other:	1) Orient to environment 2) Identify communication technique before surgery 3) Maintain quiet atmosphere 4) Other:			Prevent/reduce fear and anxiety Other:_____ Resolved: Date____ Time____ Init____
	Knowledge Deficit 1) Fear of unknown 2) Other:	1) Assess level of knowledge 2) Initiate pre- and postop teaching 3) Explain and review discharge instructions 4) Answer questions thoroughly 5) Initiate discharge planning 6) Other:			Prevent/reduce fear and anxiety Other:_____ Resolved: Date____ Time____ Init____
	Self-Concept: Disturbance in Body Image 1) Surgical procedure 2) Disfigurement 3) Other:	1) Encourage verbalization of feelings 2) Stress patient's strengths 3) Allow patient to express and discuss anger and grief 4) Encourage questions about incision, scar, future 5) Discuss and refer to support groups 6) Other:			Communicate realistic body image Other:_____ Resolved: Date____ Time____ Init____
	Communication Impaired: Verbal 1) Deafness 2) Speech impediment 3) Language barrier 4) Other:	1) Provide materials/tools necessary for communication 2) Allow adequate time for communication 3) Allow family member to assist with communication 4) Provide person to use sign language or translate for patient 5) Other:			Identify effective communication technique Other:_____ Resolved: Date____ Time____ Init____
	Fluid Volume Deficit 1) Dehydration 2) Fluid loss in surgery 3) Nausea/vomiting 4) Other:	1) Monitor intake and output 2) Maintain IV infusion as ordered 3) Provide comfort measures/ medication relative to N/V 4) Monitor vital signs 5) Monitor dressing 6) Other:			Exhibit adequate hydration - nausea/ vomiting minimal Other:_____ Resolved: Date____ Time____ Init____

Signature _____ Init. _____   Signature _____ Init. _____   Signature _____ Init. _____

Exhibit 9-4 (Continued)

Page 2

DATE TIME INIT	NURSING DIAGNOSIS/ ETIOLOGY	NURSING INTERVENTION	DATE TIME INIT	COMMENTS (Date, time and initial each comment)	OUTCOME
	Infection Potential 1) Trauma 2) Decreased body resistance 3) Postsurgery 4) Other	1) Monitor for signs and symptoms of (S/S) infection 2) Reinforce hygiene behavior 3) Teach S/S of infection 4) Monitor vital signs 5) Use isolation precautions as infectious agent indicates 6) Other:			Establish decreased potential for infection Demonstrate optimal hygiene techniques____ Other:____ Resolved:____ Date____ Time____ Init____
	Potential for Injury 1) Postanesthesia drug influence 2) Age 3) Physical disability 4) Medicated 5) Other:	1) Give instructions to patient/family 2) Assist with ambulation 3) Keep side rails up, bed in low position 4) Other:			No injury occurs Other:____ Resolved:____ Date____ Time____ Init____
	Sensory Perception Alteration 1) Surgical procedure 2) Visual or hearing impaired 3) Paralysis 4) Other:	1) Give clear, concise explanations 2) Introduce self frequently 3) Place call light within reach 4) Point out surroundings 5) Stay close to patient pre- and postop 6) Maintain safety precautions 7) Explain procedures beforehand 8) Identify communication technique before surgery 9) Other:			Experience minimal adverse reactions due to sensory limitations Other:____ Resolved:____ Date____ Time____ Init____
	Comfort Altered: Pain Acute 1) Surgical incision 2) Decreased body temperature 3) Other:	1) Teach to notify 2) Monitor response to analgesia 3) Monitor type/quality/intensity of pain 4) Offer comfort of warm blankets 5) Other:			Verbalize reduction or alleviation of pain/ discomfort____ Other:____ Resolved:____ Date____ Time____ Init____
	Tissue Perfusion Altered 1) Reduced venous flow 2) Other:	1) Position for maximum circulation 2) Monitor pulses/color/sensation to operative site 3) Monitor cast/dressing 4) Other:			Exhibit adequate tissue perfusion____ Other:____ Resolved:____ Date____ Time____ Init____
	Other				

Patient Name____

182

Exhibit 9-5 Instructions for home care following D & C.

INSTRUCTIONS FOR HOME CARE FOLLOWING
D & C (DILATATION AND CURETTAGE)

1. <u>ACTIVITY</u>: Rest in bed the day of your surgery. You may resume normal activities as soon as you are comfortable doing so beginning the day after surgery.

2. <u>VAGINAL DISCHARGE</u>: There will probably be a small amount of bleeding from the vagina (birth canal) for a couple of days. If excessive amounts of bright red bleeding occurs, you should notify your doctor. Use pads rather than tampons. Do no douche until seen by your doctor.

3. <u>SEXUAL RELATIONS</u>: You should not have sexual intercourse until the vaginal bleeding has stopped.

4. <u>PAIN</u>: You may experience mild uterine cramping. Use acetaminophen (examples: Tylenol, Panadol) or ibruprofen (examples: Advil or Nuprin).

5. <u>DIET</u>: For the first few hours, limit your diet to liquids. After tolerating fluids well, you may eat bland foods. By the day after your surgery, you should be eating normally.

6. <u>POSTOPERATIVE CHECK-UP</u>: Please call the office the day after surgery to make an appointment to be seen by your doctor for a check-up 2 weeks after your surgery. The office number is 843-0677.

7. <u>AFTER LEAVING THE HOSPITAL</u>: Call your doctor if you have:

   * Heavy vaginal bleeding (Heavier than a regular period).

   * Chills or fever or 100 degrees.

   * Frequency and burning with urination.

   * A red, hard, tender, or hot area along the leg veins or calves.

   * Chest pain - sharp, stabbing pain or difficulty breathing.

   * Persistent nausea and vomiting.

   * Any other unexplained signs or symptoms.

   After normal office hours you can dial the office number and reach the doctor's answering service. They will direct you as to how to get in contact with your doctor.

Exhibit 9-6 Telephone interview audit summary.

AUDIT SUMMARY   TOPIC <u>OR/PACU/SDS Post-Op Phone Call List</u>   PURPOSE <u>To monitor process of post-op phone calls,</u>
<u>appropriateness of nursing advice. To monitor</u>
<u>outcomes of SDS patients.</u>

DATE: # records reviewed: _____ ORIGINAL AUDIT: _____ RE-AUDIT: _____ NURSING UNITS IN STUDY: _____

AUDIT CRITERIA	% Standard	Compliance #	Compliance %	PROBLEM SUMMARY/ACTIONS TAKEN (When/By Whom)
1. The patient was able to eat and drink.	90%			
2. The patient did not experience nausea or vomiting.	90%			
3. The patient had taken pain medication with adequate relief of pain.	90%			
4. The patient had bleeding or drainage which was within normal limits for the surgical procedure.	90%			

_____ Assistant Executive Director/Nursing   Date _____   Q.A. Chairman _____ Date _____

_____ Executive Director   Date _____   Department Director _____ Date _____

_____ Q.A. Chairman (Nursing)   Date _____   President/Board/Trustees _____ Date _____

_____ Chief/Medical Staff   Date _____

<u>FOR INFORMATIONAL PURPOSE: SUMMARY OF PATIENTS POST-OP QUESTIONS</u>

The patient had the following questions: **Advice given by nurse. Was advice**
   (space to record patient's questions)   **appropriate?**

<u>SUMMARY OF NUMBER OF PATIENT'S QUESTIONS AND % OF APPROPRIATENESS OF NURSE'S RESPONSE</u>

Exhibit 9-7 Outpatient questionnaire. (Reprinted by permission, Lawrence Memorial Hospital, Lawrence, KS.)

Lawrence Memorial Hospital

OUTPATIENT QUESTIONNAIRE

Name _____ Date of Outpatient Surgery _____

A. ABOUT YOUR COMFORT

	YES	NO
1. Was your room comfortable?	☐	☐
2. Was parking convenient?	☐	☐
3. Was your family allowed to be sufficiently involved?	☐	☐
4. Was your privacy respected as well as possible?	☐	☐
5. Do you feel your waiting time before surgery was reasonable?	☐	☐
6. Were your clothes and personal belongings stored satisfactorily?	☐	☐

B. ABOUT YOUR CARE

1. Did you talk with a nurse from Same Day Surgery before you came in for your surgery? ☐ ☐
   Was this helpful to you? If no, what would have been more beneficial? _____

2. Did a nurse in Same Day Surgery talk with you on the day of your surgery and explain what you could expect during your visit? ☐ ☐
3. Did a member of the anesthesia team talk with you and answer your questions before surgery? ☐ ☐
4. Did your surgeon visit you before surgery? ☐ ☐
5. Was the recovery room quiet and reassuring as you awoke from your anesthetic? ☐ ☐
   If no, what was disturbing? _____

6. Did you feel that your needs were adequately met in the Recovery Room? ☐ ☐
   If not, what would have been more beneficial to you? _____

7. Did a nurse in Same Day Surgery call you the evening after your surgery? ☐ ☐
   Was this beneficial to you? ☐ ☐
   If no, what would have been more beneficial? _____

8. How would you rate the care you received?
   EXCELLENT _____
   GOOD _____
   FAIR _____
   POOR _____

C. PLEASE RATE ANY SPECIAL SERVICES YOU RECEIVED.

	EXCELLENT	GOOD	FAIR	POOR
X-RAY	☐	☐	☐	☐
LABORATORY	☐	☐	☐	☐
EKG	☐	☐	☐	☐

Comments: _____
_____
_____

D. ABOUT YOUR ADMISSION INFORMATION AND BILLING

	YES	NO
1. Were you admitted quickly and pleasantly by clerk?	☐	☐
2. Were your business office procedures handled efficiently?	☐	☐
3. If you had questions regarding your billing, were the business office personnel pleasant and courteous?	☐	☐

We are very interested in your comments about any aspect of the Outpatient Surgical Unit:
_____
_____
_____

If you wish to discuss this questionnaire about the Outpatient Surgery Unit, please feel free to call the Same Day Surgery nurse at 749-6480 or the Director of Surgery at 749-6184 on Monday-Friday between 1:00-4:00 pm. Thank You.

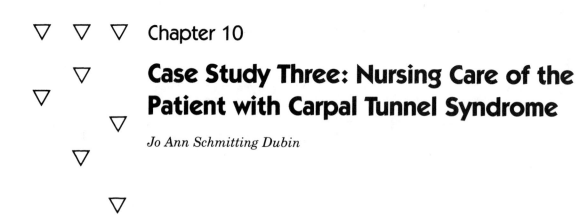

▽ ▽ ▽ Chapter 10

Case Study Three: Nursing Care of the Patient with Carpal Tunnel Syndrome

Jo Ann Schmitting Dubin

Carpal tunnel syndrome (CTS), a progressively debilitating condition, can be treated nonsurgically if diagnosed early. All too frequently, however, the symptoms of CTS are ignored or misdiagnosed until surgical intervention is required, and permanent median nerve damage has already occurred. Presently, there is strong evidence that CTS is an occupational disease.[1,2] If this is true, it follows then that the best possible treatment for CTS is education and prevention in high risk occupational settings. The purpose of this chapter is to present a discussion of the ambulatory surgical treatment of CTS and to address the following four questions:

1. What are the nursing assessment techniques that are used to assess the patient with CTS, including specific institutional forms?
2. What information from the patient assessment data can be used to formulate nursing diagnoses?
3. How can a perioperative care plan be developed for the ambulatory surgical patient with CTS?
4. What methods can be used to evaluate patient outcome based on patient education, discharge planning, and follow-up care?

Nursing Assessment Techniques

In order to provide the nurse with assessment techniques that can be used to evaluate signs and symptoms of CTS accurately, wrist/hand anatomy signs, symptoms, and etiology of the syndrome are reviewed. CTS is defined as an acute or chronic compression of the "median nerve between the inelastic carpal ligament and other structures within the carpal tunnel."[3]

Exhibits for Chapter 10 are located at the end of the chapter on pages 195–201.

Wrist/Hand Anatomy

As seen in Figure 10–1, the carpal canal is a four-sided compartment that is formed by the carpal bones on three of the sides, with the fourth structural boundary being the transverse ligament. These structures act as a protective shelter for nine ligaments and the median nerve.[2] As bone is a rigid, noncompliant material, it follows that, if there is a change in the composition of any of the structures in or around the canal, the canal structures will be squeezed and compressed, resulting in CTS.

Figure 10-1 Carpal Tunnel Anatomy. (Reprinted with permission, Dehaan, M. R., Wilson R. L. (1987). Diagnosis and management of carpal tunnel syndrome. *Journal of Musculoskeletal Medicine, 6*(2), 47–60. Illustration by Robert Margulies.)

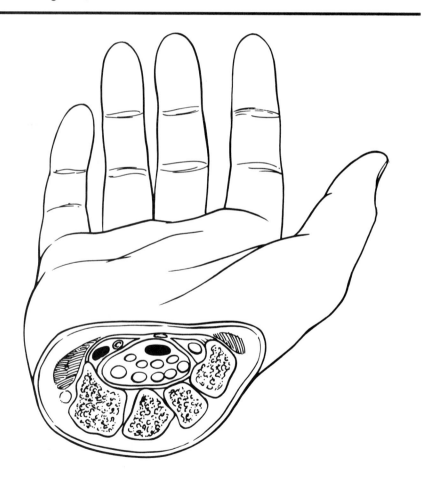

Signs and Symptoms

In understanding the symptoms of CTS, it is essential to know what structures are innervated by the median nerve. The median nerve supplies sensation to the volar portion of the thumb and most of the palm, all of the index and long finger and wrist, and almost half of the ring finger. It also facilitates flexion of the fingers, pronation of the forearm, and makes opposition of the thumb possible (Fig. 10–2). Because the median nerve innervates such a large area, CTS can become debilitating, and the symptoms are quite predictable.[4] Frequently, the patient is awakened at night by a burning pain in the hand and fingers that may be relieved temporarily by massaging and shaking of the affected hand.[1] Moreover, a tingling pain may appear in response to repetitive motions. If left untreated, symptoms can progress to loss of pincher grasp, loss of dexterity, and absent or decreased sensation on the palmar surface of the index finger. Symptoms may also progress to the development of thenar muscle atrophy, as well as possible swelling of the fingers and volar surface of the forearm. It is also possible for the pain to radiate into the elbow and forearm.

Figure 10-2 Nerve Innervation. (Reprinted with permission, Parker, B. C. Rehabilitative aspects of nerve injuries of the hand. *Orthopaedic Nursing, 7,* 29–34, 1988).

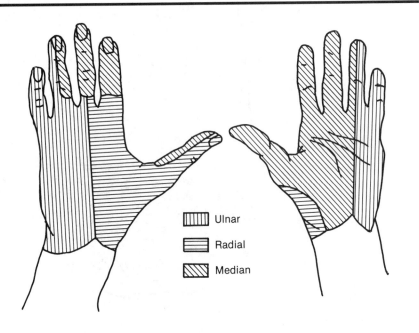

Etiology

The causes of CTS are many and, as previously stated, are frequently occupational. Some of the most common causes are repetitive motions and abnormal postures of the hand that result in wear or tear over time.[4] Colles or scaphoid fractures frequently give rise to CTS as a result of the positioning necessary to repair the fracture, as well as the fracture injury itself. The edema of pregnancy has also been implicated in the development of CTS; however, symptoms usually subside when the pregnancy is terminated. Lipomas, ganglionic cysts, and gouty trophi of the wrist are also major contributors to the development of CTS, as is rheumatoid arthritis with its accompanying synovial thickening of the flexor tendon sheaths.

Diagnosis

Frequently, subjective data obtained through a patient history lead one to suspect CTS. Physical examination may reveal decreased sensation to pin prick in the palm and fingers, positive Tinel's and Phalen's signs, and possibly loss of thenar eminence.[5] Tinel's sign is positive when there is a radiating tingling in the hand and fingers in response to percussion of the median nerve at the wrist.

Phalen's test requires the patient to extend the forearms and to flex the hands at the wrist for approximately one minute. The median nerve of the patient with CTS is already compromised, and this posture almost immediately causes pain and tingling. The final diagnostic tool is electronic nerve conduction testing to map the nerve/muscle impairment accurately.

▽

Medical and Surgical Treatment

The key to successful treatment of CTS is early diagnosis. If diagnosed early, CTS can be treated nonsurgically through the use of night and occupational splints, nonsteroidal anti-inflammatory agents, and steroidal injections.[5] If these modalities are ineffective, surgical intervention may be required. Surgical intervention requires that an incision be made to provide maximal exposure of the median nerve in the carpal canal. This is accomplished by making a small incision from the wrist flexion crease, down to the palm, and between the thenar and hypothenar muscle (Fig. 10–3). Once this incision is made, the transverse carpal ligament is sectioned to release the median nerve and to facilitate removal of lesions or to correct anatomical abnormalities. When the median nerve is severely constricted, normal saline is directly injected into the nerve to facilitate dilatation. Frequently, the patient reports immediate postoperative relief of pain.

Figure 10-3 Carpal Tunnel Incision. (Reprinted with permission, Dehaan, M. R., Wilson, R. L. (1987). Diagnosis and management of carpal tunnel syndrome. *Journal of Musculoskeletal Medicine, 6*(2), 47–60. Illustration by Robert Margulies.)

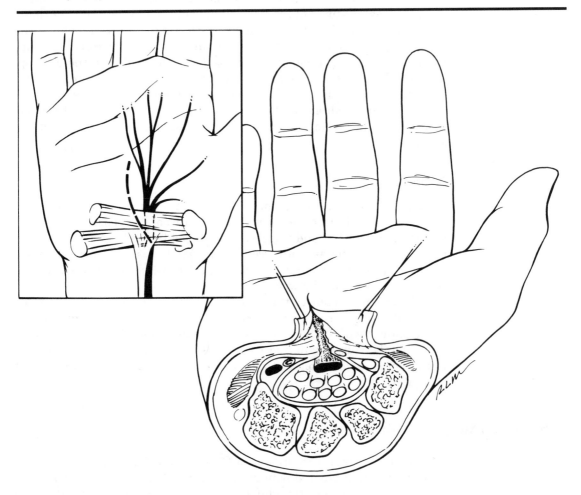

▽

Patient Anesthesia

Anesthesia is a separate process that provides its own set of interdependent nursing concerns.[5,6] Generally, patients with CTS receive some form of local anesthesia, and usually follow a predictable postoperative course. Although rare, the ambulatory surgical nurse must be alert for signs of toxicity or allergic reaction.[6] Symptoms can range from a rash to delirium—just about anything is possible. With the potential for complications, it is essential that the nurse be familiar with the two groups of agents available; the amides and esters (Table 10–1).[6] Not only is famil-

Table 10-1 Some General Nursing Concerns
Regarding Local Anesthetics

Type of Agent	Characteristics
Amides	Likely to cause toxicity Slowly metabolized in the liver Allergic reactions rare
Esters	Metabolized in the plasma Unlikely to cause toxicity Allergic reactions rare
Epinephrine	Frequently used in combination with a local anesthetic as a result of its vasoconstrictor effects Because of its vasoconstrictor effects, less bleeding and slower absorption occur, thus decreasing the amount of anesthetic necessary.

(Adapted from Burden, N., & Iyer, J. (1987). Local anesthesia not always benign. *Journal of Post Anesthesia Nursing, 2*(1), 45–50.)

iarity with these drugs essential, but it is also important to know the route, dose, and speed of administration of the drug; the preoperative anxiety level and general physical condition of the patient; and any adjuncts that may have been used. All of these factors play a role in how the patient reacts to the drug administered. Upon receiving the patient in the recovery area, a residual block will probably be present. It is essential that the extremity be protected from injury and appropriately supported. It is also essential to caution the patient about this temporary loss of sensation and any movement restrictions necessary during this early phase of recovery. If the patient is discharged with some form of residual block, it is extremely important that very specific instructions be given for appropriate care of the extremity.

Intraoperatively, it is important that the site of injection be inspected prior to cast or dressing application.[7] It is also very important that the appearance of the site be documented appropriately in the patient's record.

▽

Nursing Assessment

Knowing the general facts regarding CTS, the ambulatory surgical nurse (ASN) is now ready for the nurse–patient preoperative encounter. The following material serves as a guide for what to assess and the potential patient concerns that may arise. It is vitally important that the ASN develop a preoperative baseline, paying special attention to impairment of mobility and sensation, so that the patient's progress can accurately be assessed postoperatively.[8] In addition, the ASN needs to assess the patient's level of pain and anxiety.

Accurate and standardized assessment data are essential for the development of nursing diagnoses, care plans, and evaluation. Standardization facilitates evaluation of the effectiveness of care, as well as effective communication between care providers. Effective and accurate communication enhances continuity of care and patient recovery. Exhibit 10–1 is an example of an assessment form that can be used to assess the status of a patient with CTS appropriately, and that can facilitate accurate communication of this information to other health care providers.

In most instances, the assessment form requires that patients quantify and qualify what they are feeling. By actively including the patient in the assessment, the ASN facilitates the "diagnosis and treatment of human responses to actual or perceived potential health problems (p.9),"[9] hence providing the ASN with a definition of nursing.

The first two pages of the assessment form contain general assessment data pertinent to all patients. The last pages are specific to the patient with CTS. With computerization, specific individualized assessment forms can be generated on an as needed basis. If this is not possible, one copy of each specific medically diagnosed disease assessment may be kept on file and photocopied on an as needed basis. The value of this assessment form to the ASN is obvious when extraneous assessment data are eliminated and valuable nursing time is saved.

▽

Nursing Diagnosis and Care Plan

The purpose of the assessment form is to identify specific patient problems.[10] Nursing diagnoses are developed from these patient problems, as is the subsequent nursing care plan. The nursing diagnosis and care plan can be highly individualized to meet specific patient needs. This initial assessment also serves as a prime time to initiate patient teaching about CST and what can be expected during the perioperative experience, as well as the patient's responsibility in the recovery process. A case study is now presented to illustrate the use of the assessment form in assigning appropriate nursing diagnoses from the assessment data. These nursing diagnoses are then used in the development of the nursing care plan.

Case Study

Jill Johnson is a 40-year-old white female from Promart Industries who was referred to the surgeon as a result of pain in her right hand that had been present for approximately one month. Jill began employment at Promart seven months ago. In her job, she does a lot of repetitive work, including sewing, which requires manual dexterity of the right hand. Jill complained of pain and numbness, mostly in her third finger and in her fourth digit. She also mentioned that she experiences numbness mostly at night.

Exhibit 10–2 illustrates the utilization of the assessment form, assigning specific nursing diagnosis, and the subsequent development of a perioperative care plan from this diagnosis.

▽

Perioperative Care

The nursing diagnoses used are taken from NANDA's *Taxonomy I*.[11] By utilizing *Taxonomy I,* communication between nurses is enhanced, as all nurses then are using the same theoretical framework. Moreover, if communication is better, patient care will be enhanced. It also follows that standardized, specific guidelines lend credibility to nursing as a profession. It is easy to see how the perioperative care plan is developed using the nursing diagnosis, which is derived from the case study and assessment. The patient encounter also affords the ASN with an opportunity to instruct patients and to assess their general knowledge base regarding the disease, surgery, perioperative expectations, and daily level of functioning.

▽

Patient Education and Discharge Planning

The discharge plan should be started the minute the ASN meets the patient. The assessment again serves as a data base for organizing discharge criteria.[12–14] Discharge data are acquired by interviewing patients and eliciting a description, in their own words, of what the ASN has taught them about their disease, the treatment, and their postoperative responsibilities. It is also important that a clear outline of patient discharge criteria be explained to the patient, and that a written copy be sent home with the patient. Exhibit 10–3 is an example of a patient discharge plan that can be modified to fit an individual patient's needs.[15–17]

The discharge plan has a generic format for two reasons: (1) it clearly outlines and organizes the information the nurse must emphasize regarding the patient's discharge and successful home management; and (2) it provides the patient with a hard copy of the instructions for reference. Further, the discharge form requires patients to acknowledge that they understand their role in the recovery program. This discharge plan has a two-part format, allowing one copy to accompany the patient home and the other to become a permanent part of the patient's record.

▽

Summary

In these days of rising health care costs, there is also a concurrent movement to contain these costs. One of the ways cost containment can be accomplished is to perform more surgery on an outpatient basis.[15] It is also a fact that there is a shortage of practicing nurses, with little sign of relief in the near future. In view of these facts, it is imperative that innovative ways to meet patient needs be developed to minimize nursing time and contain health care costs. The use of standardized institutional forms eliminates unnecessary paperwork and focuses on an individual patient's problem(s). Moreover, efficient communication with other health care providers enhances both patient care and patient education. These measures ultimately result in cost containment and more efficient allocation of nursing time.

References

1. Berger, M. R., & Froimson, A. I. (1979). Hands that hurt: CTS. *American Journal of Nursing, 79*(2), 264–269.
2. Carpal Tunnel Syndrome Reported Reaching Epidemic Numbers. (1989, August). *P.T. Bulletin, 30,* 3.
3. *Mosby's Medical and Nursing Dictionary.* (1986, p. 197). St. Louis: C. V. Mosby.
4. Krames Communications. (1987). *Carpal tunnel syndrome: Relieving the pressure in your wrist.* Daily City, CA: Krames Communications.
5. Dehaan, M. R., & Wilson, R. L. (1987). Diagnosis and management of carpal tunnel syndrome. *Journal of Musculoskeletal Medicine, 6*(2), 47–60.
6. Burden, N., & Iyer, J. (1987). Local anesthesia not always benign. *Journal of Post Anesthesia Nursing, 2*(1), 45–50.
7. Zimmer Care Systems. (1984). *Getting along with your cast.* Charlotte, NC: Zimmer, Inc.
8. Lewis, J. M., & Beaulieq, J. (1987). Application of nursing diagnosis to the par scoring system. *Journal of Post Anesthesia Nursing, 2*(4), 237–243.
9. American Nurses' Association. (ANA). (1980). *ANA social policy statement.* Kansas City: American Nurses' Association, p. 9.
10. Mamaril, M. E. (1985). Stress and the ambulatory surgical unit. *Journal of Post Anesthesia Nursing, 4*(3), 172–176.
11. North American Nursing Diagnosis Association. (1990). *Taxonomy I revised 1989 with official diagnostic categories.* St. Louis: North American Nursing Diagnosis Association.
12. Mezzanotte, J. A. (1987). Checklist for better discharge planning. *Nursing '87, 17*(10), 55.
13. Miller, B. (1987). Osteoarthritis in the primary health care setting. *Orthopaedic Nursing, 6*(5), 50.
14. American Medical Association. (1984). *Guides to the evaluation of permanent impairment* (2nd ed., p. 73). Chicago: American Medical Association.
15. Miller, B. K. (1987). Hands that hurt less. *American Journal of Nursing, 87*(2), 266–267.
16. Parker, B. C. (1988). Rehabilitative aspects of nerve injuries of the hand. *Orthopaedic Nursing, 7*(1), 29–34.
17. Smith, C. W. (1988). Patient information checklist. *Orthopaedic Nursing, 7*(5), 50.

Exhibit 10-1 Patient assessment form.

```
                                          DATE  ____/____/____
                                          NAME  _____
                                          AGE ____ DOB ____/____/____
                                          SS# ____/____/____

DIAGNOSIS: _____

OPERATIVE PROCEDURE: _____

HEIGHT: _____, WEIGHT: _____, NPO: _____ YES _____ NO

ALERT & ORIENTED X'S THREE: ____ YES ____ NO. IF NOT EXPLAIN: _____


ANESTHESIA TYPE: _____   ANY PROBLEMS WITH URINATION: ____ YES ____ NO.

PRE-OP LABORATORY WORK COMPLETED: YES    NO    DATE DONE

        CBC & DIFF          ____   ____   ____/____/____

        U/A                 ____   ____   ____/____/____

        CHEST X-RAY         ____   ____   ____/____/____

        OTHER               ____   ____   ____/____/____

        ABNORMALS REPORTED TO DR. _____

HISTORY OF:____ HTN,____ CVD,____ KIDNEY DISEASE,____ DIABETES,____ ASTHMA,____ COPD,

        ____ BLEEDING DISORDER,____ OTHER: LIST: _____

MEDICATIONS PRESENTLY TAKING: _____

ALLERGIES: _____

TYPE OF EMPLOYMENT: _____

        VITAL SIGNS T _____, BP _____, P _____, R _____.

BREATH SOUNDS: _____

HEART SOUNDS: _____
```

Exhibit 10-1 (Continued)

```
INTEGUMENT:(CIRCLE ONE) WARM & DRY,  COOL & CLAMMY,  OTHER _____

COLOR: (CIRCLE ONE)

    NAIL BEDS: PINK,   DUSKY,    OTHER _____

    MUCOUS MEMBRANES:  PINK,  DUSKY,  OTHER _____

CAPILLARY REFILL: RT. HAND ____ SEC.,LT.HAND ____ SEC.,RT FOOT ____ SEC.,LT FOOT ____ SEC.

PULSES PRESENT:    YES    NO    PULSES EQUAL:    YES    NO

    RADIAL          ____   ____

    PEDAL           ____   ____

    TIBIAL          ____   ____

PAIN MEDICATION PRESENTLY TAKING: _____

FREQUENCY: _____

IS RELIEF OBTAINED: YES,  NO,  SOMETIMES.  RELIEF OBTAINED ____ % OF TIME.

PATIENTS OWN COMFORT MEASURES: _____

RATES TYPICAL PAIN AS: (CIRCLE ONE WITH 10 BEING WORSE POSSIBLE PAIN)

    1   2   3   4   5   6   7   8   9   10

ACCORDING TO PATIENT HAS PAIN: ____ % OF TIME, ____ TIME PER DAY

*   GRADE OF IMPAIRMENT: (PICK ONE)

    ____ NO LOSS OF SENSATION OR NO SPONTANEOUS ABNORMAL SENSATIONS.

    ____ DECREASED SENSATION WITH OR WITHOUT PAIN, WHICH INTERFERES WITH
         ACTIVITY.

    ____ DECREASED SENSATION WITH OR WITHOUT PAIN, WHICH MAY PREVENT ACTIVITY.

    ____ DECREASED SENSATION WITH SEVERE PAIN, WHICH MAY CAUSE OUTCRIES AS
         WELL AS PREVENT ACTIVITY.

    ____ DECREASED SENSATION WITH PAIN, WHICH MAY PREVENT ALL ACTIVITY.

*   Direct Quote Guidelines to the Evaluation of Permanent Impairment, AMA,
    1984, p.73
```

(Continued)

Exhibit 10-1 (Continued)

YES	NO	CAN IDENTIFY OBJECT BY TOUCH? (KEY, COIN)
YES	NO	CAN PICK UP OBJECT? (COIN, KEY) DESCRIBE: _____
YES	NO	CAN ACCURATELY DESCRIBE DISEASE IN OWN WORDS?
YES	NO	IF ANSWER TO ABOVE NO, INSTRUCTED PATIENT ON DISEASE AND PATIENT VERBALIZES AN UNDERSTANDING.
YES	NO	CAN ACCURATELY DESCRIBE SURGERY TO BE PERFORMED IN OWN WORDS?
YES	NO	IF ANSWER TO ABOVE NO, INSTRUCTED PATIENT ON SURGERY AND PATIENT VERBALIZES AN UNDERSTANDING.
YES	NO	VERBALIZES THAT HE UNDERSTANDS WHAT HIS RESPONSIBILITIES IN THE RECOVERY PROCESS ARE?
YES	NO	IF ANSWER TO ABOVE NO, PATIENT INSTRUCTED AND VERBALIZES IN OWN WORDS WHAT RESPONSIBILITY IS.
YES	NO	ABLE TO PERFORM ACTIVITIES OF DAILY LIVING UNASSISTED? IF NO NEEDS, ASSISTANCE WITH WHAT?

NURSING DIAGNOSIS	CARE PLAN	EVALUATION
_____	_____	_____
_____	_____	_____
_____	_____	_____
_____	_____	_____
_____	_____	_____

Exhibit 10-1 (Continued)

APPEARS RELAXED: (CIRCLE ONE) YES, NO. IF NO PLEASE EXPLAIN: _____

BRIEF DESCRIPTION OF PATIENTS APPEARANCE: _____

_____

_____

VERBALIZES CONCERNS: YES, NO. IF YES CONCERNS ARE: _____

_____

ADDITIONAL COMMENTS: _____

_____

CARPAL TUNNEL SYNDROME

RT. HAND		LT. HAND		(CIRCLE ONE)
YES	NO	YES	NO	CAN FEEL LIGHT TOUCH ON PALM?
YES	NO	YES	NO	CAN FEEL LIGHT TOUCH ON INDEX FINGER?
YES	NO	YES	NO	CAN FEEL LIGHT TOUCH ON LONG FINGER?
YES	NO	YES	NO	CAN FEEL LIGHT TOUCH ON RING FINGER?
YES	NO	YES	NO	CAN IDENTIFY SENSATION OF COLD ON PALM?
YES	NO	YES	NO	CAN IDENTIFY SENSATION OF COLD ON INDEX FINGER?
YES	NO	YES	NO	CAN IDENTIFY SENSATION OF COLD ON LONG FINGER?
YES	NO	YES	NO	CAN IDENTIFY SENSATION OF COLD ON RING FINGER?
YES	NO	YES	NO	CAN IDENTIFY SENSATION OF WARMTH ON PALM?
YES	NO	YES	NO	CAN IDENTIFY SENSATION OF WARMTH ON INDEX FINGER?
YES	NO	YES	NO	CAN IDENTIFY SENSATION OF WARMTH ON LONG FINGER?
YES	NO	YES	NO	CAN IDENTIFY SENSATION OF WARMTH ON RING FINGER?

Exhibit 10-2 Example of completed patient assessment form.

DIAGNOSIS: CTS

DATE 11 / 18 / 91

NAME JILL JOHNSON

AGE 40 DOB 12 /04 /47

SS# 408 / 84 / 0556

OPERATIVE PROCEDURE: CTS RELEASE

HEIGHT: 5' , WEIGHT: 158# , NPO: X YES NO

ALERT & ORIENTED X'S THREE: X YES NO. IF NOT EXPLAIN:

ANESTHESIA TYPE: LOCAL ANY PROBLEMS WITH URINATION: YES X NO.

PRE-OP LABORATORY WORK COMPLETED: YES NO DATE DONE

CBC & DIFF X 11 / 15 / 91

U/A X 11 / 15 / 91

CHEST X-RAY X 11 / 15 / 91

OTHER X / /

ABNORMALS REPORTED TO DR.

HISTORY OF: – HTN, – CVD, – KIDNEY DISEASE, – DIABETES, – ATHSMA, – COPD,
– BLEEDING DISORDER, – OTHER: LIST:

MEDICATIONS PRESENTLY TAKING: PREMARIN 125 MG

ALLERGIES: PNC

TYPE OF EMPLOYMENT: SEAMSTRESS

VITAL SIGNS:T 98⁸/0 F , BP 170/80 , P 100 , R 20

BREATH SOUNDS: REGULAR, UNLABORED, CLEAR TO AUSCULTATION

HEART SOUNDS: POS S1, S2, NO ABNORMAL SOUND

Exhibit 10-2 (Continued)

INTEGUMENT:(CIRCLE ONE) (WARM & DRY), COOL & CLAMMY, OTHER

COLOR: (CIRCLE ONE)

NAIL BEDS: (PINK), DUSKY, OTHER

MUCOUS MEMBRANES: (PINK), DUSKY, OTHER

CAPILLARY REFILL: RT. HAND=3SEC.,LT.HAND=3SEC.,RT FOOT=3 SEC.,LT FOOT=3 SEC.

PULSES PRESENT: YES NO PULSES EQUAL: YES NO

RADIAL X X

PEDAL X X

TIBIAL X X

PAIN MEDICATION PRESENTLY TAKING: TYLENOL #3

FREQUENCY: = 3 X'S/DAY

IS RELIEF OBTAINED: YES, NO, (SOMETIMES), RELIEF OBTAINED 25 % OF TIME.

PATIENTS OWN COMFORT MEASURES: MASSAGES HAND

RATES TYPICAL PAIN AS: (CIRCLE ONE WITH 10 BEING WORSE POSSIBLE PAIN)

1 2 3 4 5 6 7 8 9 (10)

ACCORDING TO PATIENT HAS PAIN: 90 % OF TIME, TIME PER DAY

GRADE OF IMPAIRMENT: (PICK ONE)

___ NO LOSS OF SENSATION OR NO SPONTANEOUS ABNORMAL SENSATIONS.

___ DECREASED SENSATION WITHOUT PAIN WHICH IS FORGOTTEN DURING ACTIVITY.

X DECREASED SENSATION WITH OR WITHOUT PAIN, WHICH INTERFERES WITH
ACTIVITY.

___ DECREASED SENSATION WITH OR WITHOUT PAIN, WHICH MAY PREVENT ACTIVITY.

___ DECREASED SENSATION WITH SEVERE PAIN, WHICH MAY CAUSE OUTCRIES AS
WELL AS PREVENT ACTIVITY.

___ DECREASED SENSATION WITH PAIN, WHICH MAY PREVENT ALL ACTIVITY.

(Continued)

197

Exhibit 10-2 (Continued)

APPEARS RELAXED (CIRCLE ONE): YES, (NO.) IF NO PLEASE EXPLAIN: BROW FURROWED FIDGETING WITH HANDS

BRIEF DESCRIPTION OF PATIENT'S APPEARANCE: FRIENDLY, OBESE

VERBALIZES CONCERNS: (YES,) NO. IF YES CONCERNS ARE: STATES, "I AM THE BREAD WINNER IN MY FAMILY AND I'M WORRIED I WON'T BE ABLE TO RETURN TO WORK."

ADDITIONAL COMMENTS: PAIN MOSTLY AT NIGHT

CARPAL TUNNEL SYNDROME

RT. HAND	LT. HAND	(CIRCLE ONE)
YES (NO)	YES (NO)	CAN FEEL LIGHT TOUCH ON PALM?
YES (NO)	YES (NO)	CAN FEEL LIGHT TOUCH ON INDEX FINGER?
YES (NO)	YES (NO)	CAN FEEL LIGHT TOUCH ON LONG FINGER?
YES (NO)	YES (NO)	CAN FEEL LIGHT TOUCH ON RING FINGER?
YES NO	YES NO	CAN IDENTIFY SENSATION OF COLD ON PALM?
YES NO	YES NO	CAN IDENTIFY SENSATION OF COLD ON INDEX FINGER?
YES NO	YES NO	CAN IDENTIFY SENSATION OF COLD ON LONG FINGER?
YES NO	YES NO	CAN IDENTIFY SENSATION OF COLD ON RING FINGER?
YES NO	YES NO	CAN IDENTIFY SENSATION OF WARMTH ON PALM?
YES NO	YES NO	CAN IDENTIFY SENSATION OF WARMTH ON INDEX FINGER?
YES NO	YES NO	CAN IDENTIFY SENSATION OF WARMTH ON LONG FINGER?
YES NO	YES NO	CAN IDENTIFY SENSATION OF WARMTH ON RING FINGER?

Exhibit 10-2 (Continued)

(YES) NO CAN IDENTIFY OBJECT BY TOUCH? (KEY, COIN)
(YES) NO CAN PICK UP OBJECT? (COIN, KEY) DESCRIBE: HAD SOME DIFFICULTY WITH RIGHT HAND

(YES) NO CAN ACCURATELY DESCRIBE DISEASE IN OWN WORDS?
YES NO IF ANSWER TO ABOVE NO, INSTRUCTED PATIENT ON DISEASE AND PATIENT VERBALIZES AN UNDERSTANDING.

YES (NO) CAN ACCURATELY DESCRIBE SURGERY TO BE PERFORMED IN OWN WORDS?
(YES) NO IF ANSWER TO ABOVE NO, INSTRUCTED PATIENT ON SURGERY AND PATIENT VERBALIZES AN UNDERSTANDING.

YES (NO) VERBALIZES THAT HE UNDERSTANDS WHAT HIS RESPONSIBILITIES IN THE RECOVERY PROCESS ARE?
(YES) NO IF ANSWER TO ABOVE NO, PATIENT INSTRUCTED AND VERBALIZES IN OWN WORDS WHAT RESPONSIBILITY IS.

(YES) NO ABLE TO PERFORM ACTIVITIES OF DAILY LIVING UNASSISTED? IF NO NEEDS, ASSISTANCE WITH WHAT?

(YES) NO IS PATIENT AWAKEN AT NIGHT WITH PAIN?
YES (NO) AFTER SLEEPING DOES PATIENT FEEL RESTED?
YES (NO) IS PATIENT ABLE TO PERFORM EMPLOYMENT DUTIES? IF NO HOW IS JOB PERFORMANCE AFFECTED? PAIN FREQUENTLY REQUIRES HER TO STOP SEWING NUMBNESS AND PAIN SLOWS HER UP

NURSING DIAGNOSIS	CARE PLAN	EVALUATION
1. EXCHANGING 1-1-2-1	1. INSTRUCT PATIENT	VERBALIZES SHE
HEIGHT 5' WT. 158#	ON WEIGHT LOSS	UNDERSTANDS SHE TO
	2. INSTRUCT ON	LOSE WEIGHT FOR HER
	IMPORTANCE OF	HEALTH.

Exhibit 10-2 (Continued)

DAILY EXERCISE
PROGRAM.
3. INSTRUCT ON
IMPORTANCE OF
GOOD NUTRITION.

2. FEELING PAIN 9-1-1
PAIN 90% OF TIME
T#3 3X'S/DAY.
RELIEF SOMETIMES.
1. HAVE PATIENT
ELEVATE ARM ABOVE
HEART LEVEL.
2. OCCUPATIONAL OVER
NIGHT SPLINT.
3. EXERCISE FINGERS
4. PAIN RX AS NEEDED.

VERBALIZES SHE
UNDERSTANDS SOME
THINGS SHE CAN DO.
VERBALIZES AN
UNDERSTANDING OF HOW
TO SAVE PAIN RX.

3. FEELING ANXIETY 9-3-1
BROW FURROWED
BP 70/80. "WORRIED
WON'T BE ABLE TO
RETURN TO WORK."
1. EXPLAIN SURGERY,
ANESTHESIA, POSTOP
COURSE.
2. ALLOW PATIENT TO
VERBALIZE CONCERNS.

CAN EXPLAIN DISEASE
AND POSTOP COURSE IN
OWN WORDS.
ACKNOWLEDGES SHE MAY
HAVE TO SWITCH JOBS.

4. KNOWLEDGE DEFICEIT
8-1-1 CANNOT EXPLAIN
POSTOP RESPONSIBILITY
1. INSTRUCT ON CAST
CARE.
2. INSTRUCT ON IMPORT-
ANCE OF ELEVATION.
3. INSTRUCT ON IMPORT-
ANCE OF ICE.
4. INSTRUCT ON IMPORT-
ANCE OF ANALGESTU
5. INSTRUCT ON EXERCISE

VERBALIZES SHE
UNDERSTANDS THE
REASONS AND IMPORT-
ANCE OF THESE
MEASURES.

Exhibit 10-2 (Continued)

6. INSTRUCT ON RETURN
APPOINTMENT

5. MOVING SLEEP
DISTURBANCE 6-2-1
WAKES AT NIGHT WITH
PAIN.
1. INSTRUCT ON ARM
ELEVATED ABOVE
HEART LEVEL.
2. SHOULD TAKE PAIN
RX AT NIGHT IF
HAVING PAIN.
3. ICE TO SITE.

VERBALIZES SHE
UNDERSTANDS HOW THESE
MEASURES CAN PREVENT
PAIN ALLOWING HER TO
SLEEP.

6. MOVING 6-1-1-2
ACTIVITY INTERMEDIATE
PAIN CAUSES HER TO
SLOW DOWN OR STOP
1. SPLINT.
2. SWITCH TO LIGHTER
DUTY WORK.

VERBALIZES SHE
UNDERSTANDS HER
OPTIONS AND ACCEPTS

7. EXCHANGING 1-6-2-1-2-
IMPAIRED SKIN
INTEGRITY. CTS
RELEASE.
1. MONITOR SURGICAL
PREP.
2. MONITOR DRESSING
APPLICATION.

NO BREAK IN STERILE
TECHNIQUE. NO SIGN OF
INFECTION.

8. MOVING 6-1-1-1
IMPAIRED PHYSICAL
MOBILITY. ANESTHESIA
LOCAL.
1. MONITOR INJECTION
SITE.
2. MONITOR FINGER
MOBILITY AND
SENSATION.

NO COLOR CHANGE AT
INJECTION SITE.
MOBILITY AND
SENSATION.
MONITOR FOR RETURN.
PATIENT VERBALIZES
SHE UNDERSTANDS SHE
NEEDS TO PROTECT
EXTREMITY.

9. MOVING 6-1-1-1
1. MOVE FINGERS AS
ORDERED.

VERBALIZES SHE
UNDERSTANDS THESE

(Continued)

Exhibit 10-2 (Continued)

2. EXERCISES AS ORDERED.

MEASURES WILL DECREASE SWELLING,

3. ARM ABOVE HEART LEVEL AS MUCH AS POSSIBLE.

INCREASE CIRCULATION, AND INCREASE MOBILITY

4. INSTRUCT, MAY NEED ASSISTANCE WITH ADL.

VERBALIZES SHE WILL HAVE HELP AT HOME.

10. SELFCARE DEFICIET

6-5-2

11. KNOWLEDGE DEFICIET

1. WHAT TO REPORT TO DOCTOR.

VERBALIZES SHE UNDERSTANDS WHAT TO REPORT CAN EXPLAIN

2. WHAT PAIN MED. IS HOW TO TAKE AND SIDE EFFECTS TO BE AWARE OF.

HOW TO TAKE PAIN RX AND SIDE EFFECTS,

3. CAST CARE.

VERBALIZES SHE UNDERSTANDS WHEN

4. INSTRUCT WHEN RETURN APPOINTMENT

RETURN APPOINTMENT IS AND THAT SHE IS TO

5. INSTRUCT SHE IS NOT TO RETURN TO WORK.

REMAIN OFF WORK TILL THEN.

Exhibit 10-3 Discharge plan.

DATE: ___/___/___

DISCHARGE PLAN

ACTIVITY

___ ELEVATE EXTREMITY ABOVE HEART LEVEL. ___ DAYS.

___ REST EXTREMITY FOR ___ DAYS.

___ MOVE FINGERS ___ TIMES, EVERY ___ HOURS WHILE AWAY.

___ SQUEEZE SPONGE OR BALL ___ TIMES, EVERY ___ HOURS, STARTING ___.

___ OTHER EXERCISES: ___.

PAIN

___ ELEVATE ARM ABOVE HEART LEVEL.

___ ICE BAG ___ MIN. ON ___ MIN OFF.

___ PAIN MEDICATION AS ORDERED. MEDICATION IS TO BE TAKEN ___.

___ KNOWS WHAT MEDICATION ORDERED IS. MEDICATION ORDERED IS ___.

___ KNOWS HOW MEDICATION IS TO BE TAKEN. ___.

___ KNOWS HOW MEDICATION WORKS.

___ PRECAUTIONS AND SIDE EFFECTS OF MEDICATION ___.

DRESSING

___ DO NOT CHANGE.

___ CHANGE IN ___ DAYS.

___ CLEANSE INCISION WITH ___, APPLY ___, AND REDRESS WITH ___.

CAST

___ KEEP LIMB ELEVATED.

___ DO NOT PLACE OBJECTS UNDER CAST TO SCRATCH ITCHY SKIN.

___ MOVE FINGERS FREQUENTLY TO REDUCE SWELLING AND PREVENT STIFFNESS.

___ DO NOT PUT EXTRA MATERIAL IN CAST TO PAD IT.

___ DO NOT GET CAST WET.

Exhibit 10-3 (Continued)

REPORT TO DR. ___.

___ TEMPERATURE GREATER THAN 101 F.

___ PAIN INCREASES AFTER 24 HOURS.

___ ANY FOUL ODOR OR DRAINAGE.

___ PAIN NUMBNESS OR CONTINUED TINGLING IN FINGERS.

___ EXCESSIVE PUFFINESS OR THROBBING.

___ PAIN THAT IS NOT RELIEVED BY PRESCRIBED MEDICATION.

___ COLDNESS OR DISCOLORATION OF THE SKIN OR NAILBEDS.

___ CAST FEELS TOO TIGHT.

___ CAST IS BROKEN.

___ IF YOU HAVE A PROBLEM AND NEED TO REACH DR. ___ THE OFFICE NUMBER IS ___.

EMPLOYMENT

___ MAY RETURN TO WORK ON ___.

___ MAY RETURN TO LIGHT DUTY ON ___.

___ MUST REMAIN OFF FROM WORK UNTIL SEEN BY DR. ___.

RETURN APPOINTMENT

___ CALL DR. ___ AT ___ AND MAKE APPOINTMENT TO BE SEEN IN ___.

___ RETURN APPOINTMENT WITH DR. ___ IS ON ___ AT ___:___.

OTHER INSTRUCTIONS: ___.

_____

_____

I HAVE READ AND UNDERSTAND THE ABOVE INFORMATION GIVEN TO ME BY ___.

IF I HAVE ANY QUESTIONS REGARDING THE ABOVE I AM TO CALL ___.

SIGNED _____ WITNESS _____ DATE _____

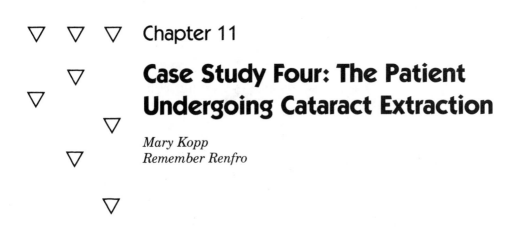

∇ ∇ ∇ Chapter 11

∇

∇

∇

∇

Case Study Four: The Patient Undergoing Cataract Extraction

Mary Kopp
Remember Renfro

∇

∇

Within the past decade, ophthalmology shifted the approach to cataract management from an inpatient to an outpatient surgical procedure. In the United States, more than 90% of all cataract surgeries are performed in outpatient settings.[1] This change in approach occurred as a result of advancements in technology, and was greatly influenced by the development of stringent health care insurance guidelines. Nursing care standards related to the management of the patient undergoing cataract extraction have also shifted, exemplifying an expanding nursing role and an evolving surgical management approach.

The ambulatory surgical unit (ASU) perioperative nurse is faced with wide-ranging responsibilities in providing care for the patient with cataracts. The nurse functions interdependently in implementing medical orders related to the medical management of the surgery patient. Simultaneously, the nurse applies the nursing process to identify patient needs and implement nursing orders to achieve specific outcomes. These responsibilities must all be completed in a matter of hours due to the brief patient stay in ASUs.

The goal of this chapter is to identify nursing care issues related to the patient with cataracts and to apply the nursing process in the development of a perioperative plan of care for patients undergoing ambulatory cataract extraction. This chapter answers the following questions:

1. What are the nursing assessment techniques and forms needed to assess the ophthalmic patient?
2. What information from the patient assessment data can be used to formulate nursing diagnoses?
3. How can a perioperative care plan be developed for this type of ambulatory surgical patient?
4. What methods can be used to evaluate patient outcomes based on patient education, discharge planning, and follow-up care?

Exhibits for Chapter 11 are located at the end of the chapter on pages 215–226.

▽

Changing Times and the Impact on Nursing Care

Because of advancements in procedural techniques and the increased sophistication of implant design, the perioperative medical management of the patient with cataracts has changed dramatically. A prime example of this evolution in patient care is the postoperative regimen for such patients. Fifteen years ago, cataract surgery was performed on inpatients who then underwent a postoperative regimen of strict bed rest, with sand bag support to the head, for several days. Nursing care issues revolved around possible complications relating to extended bed rest, alterations in nutrition, and an interruption in self-care capabilities.

Today, the length of stay for the patient undergoing cataract surgery is only a matter of hours. These patients are encouraged to sit up immediately following surgery, take nourishment, and ambulate to the bathroom. Their activity level is usually only slightly limited, with instructions to avoid heavy lifting and bending with the head below the waist. These patients are often dismissed within an hour following the procedure, and thereafter are responsible for medication administration, dressing changes, and evaluation of their own postoperative process. Because of the self-care responsibilities of these patients, nursing care focuses on preparing the patient for self-care management upon discharge. Nursing documentation reflects a plan of care, based on the nursing process, that addresses immediate perioperative concerns and prepares the patient for discharge and home management.

Nursing care of the patient undergoing cataract surgery is impacted by the approach to medical management and by the characteristics of the specific patient population. Typically, such patients are elderly, and often live alone. Activity levels may be limited by decreased mobility, altered sensory perception, and a decline in energy level. The patient's cognitive level may be affected by senile dementia. The factors just mentioned, combined with the sophistication of today's approach to cataract management, present the nurse with a number of challenges. The nursing process is the perfect tool for meeting this challenge, and that process begins with assessment.

▽

Nursing Assessment Techniques

Assessment information for ASU admission can be obtained through a number of approaches. One approach is the preadmission phone interview, which allows the nurse to gather health information regarding the upcoming surgical admission in a manner and at a time that is convenient for both the patient and the nurse. Miller, Bristol, Sepulveda, and

Lyon indicated that the time element involved in completing a nursing assessment was both challenging and necessary, and confirmed that a preadmission nursing assessment by phone was a reasonable option.[2,3] A questionnaire that demonstrates one format for gathering and recording preadmission assessment information is depicted in Exhibit 11–1.[4] This particular form could be mailed to the patient preoperatively, or completed through a phone interview.

During the initial interview, the nurse collects information from the patient that will be used to formulate nursing diagnoses. Preoperative instructions from the surgeon and clinic are also confirmed by phone. The nurse would assess patient concerns that would indicate an unfamiliarity with clinic routine or the surgical procedure. The nurse could also identify risk factors, such as a lack of assistance in the home, medical complications (e.g., glaucoma, hypertension, diabetes mellitus), or blindness in the fellow eye. The preadmission nurse initiates the care plan based on the problems identified and the nursing diagnoses formulated through the phone interview. The nursing staff continues the assessment phase of the nursing process when the patient arrives the next morning for the surgical procedure.

On the day of surgery, the preoperative nurse admits the patient to the ASU. The nurse briefly reviews the preadmission information and assesses the patient's understanding of the procedure and the disease, as well as the patient's level of compliance with the preoperative instructions (e.g., NPO status). Several institutional assessment forms are included for review (Exhibits 11–2 and 11–3).[4,5]

The nurse assesses the patient for physiological, psychological, or behavioral traits that might indicate a problem or concern. According to Kopp, in an experimentally designed study, an ambulatory surgical patient elicits numerous behavioral responses while under the stress of an impending surgical procedure.[6] Kopp developed a tool, The Ambulatory Care Reaction Rating Scale (ACRRS) that measured patient responses elicited during the total perioperative surgical experience. The study indicates that people under stress frequently elicit various facial expressions and unusual body movements.[6] Kopp also noted that patients under stress shift their position, wiggle their toes, and maintain an extremely stiff position. Observed patients often frowned; had a reddened or blotchy neck and face; talked with a rapid, shakey, or high-pitched voice giving brisk responses; or gave no verbal response at all.[6] These identified stress-related behaviors are cues for the nurse in identifying specific nursing diagnoses.

Admission assessment forms for the ambulatory surgical patient vary from one institution to another. An assessment form using nursing diagnoses emphasizes nursing care issues. An example of a general nursing assessment form is given in Chapter 4. Exhibit 11–4 shows an ophthalmic admission assessment form that was developed in 1989 by the authors using the North American Nursing Diagnosis Association

(NANDA) patterns.[7] The form supports the use of nursing diagnoses and leads to a plan of care structured around those diagnoses. To demonstrate the form's application, a specific patient profile was developed. The identified needs of this patient (Mrs. Clark) will also be incorporated into a nursing care plan that appears later in this chapter.

> Mrs. Ethel Clark is a 64-year-old woman with bilateral cataracts. Her visual acuity is 20/50 *oculus dexter* (OD) (right eye) and 20/200 *oculus sinister* (OS) (left eye). Mrs. Clark has hypertension which is controlled by medication. She is a widow who is accompanied to the clinic by her daughter. The daughter lives nearby and is involved with Ethel on a daily basis.

▽

Formulating Nursing Diagnoses

A narrative explanation of the perioperative nursing care of the patient with cataracts is included to emphasize the value of the nursing process format, including nursing diagnosis formulation, and to enhance the reader's understanding of the special care needs of such patients. The following narrative pertains to the case study just presented and is structured according to the three perioperative phases: preoperative, intraoperative, and postoperative. A nursing care plan for Mrs. Clark appears at the conclusion of the narrative.

Preoperative Nursing Intervention

Mr. Jones, RN, is assigned to circulate for Mrs. Clark's surgical procedure on the day of surgery. He learns from the operative schedule that Mrs. Clark is 64 years old and is to undergo an extracapsular cataract extraction (ECCEPC) with placement of a posterior chamber intraocular lens of the left eye (OS) under monitored anesthesia control. The surgery is to be completed by Dr. Smile at 8:00 AM the following morning.

The afternoon before the planned surgery, Mr. Jones calls Mrs. Clark at home and explains that he will be taking care of her on the day of her surgery. He then asks the patient to express her understanding of the purpose of the surgery, as well as how the surgery is likely to affect her daily routine at home. The time and date of her arrival at the ASU are verified, and the NPO routine, as well as her routine medications and allergies, are reviewed. A nursing history is recorded, and the phone interview is ended after Mr. Jones offers emotional support, reassuring Mrs. Clark that the staff will take every action to ensure her welfare and comfort during her stay at the ASU.

Upon admission, Mr. Jones completes the admission assessment form, building on the plan of care initiated the preceding day, and formulates the nursing diagnoses (see Exhibit 11–4). Mrs. Clark is oriented to the unit, at which time there is a discussion of the coolness and noises of the operating room (OR), the rationale for monitoring blood pressure, the use of a cardiac monitor and the pulse oximeter. Mr. Jones explains the purpose of all preoperative medications, including the dilating drops that will stimulate photophobia and blur the patient's vision (Figs. 11–1 and 11–2).

The type of anesthetic to be used is discussed, and the importance of the patient's lack of movement during the operation is emphasized. Mr. Jones instructs Mrs. Clark to squeeze his hand, or that of the anesthetist, if she needs something during the procedure. Mr. Jones explains the purpose of the Honan cuff (or "Super Pinky") during its application (Fig. 11–3).

During the preoperative period, Mrs. Clark expresses concerns regarding the potential for postoperative pain. In response, Mr. Jones reviews the surgeon's routine procedures for pain management. Mrs. Clark also expresses a high level of concern for her visual future, stating that she has to live alone. Based on the information and observations gathered during this preoperative assessment, Mr. Jones identifies a number of nursing diagnoses that are included in the nursing care plan that follows (Exhibit 11–5).

Intraoperative Nursing Intervention

After carefully transferring Mrs. Clark to the OR, meticulous attention is paid to her position and comfort. The staff follows institutional policy

Figure 11-1 Preoperative teaching.

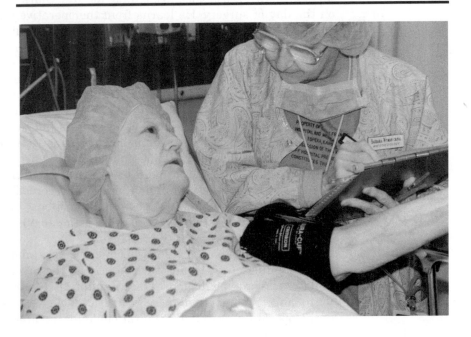

Figure 11-2 Eyedrop instillation.

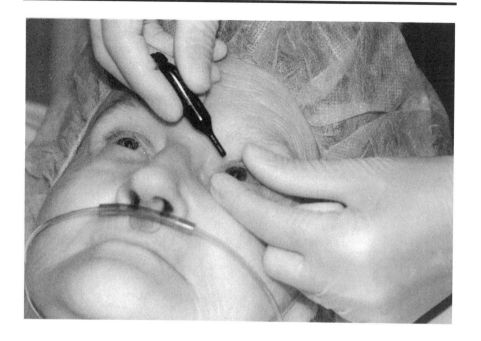

Figure 11-3 Honan cuff application.

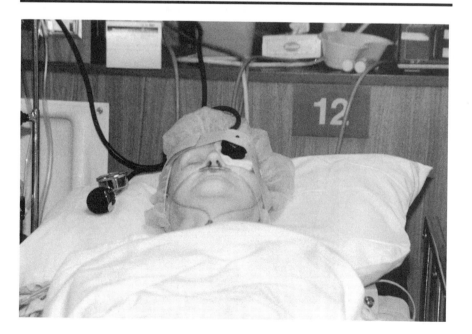

in using safety straps, padding, and the application of oxygen cannula (Fig. 11–4). Mr. Jones encourages feedback from Mrs. Clark to ensure compliance with the "no motion" request during the procedure.

Careful attention during patient preparation and draping ensures patient safety and provides emotional support (Fig. 11–5). As the drape isolates the patient, it may present a severe challenge for the claustrophobic individual (Fig. 11–6). Mr. Jones again reassures Mrs. Clark that she will be attended and monitored continuously throughout the procedure.

The surgical procedure is completed without complication (Fig. 11–7). The circulating nurse must constantly be aware of potential surgical complications that would require interdependent nursing actions, such as the administration of intravenous acetazolamide (Diamox) to reduce an elevation in intraocular pressure. In anticipation of possible vitreous loss, the nursing staff ensures that the equipment and supplies needed for an anterior vitrectomy are readily available. At the close of the procedure, the dressing is applied using strict aseptic technique and ensuring that the globe of the eye is free from external pressure (Fig. 11–8).

Postoperative Nursing Intervention

Mrs. Clark is reunited with her daughter for her postoperative recovery and is encouraged to take fluids by mouth (Fig. 11–9). Mr. Jones reviews

(text continues on page 212)

Figure 11-4 Proper positioning of patient.

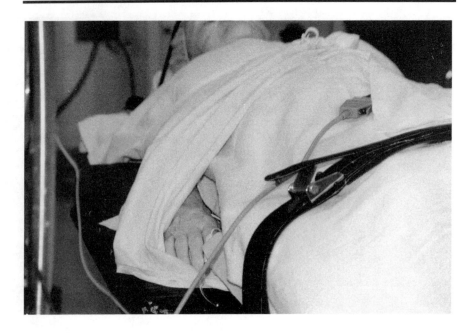

Figure 11-5 Prepping the patient.

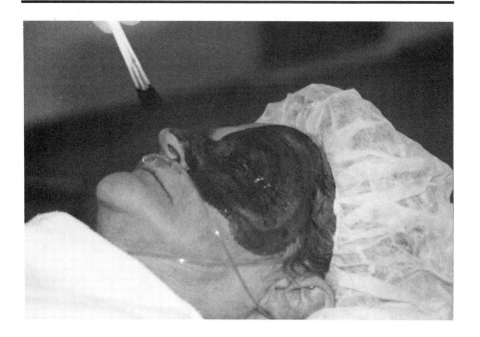

Figure 11-6 Draping the patient.

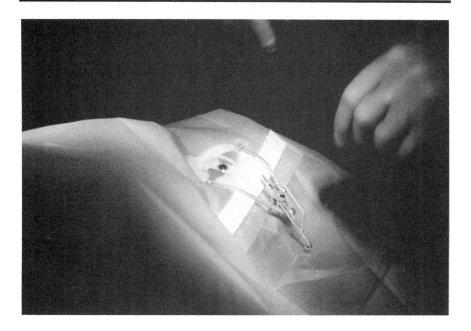

Figure 11-7 Procedure for cataract extraction. *A,* Removal of lens nucleus. *B,* Stripping of lens cortex. *C,* Intraocular lens insertion. Reproduced by permission from Jaffe, Norman S., Jaffe, Mark S., and Jaffe, Gary F.: Cataract surgery and its complications, ed. 5, St. Louis, 1990, The C. V. Mosby Co.

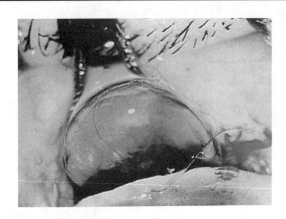

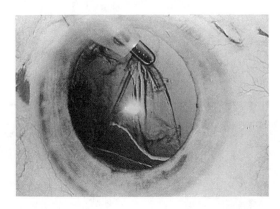

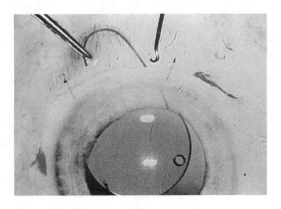

Figure 11-8 Placement of eye dressing.

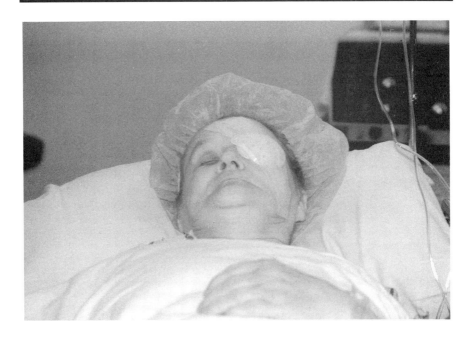

Figure 11-9 Fluid intake is encouraged postoperatively.

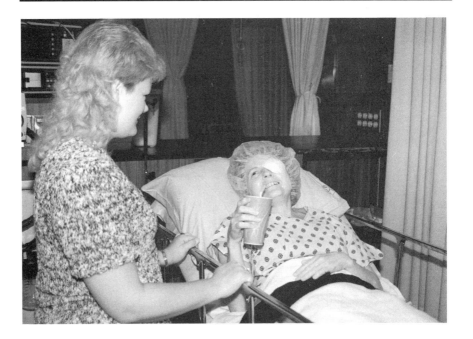

postoperative medications and activity restrictions with Mrs. Clark and her daughter according to surgeon preference. Mrs. Clark is given written instructions, which include the date and time for her next appointment with Dr. Smile. Mr. Jones advises the patient that he will call the following day to check on her progress. He emphasizes that recovery from cataract surgery requires several weeks and encourages Mrs. Clark to be patient with her progress and to call the doctor's office with any questions or concerns. Special attention is given to reviewing with the patient those postoperative sensations that might indicate a problem (e.g., flashing lights, a decline in vision or visual field, or severe pain). Mrs. Clark is also provided with emergency phone numbers.

The nursing care plan that Mr. Jones developed for Mrs. Clark is presented in Exhibit 11–5. Many of the nursing diagnoses and nursing orders noted are applicable to most ambulatory surgical patients with cataracts, which makes it easy to individualize quality care plans from a standard plan of care.

▽

Evaluating Patient Outcomes

To ensure that the nursing process has influenced the patient experience, it is necessary to evaluate the end result, or patient outcome. Patient outcome is influenced by patient education, discharge planning, and follow-up care. The method that is most commonly used to evaluate patient outcomes is the patient's verbal or written self-report of postoperative progress. This can be accomplished with a postoperative phone call or through a mailed questionnaire.

The nursing care plan is also an effective method for evaluating patient outcomes because these outcomes are the very essence of applied nursing care. Each nursing diagnosis is evaluated as to whether the expected outcome was met; if not, additional nursing orders are implemented. Unlike medical diagnoses that remain the same throughout the patient treatment program, nursing diagnoses change as the patient's status changes. Thus, it is easy to evaluate the care of Mrs. Clark as outlined in the nursing care plan presented in Exhibit 11–5.

Patient education issues can be summarized on a home instruction sheet, which can then be reviewed with patients and their supportive caregiver upon discharge (Exhibits 11–6 and 11–7). It is helpful to have home instruction sheets written with a black felt-tipped pen for sharp contrast. Important points to emphasize are activity limitations, the proper use of medications and appropriate eye care, and the prompt reporting of unusual postoperative signs and symptoms. The effectiveness of patient education can be evaluated by determining the patient's degree of adherence to the postoperative regimen.

Discharge planning usually begins during the early phases of the admission assessment process at the time of the initial nurse-patient interaction. The nurse can help the patient identify needs, and can assist the patient in making specific arrangements to meet those needs. For example, one nursing diagnosis identified by Mr. Jones was impaired home maintenance management. In response to this diagnosis, plans were made for the patient's daughter to stay at Mrs. Clark's home for one week following surgery.

As with the effectiveness of patient education, the impact of discharge planning can be evaluated only by assessing patient outcomes. For a patient who has undergone cataract extraction, one follow-up method is a phone interview conducted one to two days after surgery. Postoperative assessment forms, as depicted in Exhibits 11–8 through 11–10, may facilitate telephone follow-up.[5–8]

▽
Summary

In today's fast-paced ambulatory surgical setting, nurses are challenged to provide comprehensive care of unwaveringly high quality. The nursing process provides the perioperative nurse with an organized approach to patient care and a structure that promotes consistent care and precise documentation. The goal of this chapter was to familiarize the nurse with various techniques that might be used to develop a nursing care plan for a patient undergoing cataract extraction. The care plan presented in this chapter provided a specific example of the application of the nursing process to the care of such patients. The reader is encouraged to review additional reading materials regarding the technological aspects of cataract management.

References

1. U.S. Department of Health and Human Services. (1989). *Vital and health statistics: Detailed diagnoses and procedures, national hospital discharge survey, 1987*. (Series 13: Data from the National Health Survey, No. 100). Hyattsville, MD.
2. Miller, D. (1988). The rationale and benefits of a required preadmission ambulatory surgery program. *Journal of Post Anesthesia Nursing, 3*(1), 39–42.
3. Bristol, I., Sepulveda, T., & Lyon, M. (1989). Streamlining the preop process. *Health Progress, 70*(1), 86–87.
4. Wills Eye Hospital. *Nursing assessment: Day surgery unit*. Philadelphia: Wills Eye Hospital.
5. Baptist Medical Center, Kansas City, MO, Center for Eye Research.
6. Kopp, M. (1987). *The effects of sedative music on surgical outpatients*. Unpublished master's thesis, University of Kansas, Kansas City, KS.
7. Classification of Nursing Diagnosis: Proceedings of the eighth conference (1989). (Ed.) Rosemary Carroll-Johnson. Philadelphia: J. B. Lippincott.
8. St. Francis Hospital Post Operative Questionnaire, Topeka, KS.

Bibliography

Brunner, L. S., & Suddarth, D. S. *Textbook of medical-surgical nursing* (6th ed.). Philadelphia: J. B. Lippincott.

Carpenito, L. J. (1989). *Nursing diagnosis, application to clinical practice.* Philadelphia: J. B. Lippincott.

Hunt, L. (1988). Use of the Honan intraocular pressure reducer. *Journal of Ophthalmic Nursing and Technology, 7*(2), 59–61.

Hersh, P. (1988). *Opthalmic Surgical Procedures.* Boston: Little Brown and Co.

Jaffe, N. (1984). Cataract Surgery and Its Complications. St. Louis: C. V. Mosby Co.

Monk-Boyd, H. (1987). *Nursing care of the eye.* Norwalk, CT: Appleton & Lange.

Thompson, J. M., McFarland, G. K., Hirsch, J. E., Tucker, S. M., & Bowers, A. C. (1989). *Mosby's manual of clinical nursing* (2nd ed.). Philadelphia: C. V. Mosby.

Exhibit 11-1 Preoperative assessment questionnaire. (Courtesy of Wills Eye Hospital, Philadelphia, PA).

JJJWills Eye Hospital

HEALTH QUESTIONNAIRE/ ASSESSMENT FORM

Patient's Name: _____

Sex: M   F

Street Address: _____

City: _____

State: _____   Zip: _____

Home Phone # _____ Work (Other) Phone # _____

Ht: _____   Wt: _____

Age: _____   D.O.B.: _____

Name of relative completing this report (If Applicable): _____

Relationship to Patient: _____

Circle appropriate answer (Y for Yes and N for No) Some questions may also require comments.

1. Do you have a history of high blood pressure (hypertension)? . . . . Y N
2. Have you been hospitalized for a medical emergency within the past 6 month?   . . . . Y N
   If Yes, when and why: _____
3. Do you have a history of angina or chest pain?   . . . . Y N
   If Yes, do you take nitroglycerin or other medication as needed for chest pain
   2 or more times a week? . . . . Y N
4. Have you had a heart attack or cardiac arrest?   . . . . Y N
   If yes, when: _____
5. Have you had a stroke?   . . . . Y N
   If yes, when: _____
6. Do you have a history of asthma, emphysema, or other respiratory problems?   . . . . Y N
   If Yes, circle the medication(s) you take: ·
       Theodur   Slobid   Alupent   Vanceril   O2
       Quibron   Elixophyllin   Brethine   Ventolin   Cromolyn Na+
       Other: _____
7. Have you had an asthmatic attack or increasing shortness of breath in the last 3 months?   . . . Y N
8. Do you take Prednisone or other steroids?   . . . . Y N
   If Yes, how much and why: _____
   How long have you been taking it: _____
9. Do you take Coumadin, Persantine, Aspirin or other blood thinners?   . . . . . . Y N
   If Yes, which one and how often: _____
10. Have you ever had a seizure? . . . . Y N
    If Yes, are the seizures controlled with medication?   . . . . Y N
    Have you had a seizure in the last three months?   . . . . Y N
    When: _____
11. Are you a diabetic?   . .   . . Y N
    If Yes, do you take Insulin?   . .   . . Y N
    Types and Doses: AM _____   PM _____
                              AM _____   PM _____
    Has your Insulin been adjusted in the last month?   . .   . . Y N
    What was your most recent blood sugar: _____ Random _____ Fasting
12. Have you ever been treated for anxiety, depression or psychiatric problems?   . . . . . . Y N
13. Have you ever smoked cigarettes?   . . . . Y N
    How much: _____
    When did you have your last cigarette: _____
14. Do you drink alcoholic beverages?   . . . . Y N
    How much and how often: _____

(Continued)

Exhibit 11-1 (Continued)

15. Do you currently, or have you in the past, abused prescription medication or used street drugs? Y N
16. Have you been exposed to or treated for any of the following:
        ( ) T.B.   Date of Exposure: _._____ Treatment Date:_____
        ( ) AIDS   Date of Exposure: _____ Treatment Date:_____
        ( ) Hepatitis   Date of Exposure: _____ Treatment Date:_____
        ( ) Other Infectious Disease: _____
17. If you are Female, when was your last menstrual period? _____
      Could you be pregnant?   . . . . Y N
18. Do you have a history of any of the following:
        Eczema   Y N   If Yes, when: _____
        Shingles   Y N   If Yes, when: _____
        Cold Sores Y N   If Yes, when: _____
19. Do you have a history of kidney or bladder problems? . . . . Y N
    If Yes, what and when: _____
20. Have you been treated for cancer? . . . . Y N
    If Yes, what type and when: _____
21. Do you have any physical disabilities? (Including arthritis, hearing difficulties, need to use cane/ wheelchair) Y N
    If Yes, what type:_____
22. Have you, or any member of your family, had difficulties with anesthesia? . . . . Y N
    If yes, explain: _____
23. Do you have a history of ulcer disease? . . . . Y N
24. Do you have a bleeding disorder? . . . . Y N
25. If the patient is under 2 years old was he/she premature . . . . Y N
    If yes, birth weight: _____
    Was he/she on a respirator . . . . Y N
    Does he/she have a history of apnea? . . . . Y N
    Does he/she have a broncopulmonary dysplasia or frequent lung infections? . . . . . Y N

GENERAL HEALTH

26. Do you get short-of-breath walking up one flight of stairs? . . . . Y N
27. Have you had a cold in the last month . . . . Y N
28. Do you get palpitations (feeling of heart flutter in chest)? . . . . Y N
29. Do you have episodes of dizziness? . . . . Y N
30. Do you get short-of-breath easily . . . . Y N
31. Are you on a special diet? . . . . Y N
32. Have you had an unexplained weight loss or gain recently? . . . . Y N
33. Do you have dentures or capped teeth? . . . . Y N
34. Are you anemic? . . . . Y N
35. List all medications that you now take or have taken within the last month (Dose and times if available):
_____
36. List all allergies: _____
37. List all past hospital admissions and surgeries (reason and approximate date):_____
_____
38. Please list any medical conditions that were not mentioned above: _____
_____
39. Do you live alone? . . . . Y N
40. Name of the person who will take you home after surgery: _____
    Relationship:_____Phone#: _____.
41. Phone number you can be reached at the day prior to surgery (if different from numbers already listed):
    #_____
42. Comments:_____
_____
_____

Signature of Patient: _____ Date: _____

Signature of Relative (If applicable): _____ Date: _____

Signature of Nurse: _____ Date: _____

Exhibit 11-2 Example one: Preoperative assessment form. (Courtesy of Wills Eye Hospital, Philadelphia, PA).

```
                                          NURSING ASSESSMENT
                                          DAY SURGICAL UNIT

                              PATIENT NAME_____
                              PATIENT HOME PHONE#_____ WORK#_____
                              PATIENT PHONE# DAY BEFORE SURGERY_____
                              PROCEDURE_____
                              SURGEON_____
DOCUMENTATION OF INABILITY TO CONTACT PATIENT  ANESTHESIA      GENERAL      LOCAL
                         R.N. DAY SURGERY_____ AM ADMISSION_____
____ ____ _____
Date  Time   Signature
                         R.N.
____ ____ _____           ____ ____ _____
Date  Time   Signature                 Date  Time   Signature
```

PRE-ADMISSION ASSESSMENT

INTERVIEW DATE_____ INFORMANT_____

AGE_____ SEX_____ ALLERGIES_____

REASON FOR ADMISSION_____

CARDIOVASCULAR	RESPIRATORY	NEURO/PSYCH	MISCELLANEOUS
CAD PACEMAKER	COPD	SEIZURES	DIABETES CANCER
CHF MI	ASTHMA	CVA	BPH ULCER
ANGINA HYPERTENSION	TB	DEPRESSION/ ANXIOUS	RENAL FAILURE AIDS
BLEEDING DISORDER	ECZEMA		HSV/HZV ARTHRITIS
DATE OF LMP_____			HARD OF HEARING

_____
_____
_____

RECENT EXPOSURE TO INFECTION_____ RECENT URI_____

DID YOU OR ANY MEMBER OF YOUR FAMILY EVER HAVE ANY ADVERSE REACTION TO ANESTHESIA?   YES   NO

If YES, explain_____

PREMATURE BIRTH_____ AGE OF GESTATION_____ BIRTH WEIGHT_____

SURGICAL HISTORY	CURRENT EYE & SYSTEMIC MEDICATIONS	SOCIAL HISTORY
		Lives with:_____
		Ambulation needs:_____
		Transportation plans:___

SMOKES: YES   NO   How much?_____ ALCOHOL: YES   NO   How much?_____

DIET_____

                              SIGNATURE_____ R.N.

(Continued)

Exhibit 11-2 (Continued)

PRE-OPERATIVE INSTRUCTIONS

PATIENT CONTACTED   YES   NO

If NO, reported to _____

NPO INSTRUCTIONS _____

_____

INSTRUCTED ARRIVAL TIME _____

_____

_____

SIGNATURE _____

ADMISSION ASSESSMENT

ADMISSION DATE _____ _____

VITAL SIGNS   T_____   P_____   R_____   B/P_____   Wt._____   Ht._____

MENTAL STATUS_____ LEVEL OF COMPREHENSION_____

FUNCTIONAL VISION:

           OD_____

           OS_____

GLASSES_____ CONTACTS_____ PROTHESIS_____

DENTURES: FULL   PARTIAL   NONE

LAST ORAL INTAKE:

       FOOD   WHAT_____

                 WHEN_____

       FLUID   WHAT_____

                 WHEN_____

   MEDICATION   WHAT_____

                 WHEN_____

VALUABLES_____

_____

_____

_____

_____

_____

SIGNATURE _____

Exhibit 11-3 Example two: Preoperative assessment form. (Courtesy of Baptist Medical Center, Center for Eye Surgery, Kansas City, MO).

CENTER FOR EYE SURGERY
KANSAS CITY, MISSOURI

PRE-OPERATIVE ASSESSMENT/PHONE CALL   DATE: _____ TIME: _____
PATIENT NAME: _____ SEX ____ AGE ____
PHYSICIAN NAME: _____
PROPOSED PROCEDURE: _____ DIAGNOSIS: _____
UNABLE TO CONTACT PATIENT _____ PHYSICIAN'S OFFICE NOTIFIED: _____ DATE: _____ TIME: ____

1. HISTORY OF DISEASE: DO YOU HAVE ANY OF THE FOLLOWING?

A. LUNG	B. VASCULAR	C. SYSTEMIC
____Bronchitis	____High Blood Pressure	____Diabetes
____Emphysema	____Heart Attack	____Thyroid Trouble
____Asthma	____Heart Murmur	____Kidney/Bladder Problems
____Chronic or A.M. Cough	____Palpitation/Irregular	____Stomach/Bowel Problems
____Sinusitis/Pneumonia	or Fast Heart Beats	____Hepatitis/Yellow Jaundice
____Shortness of Breath	____Heart Disease/Chest Pain	____Convulsions/Epilepsy
____Smoking History		____Bleeding Tendency
		____Glaucoma

    D. OTHER ILLNESSES: _____
    E. ALLERGIES: _____
        ROUTINE MEDS:

    _____   _____   _____
    _____   _____   _____
    _____

3. PERSONAL HISTORY:
    A. Physical Limitations: _____
    B. Prior Surgery (Last 5 yrs): _____
    C. Prior Anesthesia: Dates(s): _____
    D. Have You or Your Family Had Unusual Reaction to Anesthesia? _____
    E. Do You Have Dentures?: _____
    F. Do You Wear a Hearing Aid: _____

PRE-OPERATIVE PHONE CHECK LIST:

  1. Time of Arrival: _____.
  2. Proper Dress Attire Discussed: __ NA __
  3. No Eye or Face Make-Up   __ NA __
  4. Valuables/Jewlery At Home: __ NA __
  5. Bring Insurance Cards: __ NA __
  6. Responsible Adult to Drive Home __ NA __
  7. Diet Restrictions:
      a. NPO After Midnight: __ NA __
      b. No Solid Foods: __ NA __
      c. Clear Liq. Brkfst. Before 0600 __ NA __
      d. Clear Liq. Brkfst. Before 0900 __ __
  8. Take Routine Meds with Sip of Water: __ NA __

  9. Coumadin Stopped: __ NA __
10. Bring Inhaler: __ NA __
11. Insulin Dependent Diabetic
    a. Hold Regular Insulin   __ NA __
    b. LENTE/NPH: Take 1/2 Dose with
       6 oz. APPLE JUICE AT:
      (1) 0800-1000 – AT 0600   __ NA __
      (2) 1000-1300 – AT 0600   __ NA __
      (3) 1300-1600 – AT 0900   __ NA __
    c. BRING INSULIN WITH THEM: __ NA __

_____
                Signature of R.N.

ANESTHESIA EVALUATION

    A. ASA Classification: _____
    B. Anesthesia Plan: _____
        _____
        _____

_____
             Signature of Anesthesiologist

PC 800 (6/16/89)
70291/00281

Exhibit 11-4 (Continued)

MOVING

Ambulates: (prosthesis, cane, walker, wheelchair, unsteady
gait, tires easily)
Home activity changes postoperatively: Yes/No
Self care assistance: (does not: feed, bathe, dress self)
Comment: I live alone
Nursing Diagnosis Altered health maintenance R/T
postoperative care regime

PERCEIVING

Eye contact: (downcast, staring, off-centered gaze)
Pupils: (opaque, unequal)
Visual acuity: O.D. 20/50 O.S. 20/200 (contacts,
prosthesis, corrective lenses)
Hearing impaired: lt/rt ear, hearing aid lt/rt ear
Mental status: disoriented, confused, anxious, nervous,
fearful, depressed)
Body posture: (stooped, rigid/tense)
Cognition: (inability to follow simple commands)
Nursing Diagnosis altered communication R/T sensory
deprivation from surgical drapes

PAIN MANAGEMENT

How pain managed: (non-, prescription)
Nursing Diagnosis -0-

Exhibit 11-4 Ophthalmic admission assessment.

Name Ethel Clark   Date 9-28-89
Address 1303 Cedar Road   City Timberville State KS
Phone(H) 233-3333 (W) -0-   SSN 512-66-8899
Surgical Diagnosis cataract left eye
Procedure extracapacular extraction with posterior intraocular
lens implant   Surgeon Dr. Smile
Anesthesia local with monitored anesthesia control
Sex female Age 64 Known Allergies none
Medications hydrochlorothyzide – BID
Surgical/Medical Past Hx: hypertension

INSTRUCTIONS: Document by circling abnormalities only.

NUTRITION
Oral mucosa: (dry, lesions) other
Teeth– dentures: (uppers, lowers, partial crowns)
Diet Restrictions: (diabetic, low sodium) other
Skin: (lesions, diaphoresis, dry) other
Nursing Diagnosis alterations in mucous membranes R/T NPO

CIRCULATION/RESPIRATORY
Temp 98^6 Pulse 80 Bp 138/90 Resp.
Extremities: (cold, cyanotic) other
Respirations: (wheeze, positional dyspnea)
Nursing Diagnosis ineffective breathing patterns R/T sedation
and draping in OR

RELATING/CHOOSING
Marital Status: M S W X D
Number of children 1 Dependents 0
Occupation retired
Lives alone yes
Support system: Relative daughter   Friend
Family concerned about hospitalization yes, first outpatient
surgery
Gets along with support system yes
Coping with vision handicap – Y/N comments
Verbalizes problems – Y/N comments
Nursing Diagnosis anxiety, R/T unfamiliar surroundings

Exhibit 11-5 Preoperative nursing care plan.

Nursing Diagnosis	Patient Goal	Nursing Orders	Evaluation
Preoperative			
Anxiety R/T unfamiliar surroundings and surgical procedure	Patient will express an understanding of surgical procedure, preparatory actions, and surroundings.	Review sequence of and rationale for perioperative events. Encourage verbalization of questions and concerns. Provide noninvasive relaxation techniques. Give emotional support. Review anticipated effects/sensations of preparatory medications. Assure patient of constant care and monitoring.	Patient expressed an understanding of the sequence and purpose of events.
Sensory/perceptual alterations R/T loss of vision after block and postoperatively	Patient will verbalize expectation of temporary vision loss and alteration in depth perception.	Describe blocking procedure and the resulting loss of vision in the operative eye. Review the doctor's routine for postoperative patching. Discuss the perceptual alteration resulting from monocular vision (lack of depth perception, decrease in field). Approach patient from noneffected side.	Patient anticipated loss of vision after block and expressed an understanding of monocular vision.
High risk for injury R/T sedation and impaired sensory/perceptual functioning	Patient will remain injury free.	Provide continuous orientation to environment. Keep side rails up and safety strap on. Assess ROM and position of patient for comfort throughout perioperative stay. Supervise patient during all transfers.	Patient was free from any injury related to transfers or positioning.
Intraoperative			
High risk for injury R/T infection	Patient will remain free of infection.	Monitor aseptic technique throughout perioperative period. Educate patient postoperatively regarding signs and symptoms of infection (fever, drainage).	Patent was free of signs and symptoms of infection postoperatively.
Potential for ineffective breathing pattern RT sedation, draping	Patient will maintain adequate oxygen exchange.	Review rationale for administering oxygen while applying patient's cannula. Explain purpose of oxygen monitor. Check drape position to ensure proper cannula positioning and patient comfort.	Adequate respiratory exchange was maintained throughout procedure.

(Continued)

Exhibit 11-5 (Continued)

Nursing Diagnosis	Patient Goal	Nursing Orders	Evaluation
High risk for injury R/T positioning, prepping solution, and alterations in skin integrity	Patient will remain free from injury related to positioning or physical hazards.	Encourage patient to provide feedback so as to ensure comfortable positioning; position patient according to policy and procedure. Assess skin integrity and pressure points. Cleanse patient's skin of residual prepping solution prior to discharge from OR.	Patient remained injury free and comfortable in relation to alterations in skin integrity and reactions to prepping solutions.
Altered communication R/T sensory deprivation secondary to draping	Patient will continue to express needs and concerns intraoperatively.	Discuss with the patient the need to remain quiet with minimal movement during the procedure. Implement a communication system (i.e., patient will move exposed hand, not head, when needing to speak).	Patient squeezed nurse's hand before speaking.
Altered oral mucous membranes (dryness) R/T NPO status and use of diuretics, hyper-osmotics.	Patient will remain comfortable.	Explain the drying effects of NPO and medications. Moisten lips with water or lemon glycerin swab prior to procedure.	Patient verified increased comfort after nursing intervention.
Postoperative			
Altered health maintenance R/T postoperative care regimen.	Patient will express an understanding of postoperative regime.	Review postoperative activity restrictions and medication instructions. Provide large-print written instruction sheet. Provide time for and encourage patient questions. Demonstrate eye drop instillation and bandaging technique. Discuss pain management. Explain importance of protecting operative eye (shield, glasses). Review normal and abnormal signs and symptoms. Make follow-up call to patient two days after surgery.	Patient expressed an understanding of instructions and expectations prior to discharge from unit. Patient repeated eyedrop instructions.
Altered home maintenance management R/T change in vision and activity levels	Effective plan for patient's home management will be in place prior to discharge.	Review importance of compliance with activity restrictions. Emphasize the perceptual impact of monocular vision. Facilitate involvement of patient's support system.	Patient and support system had an understanding of the need for assistance and participated in formation of a plan for dealing with alteration in visual acuity and activity levels. Follow-up phone call was made to evaluate effectiveness of plan.

Exhibit 11-6 Postoperative self-care instructions for the patient undergoing cataract surgery.

ACTIVITIES

Do's   Don'ts
Watch TV   Rub Eye

Any activity in moderation   Strain

Wash hair in ___ days; lean   Bend with head below
      back, not forward   waist

Wear shield or eye glasses   Lift items over 20
      for ___ weeks; sunglasses   pounds
      for comfort
                                              Indulge in sexual
Drive only with doctor's   relations
      permission   ___ weeks

MEDICATIONS AND EYE CARE

Drops: _____   Medications: _____

       _____   _____

*   Wash hands before and after close contact with eye

*   To instill eye medications, tilt head back, gaze at the
      ceiling, and gently pull the lower lid down

*   Take all eye medications to follow-up appointments

Next Doctor's Appointment: _____

Emergency Phone Number: _____

Exhibit 11-7 Postoperative call questionnaire. (Courtesy of St. Francis Hospital, Topeka, KS).

POST OP CALL QUESTIONNAIRE

PATIENT'S NAME _____ AGE _____
SURGEON _____ TYPE OF ANESTHESIA _____
DATE _____ PROCEDURE _____
PHONE NUMBER (home) _____ (work) _____
PERSON MAKING CALL _____ DATE _____
TIME OF CALL (1st attempt) _____ (2nd attempt) _____

1. How did your feel when you got home? _____ Explain _____
    _____

2. Did you require medication for pain or nausea? _____ Explain _____
    _____

3. Regarding anesthesia - How long did your numbness last? _____
    _____

4. Did you experience any bleeding, drainage or swelling at your incision
    site? _____
    _____

5. Did you run a fever? _____ Do you remember what it was? _____ Did you
    take anything for it?_____
    ** Please call us in the next week if you run a temperature over 100
    degrees that requires medication.

6. Did you have an IV? _____ Did you notice any redness or swelling at the
    IV site? _____ Did you use warm moist packs? _____

7. Did you call your physician or the hospital for any reason? _____
    _____

8. Do you have any questions regarding your care or discharge instruction?
    _____

9. Was this your first time to use our Outpatient Surgery Department?
    _____

10. Could we have done anything to make your stay more comfortable?
    _____

11. Did you feel the amount of time you were allowed to spend with your
    family/friends before and after surgery was enough? _____
    _____

    Additional comments _____
    _____
    _____

Exhibit 11-8 Postoperative survey phone call form. (Courtesy of Baptist Medical Center, Center for Eye Surgery, Kansas City, MO).

POSTOPERATIVE SURVEY/PHONE CALL

PATIENT NAME: _____

PROCEDURE: _____

DATE OF PROCEDURE: _____ DATE PATIENT CALLED: _____ A.M.__ P.M.__

PHYSICIAN: _____

MENTAL STATUS: __AWAKE/ALERT __ORIENTED __CONFUSED __DROWSY

    NOTE: _____

_____

GENERAL CONDITION:

    APPETITE   __YES __NO SPECIFY:_____

    EYE DISCOMFORT __YES __NO SPECIFY:_____

ACTIVITY:

    AMBULATING   __YES __NO SPECIFY:_____

    RESTING   __YES __NO SPECIFY:_____

SHIELD/PATCH:

    DRY/INTACT   __YES __NO SPECIFY:_____

    DRAINAGE   __YES __NO SPECIFY:_____

POST-OP INSTRUCTIONS:

1. COMPLAINT WITH DISCHARGE INSTRUCTIONS:

    a. Physician Follow-up Visit:_____

    b. Handwashing Technique:__ NA __

                          _____

                             Signature of RN

Exhibit 11-9 Combined discharge instructions and follow-up questionnaire. (Courtesy of Wills Eye Hospital, Philadelphia, PA).

))) Wills Eye Hospital

DAY SURGERY UNIT

DISCHARGE INSTRUCTIONS

SURGICAL PROCEDURE _____ ANESTHETIC: Local ____ Gen. ____

1. Do not drive or operate hazardous machinery for 24 hours.
2. Do not make important personal or business decisions for 24 hours.
3. Eat light foods as you can tolerate them (water, jello, soups, cola, 7-Up, etc.), if you've had general anesthesia.
4. No alcoholic beverages should be taken for 24 hours.
5. Because you will have periods of sleepiness or feeling tired, it is not advisable to engage in strenuous activities. Rest when you are tired.
6. Tylenol may be taken every 4 hours for pain. Follow prescribed dosage on bottle.
7. Call your surgeon if you should become ill or develop a high fever. If a child, call pediatrician. If he can't be reached, Dr. _____ from the anesthesia department will be available tonight at phone number _____ .

PATIENT POST-OP FOLLOW-UP

Nausea	☐ severe	☐ moderate	☐ slight	☐ none
Pain	☐ severe	☐ moderate	☐ slight	☐ none
Fever	☐ severe	☐ moderate	☐ slight	☐ none

If general anesthesia

Sore Throat Hoarseness Cough	☐ severe	☐ moderate	☐ slight	☐ none
Muscle Aches	☐ severe	☐ moderate	☐ slight	☐ none

If so, is it getting better?_____

| RED | DRAINAGE | USE OF EYE MEDS |

Condition of eye:_____ _____ _____

General Condition of Patient: ☐ excellent ☐ good ☐ fair ☐ poor

Patient General Comments:_____

_____

_____

Date and Time Called_____ Nurse_____

WEH 192 REV. 1/86

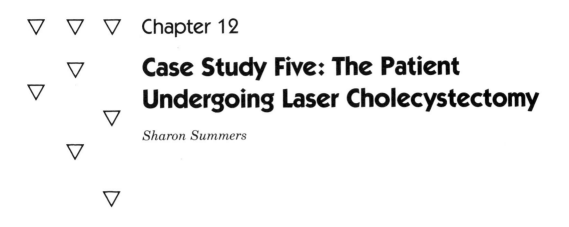

Chapter 12

Case Study Five: The Patient Undergoing Laser Cholecystectomy

Sharon Summers

Advances in surgical procedures have resulted in dramatic changes in how and where surgery is performed. Perhaps the most dramatic change has been in the use of laser technology and the increase in major procedures performed in the ambulatory surgical unit (ASU). Prior to the use of laser technology in surgery and patients' now-common shortened lengths of stay, procedures such as a cholecystectomy were only performed in the main operating room (OR), and recovery usually spanned a period of weeks, with patients frequently experiencing a great deal of pain. With the use of laser technology, cholecystectomy can be performed safely in the ASU and patients can quickly resume their usual activities with minimal postoperative pain. The purpose of this chapter is to examine laser cholecystectomy in the ASU by answering the following questions:

1. Why is the laser cholecystectomy procedure appropriate for the ASU?
2. What information is necessary to prepare the patient for the laser cholecystectomy procedure?
3. What are the nursing assessment techniques needed to establish nursing diagnoses for the laser cholecystectomy patient?
4. How can a nursing-diagnosis–based, perioperative care plan be developed for the ambulatory cholecystectomy patient?
5. What methods can be used to evaluate patient outcomes based on patient education, discharge planning, and follow-up care?

Laser Procedure in the Ambulatory Surgical Unit

Laser is an acronym for *l*ight *a*mplification by *s*timulated *e*mission of *r*adiation.[1] In 1917, Einstein hypothesized that, if a pure medium were bombarded with electrical charge, then electrons might be stimulated

Exhibits for Chapter 12 are located at the end of the chapter on pages 234–245.

and, in returning to the nonstimulated state, they might emit a given light wave.[1] If this process is enhanced in a system with mirrors, and the light waves are channeled through a narrow opening, then an intense beam of electromagnetic radiation is emitted.[1-3]

Today, there are two primary types of laser media used for electrical bombardment: gas and solid.[2] The gas media that are most commonly used are carbon dioxide (CO_2) and argon. The end result of CO_2 laser utilization is surgical excision and/or vaporization of tissue.[3] Argon emits a blue-green light through clear tissue, and this light is absorbed by pigmented tissues, such as melanin or hemoglobin.[3] The solid crystal media commonly used for laser procedures are neodymium yttrium-aluminum-garnet (ND:YAG) and ruby. In this instance, the physiological response of the light beam on tissue is thermal coagulation, rather than excision, which is appropriate for procedures such as cholecystectomy and tumor debulking.[3]

Regardless of the type of laser medium used, the physiological responses are similar. As tissue temperatures approach 50°C, the cells are destroyed; at 100°C, heating the tissue fluid will produce steam and sear and vaporize tissue, resulting in a plume of coagulated cellular products or carbonization.[4,5] Table 12–1 refers to the types of surgery that are appropriate for both types of lasers. Because the gas laser beams are narrow and precise, there is less surrounding tissue destruction and less pain than with conventional surgical trauma. Microscopic examination of tissue cut with a scalpel reveals inflammation and edema as traditional methods of hemostasis allow oozing of cellular products into the surrounding tissue.[1,5,6] Because lasers coagulate capillaries and lymphatics, there is little edema, little inflammation, and little stimulation of pain receptors. Laser cholecystectomy can be performed using the traditional supine position and the Kocher or midline incision; the primary differences lie in using a scalpel for the dissection and the Bovie for dissection, or using coagulation or laser technology for these same approaches.[7] In addition, laser cholecystectomy can also be performed using the supine

Table 12-1 Laser Uses and Safety

Type of Laser	Characteristics	Safety Education

CO_2/Argon
  Vascular
  Orthopedic
  Dermatologic
  Ophthalmologic
  Gynecologic
	Fine beam
	Precise dissection
	Coagulates and vaporizes
		Protective eye covers
		Protective skin covers
		Protect from plume inhalation
		Patient must lay still for precise
		  dissection.

ND:YAG
  Gynecologic
  Vascular
  Urologic
	Wide beam, scattering to surrounding
	  tissue
	Deep penetration of tissue
	Coagulates and vaporizes
		Protective eye covers
		Protective skin covers
		Protect from plume inhalation

position and small laparoscopy-size incisions, with dissection and coagulation processes being accomplished by laser, usually the ND:YAG.[8] Thus, laser technology is well suited for use in the ASU in patients who are ill with cholecystitis and who are expected to return home within a short period of time to resume self-care. The diversity in laser use and surgical procedures mandates special attention to patient information needs.

▽

Patient Information Needs

Patient information needs must be met to ensure a smooth perioperative experience during laser cholecystectomy in the ASU. In the past, when patients were admitted to the hospital the day before surgery, there was time to conduct patient education sessions and to prepare patients for surgery. Today, when many procedures are performed in the ASU, there is little time to teach patients prior to the surgical procedure. Several of the contributing authors in this book support the need to teach patients prior to the day of surgery using a variety of educational materials, including commercially printed pamphlets, institutionally developed written pamphlets, and audiovisual media. Whatever the format, certain information must be presented to patients undergoing laser procedures to ensure a safe, smooth recovery.

The usual preoperative teaching plan includes instructions about the procedure; the need to cough, turn, and deep breathe; the need for early ambulation; methods to alleviate anxiety; and beginning discharge planning. These instructions are also appropriate for the patient scheduled for laser cholecystectomy. In addition, there are safety measures that must be considered related to the use of the laser (Table 12-1). These laser-specific instructions are based on the type of laser used for the procedure. To decrease patient anxiety, patients should be informed as to the rationale for the OR staff's special apparel. Particular attention must be given the establishment of baseline assessment data in patients admitted to the ASU for cholecystectomy so that the nurse can validate their readiness for self-care.

▽

Nursing Assessment Techniques

Patients who are admitted to the ASU for laser cholecystectomy are decidedly different from the usual ASU patients, as they frequently have been ill preoperatively. It is important to assess these patients thoroughly to identify baseline and preexisting problems. It is recommended that the assessment form discussed in Chapter 4 be used to assess the patient and identify pertinent nursing diagnoses. It is also important that this form be completed prior to the day of surgery so that nursing interventions and patient teaching can be instituted before admission, and so that they are in place in preparation for the patient's rapid progression through the ASU. The assessment approach and nursing diagnoses appropriate for the ASU patient undergoing cholecystectomy are presented in the following case study.

Case Study

Cynthia MacDonald, a 45-year-old executive owner of MacDonald Computer Industries, LTD, has a two-month history of fatty food intolerance and colicky right upper quadrant pain. Mrs. MacDonald was seen by Dr. White two weeks ago, at which time x-ray studies revealed gallstones. She was placed on antibiotics and laser cholecystectomy was scheduled in the ASU. Mrs. MacDonald was instructed to attend an evening class three days before surgery so that blood could be drawn for baseline laboratory tests and so that the nurse could assess the patient, formulate nursing diagnoses, and develop and begin to implement the nursing care plan.

The purpose of identifying the nursing diagnoses during this preoperative visit is to meet patient needs regarding the procedure, to inform them as to what to expect during the perioperative period, and to discuss how Mrs. MacDonald can assist in self-care after discharge. As discussed in Chapter 7, patient needs are best met when they are identified by the patient, rather than using the maternalistic approach of the nurse deciding what patients need.

Following the drawing of blood for laboratory tests, the nurse can then proceed with the assessment. As seen in Exhibit 12–1, the nurse assesses Mrs. MacDonald and identifies several nursing diagnoses that can be used to plan patient care and develop the care plan, determine patient education needs, and establish criteria for discharge planning. This assessment and care plan should not be developed and then ignored; rather, it should be placed in the patient's chart where nurses can plan care based on the patient's stated needs as the patient progresses through the perioperative experience. This process prevents the needless procedure of asking the patient the same questions repeatedly. This approach to nursing care enhances the image of the professional nurse as nurses work as a team to ensure the patient's smooth perioperative progression.

The following list of nursing diagnoses is derived from the patient assessment and serves to individualize patient care (Numbers 1–5). Standard intraoperative nursing diagnoses[9] (Numbers 6–10) for surgical patients can be added to those specific to Mrs. MacDonald's assessment data, as can standard postoperative nursing diagnoses[9] (Numbers 11–14).

1. Altered nutrition, more than body requirement, R / T eating habits
2. Anxiety R / T impending procedure
3. Pain R / T disease process
4. Knowledge deficit R / T assuming patient role
5. Powerlessness R / T inability to control illness process
6. High risk for injury R / T intense light waves

7. Impaired skin integrity R / T the surgical incision
8. Hypothermia R / T exposure to coolants and/or cool environment
9. Altered fluid volume (excess or deficit)
10. High risk for injury R / T hemorrhage, trauma, falling, Bovie burns, and foreign bodies (instruments, needles, sponges, etc.)
11. Pain R / T surgical intervention
12. High risk for infection R / T surgical procedure
13. High risk for injury R / T blood loss
14. Activity intolerance R / T surgical intervention

After the patient is assessed during the preadmission visit and nursing diagnoses have been identified, the nursing care plan can be developed to ensure that Mrs. MacDonald has a smooth perioperative progression. As discussed in Chapter 3, if these data are stored on the computer, formulation of a care plan requires only a very rapid process of electronic "cutting and pasting." Thus, the perioperative care plan can be developed and edited, with nurses working as a team to meet patient needs. Nurses then can document whether nursing diagnoses are resolved. The following provides an example of appropriate additions and deletions to the care plan.

On the day of surgery, the patient is admitted to the ASU and the chart containing the preadmission care plan accompanies the patient to the holding area. The nurse reviews and verifies the preadmission assessment data (Exhibit 12–2) and evaluates which nursing diagnoses have been resolved and which need further nursing attention. For the purposes of discussion, all nursing diagnoses/care plans are included in each figure that follows so the reader can see the progression of documentation and methods for evaluation of care. As seen in all of these care plans, both independent and interdependent nursing actions are detailed (see Chapter 4 for an indepth discussion of these concepts).

Exhibit 12–3 includes care plans for interdependent and independent nursing care undertaken during the preoperative phase. Exhibit 12–4 presents care plans for interdependent and independent nursing actions taken during the intraoperative phase. During this intraoperative period, additional nursing diagnoses may be appropriate for guiding nursing care. Items 7 through 10, mentioned earlier, have been identified by Kleinbeck as pertinent to the intraoperative experience.[9]

Care plans for interdependent and independent nursing activities implemented during the postoperative phase are presented in Exhibit 12–5. This portion of the care plan is based on nursing diagnoses identified by Kleinbeck as being pertinent to the postanesthesia phase (items 11–14 of previous list).

With the exception of the first nursing diagnosis identified for Mrs. MacDonald, the nursing diagnoses listed are commonly seen in any surgical patient. Therefore, to save time, these care plans could be standardized, printed, and easily attached to the preadmission care plan for evaluation. For example, Mrs. MacDonald's nursing diagnoses, with the exception of the first nursing diagnosis listed, describe and help to organize her ASU care. This care plan differs little from that which would be appropriate for most ASU patients, and so these commonly encountered nursing diagnoses and care plans could be printed for quick inclusion into the existing care plan or chart. Use of the care plan can then facilitate the evaluation of patient outcomes and discharge planning.

▽

Evaluation of Patient Outcomes

During discharge planning, a quick review of the care plans can assist the ASU nurse in identifying the independent and interdependent nursing actions that have effectively resolved the identified nursing diagnoses and which remain unresolved. This evaluation process provides the nurse with guidelines for developing routine ASU discharge instructions and enhancing overall nursing actions. Nurses in the ASU need to develop discharge materials that can be sent home with patients. For example, Mrs. MacDonald's first nursing diagnosis—altered nutrition, more than body requirements, R / T eating habits— can be resolved with written instructions on diet and exercise for health promotion. Nursing diagnosis #7—impaired skin integrity R / T the surgical incision—can be resolved with written instructions on home care of the surgical wound. In the busy ASU setting, the nurse needs to work smarter, not harder, and printed information for repetitive procedures is vital for professional nursing practice.

Postdischarge evaluation of patient care can be accomplished by the ASU nurse using telephone interviews for three purposes. First, questions can be asked about physical needs (e.g., wound healing/drainage, pain, ambulation, etc). Second, questions can be asked about psychological needs, such as how the patient is coping and whether support systems are helpful. Third, inquiries can be made as to the nursing care received during the ASU experience (i.e., whether the nurses could have done anything to make the surgical experience less stressful). Attention to all three of these purposes can convey to the patient a sense of caring nurses who work in a caring institution. A caring reputation for the health care setting can only enhance the public relations of the institution, and are excellent marketing techniques for the ASU.

▽

Summary

The use of laser technology in the ASU will no doubt increase, as patients seem to recover quickly from the procedure with minimal discomfort. The complexity of ASU procedures will no doubt escalate in the future, leading to increased demands on the ASU staff. ASU nurses can prepare to meet patient needs by using nursing-diagnosis–based care plans to document which nursing interventions were implemented so that professional nursing practice can be validated. In addition, patient evaluation of ASU experiences can also validate the effectiveness of nursing care. Telephone evaluation is suggested for documenting the level of patient or "customer" satisfaction. Data collected during these evaluations should then be examined for both positive and negative comments, and that data used to guide the future policies and practices of the professional nurse in the ASU.

References

1. Davis, C. (1988). Beyond the blade. *Popular Mechanics, 10,* 75–77, 100.
2. Lehr, P. S. (1989). Surgical lasers. *AORN Journal, 50,*(5), 972–977.
3. Absten, G. T. (1989). Laser biophysics for the physician. In J. L. Ratz (Ed.), *Lasers in cutaneous medicine and surgery* (pp. 1–30). Chicago: Year Book Medical Publishers.
4. Fuller, T. (1989). *Surgical lasers: A clinical guide.* New York: Macmillan Publishing Co.
5. Joffe, S. N. (1989). *Lasers in general surgery.* Baltimore: Williams & Wilkins.
6. Association of Operating Room Nurses. (1989). Recommended practices: Laser safety in the practice setting. *AORN Journal, 50,*(5), 1015–1020.
7. Daly, C. J. (1989). Laser cholecystectomy. In S. N. Joffe (Ed.), *Lasers in general surgery* (pp. 40–46). Baltimore: Williams & Wilkins.
8. Swazuk, K. J., Meuller, B. G., & Daly, C. J. (1989). Laser cholecystectomy. *AORN Journal, 50*(5), 998–1005.
9. Kleinbeck, S. V. M. (1990, March 19). *In search of perioperative nursing diagnosis, A preliminary report.* Poster Presentation, North American Nursing Diagnosis Association, Orlando, FL.

Bibliography

Dixon, J. A. (1989). *Surgical applications of lasers.* Chicago: Year Book Medical Publishers.

Goldman, L. (1990). *The biomedical laser: Technology and clinical applications.* New York: Springer-Verlag.

Jackson, D. C., Martin, T., Evans, M. M., & Rubio, P. A. (1990). Endoscopic laser cholecystectomy. *AORN Journal, 51*(6), 1546–1552.

Mackety, C. J. (1989). Nursing care for patients having general surgery laser procedures. In S. N. Joffe (Ed.), *Lasers in general surgery* (pp. 296–301). Baltimore: Williams & Wilkins.

Owens, P. A. (1990). Perioperative laser nurse's role in patient education. *Laser Nursing, 4*(1), 7–12.

Ratz, J. L. (1989). *Lasers in cutaneous medicine and surgery.* Chicago: Year Book Medical Publishers.

Exhibit 12-1 Ambulatory surgical nursing diagnosis assessment form based on the nine NANDA patterns*.

Name: __Cynthia MacDonald__ Date: __9/3/91__

Address: __45 Evergreen Circle__ City: __Evergreen__ State: __MI__

Phone: __(H) 776-8132__ __(W) 776-3294__ SS#: __999-22-9999__

Surgical Diagnosis: _____

Medical Diagnosis: __Cholecystitis with cholelithiasis__

Sex: __F__ Age: __45__ Known Allergies: __O__

EXCHANGING

Color oral mucosa: __Pink__ Moist __Dry__ + Lesions

Teeth: _____ Missing: _____

Appearance: Well nourished __+__ Obese _____ Emaciated

Weight: __155__ Height: __5'5"__ Weight Gain: __20#__ Weight Loss: _____

Diet Restrictions: __Fat intolerance__ Alcohol Intake: _____

Feeding Tubes: _____ Hyperalimentation: _____

Skin: Turgor __+__ Intact _____ Lesions _____ Color _____ Temp _____

Fluid Intake: _____

Nursing Diagnosis: __Alteration in Nutrition: More than Body__
__Requirement R/T eating habits__

Circulation

Temp: __98.8__ Pulse: __92__ BP (Rt arm): __130/84__ (Lt arm): _____

Sitting: _____ Standing: _____

Exhibit 12-1 (Continued)

Apical rate: __90__ Rhythm: Regular __+__ Irregular

Heart sounds: S1 __+__ S2 __+__ S3 __O__ S4 __O__

Neck veins distended: _____

Peripheral Edema: _____ Location: _____

Pedal Pulse: Rt _____ Lt _____

Calf Tenderness: _____

Extremities: Color: _____ Temp changes: _____

History of: Pacemaker _____ Chest pain _____

Blood Clots: _____ Edema _____

Nursing Diagnosis

Respiration

Resp rate __16__ Breath sounds __WNL__ Skin Color _____

Cough __O__ Productive _____ Sputum Color _____

Smoker __O__ Pack years _____

Dyspnea __O__ On exertion _____

Nursing Diagnosis

Exhibit 12-1 (Continued)

Elimination

Abdomen: Soft_____ Firm_____ Tender _+_ Distended _+_

Ostomies_____ Bowel sounds present_____

Stool/day_____ Color_____ Constipation_____ Diarrhea_____ Laxative

use_____ Enema use_____ Incontinence of stool_____

Urine output/day_____ Color_____

Odor_____ Urgency_____

Frequency_____ Nocturia_____ Dysuria_____ Hematuria_____

Incontinent_____ Stress Incontinence_____

Nursing Diagnosis_____

COMMUNICATING

Understands spoken language _+_ Reads _+_

Writes _+_ Reads Lips_____ Hearing intact_____

Vision intact _+_

Nursing Diagnosis_____

RELATING

Marital Status: M___ S___ W___ D _+_ Children _+_

Number of Children_____ 2 _ Dependents_____

Occupation_____ **Executive/owner of own business**

Living Arrangements: Home Owner _+_ Rent_____ Others in

the home_____

Support system: Relative_____ Friend _+_

Exhibit 12-1 (Continued)

Family concerned about hospitalization _+_

Gets along with support system_____

Personal Behavior: Passive_____ Aggressive_____ Assertive _+_

Parent_____ Parenting Problems_____

Last Menstrual Period_____ Menstrual Problems_____

Birth Control Methods_____ Number of Pregnancies _+_

Complications of Pregnancies_____

Sexual Preference_____

Sexual concerns _O_ History of STD_____

Sexually active_____

Nursing Diagnosis_____

VALUING

Religious Affiliation_____ Religious Restrictions_____

Would you like minister: To visit_____ To be called_____

Cultural concerns_____

Religious concerns_____

Nursing Diagnosis_____

(Continued)

235

Exhibit 12-1 (Continued)

PERCEIVING

Body Image Changes __0__

Eye contact: Appropriate _+_ Downcast ___ Staring ___

Body Posture: Relaxed ___ Stooped ___ Rigid/tense _+_

Level of consciousness: Alert _+_ Responds to Pain ___

Oriented to: Time _+_ Place _+_ Person _+_

Mood: Calm ___ Sad ___ Angry ___ Withdrawn ___ Other ___

Early a.m. awakening ___

Pupils: Equal ___ Reactive ___

Cognition: Able to follow simple commands ___

Hearing: Normal ___ Impaired ___ Left Ear ___ Right Ear ___

Vision: Normal ___ Corrected with glasses ___ Prosthesis ___

Unilateral Neglect ___

Diversional Activities ___

Hopelessness ___ Powerlessness ___

Nursing Diagnosis **Powerlessness R/T Inability to control disease process**

Exhibit 12-1 (Continued)

CHOOSING

Coping with health problems _+_ Verbalizes problems ___

Uses defense mechanisms ___ Can meet role expectations ___

Family coping: Effective _+_ Ineffective ___

Neglectful ___ Self ___ Others ___

Complies with care: ___ Seeks Preventive care: ___

Decision maker: Yes ___ No ___

Nursing Diagnosis ___

MOVING

Ambulates _+_ Climbs Stairs ___

Gait: Steady _+_ Unsteady ___ Limp ___ Able to walk ___

Prosthesis ___ Aids: Cane ___ Walker ___ Wheelchair ___

Fatigue: ___ Tires easily ___

Feels rested after sleep ___ Trouble falling asleep ___

Maintains own home ___

Able to: Feed Self ___ Bathe Self ___

Needs Help: Feeding ___ Bathing ___ Dressing ___

Going to bathroom ___

Growth/development problems ___

Nursing Diagnosis ___

Exhibit 12-1 (Continued)

KNOWING

Cognition Intact __+__ Recent Memory Change//Deficit _____

Difficulty Learning __O__

Education level __**BA, MBA**__

Knowledge deficit:

    Regarding Illness: __+__ Condition: _____

    Altered thought process _____

Nursing Diagnosis __**Knowledge deficit R/T assuming patient role**__

FEELING

Acute pain __+__ Chronic pain _____

How pain managed __**Tylenol # 3 q4 h prn**__

Anxiety __+__

Recent Loss/grief _____ Potential Loss/grief _____

Potential for violence: Self _____ Others _____

Fearful _____ Post Trauma Experiences _____

Post Rape Syndrome: Silent _____ Verbalized _____

Nursing Diagnosis __**Alteration in Comfort: Pain R/T disease process**__

    __**Anxiety R/T impending procedure**__

Exhibit 12-2 Preadmission nursing care plan.

Interdependent Nursing Actions:
NAME: Cynthia MacDonald
DATE: 9/5/91
MEDICAL DIAGNOSIS: Cholecystitis with Cholelithiasis
RESOLVED: ___ Yes ___ No   DATE: 9/9/91

Medical Orders	Implementation	Evaluation
1. Schedule for laser cholecystectomy ASU for 9/12/91, 09:30	1. Case scheduled	1. Case scheduled
2. Order admitting lab tests on 9/9/91		

Independent Nursing Actions:
NAME: Cynthia MacDonald
DATE: 9/9/91
NURSING DIAGNOSIS: Altered nutrition, more than body requirements, R/T rating habits
RESOLVED: ___ Yes ___ No   DATE: _____

Assessment	Nursing Orders	Implementation	Evaluation
1. Ht. 5'5" Wt. 155 20# wt. gain	1. Educate as to diet/exercise for health promotion at time of discharge		

Independent Nursing Actions:
NAME: Cynthia MacDonald
DATE: 9/9/91
NURSING DIAGNOSIS: Knowledge deficit R/T assuming patient role
RESOLVED: _X_ Yes ___ No   DATE: 9/9/91

Assessment	Nursing Orders	Implementation	Evaluation
1. Stated "I am totally ignorant about what will happen to me."	1. Educate patient as to perioperative routine and laser procedure	1. Patient will view perioperative video and laser procedure video, booklets sent home with patient	1. Patient asked many questions after viewing the video tapes and thanked the staff for the written information.

Independent Nursing Actions:
NAME: Cynthia MacDonald
DATE: 9/9/91
NURSING DIAGNOSIS: Anxiety R/T impending procedure
RESOLVED: ___ Yes ___ No   DATE: _____

Assessment	Nursing Orders	Implementation	Evaluation
1. Verbalized anxiety about impending procedure	1. Provide support. Explain the procedure and the perioperative routine.	1. Staff will provide emotional support during all routine procedures and will provide explanations before procedures.	

Exhibit 12-2 (Continued)

Independent Nursing Actions:
NAME: Cynthia MacDonald
DATE: 9/9/91
NURSING DIAGNOSIS: Pain R/T disease process
RESOLVED: ___ Yes ___ No   DATE: _____

Assessment	**Nursing Orders**	**Implementation**	**Evaluation**
1. Abdomen tender on palpation 2. Abdomen distended; circumference 42 in.	1. Give pain med prn. 2. Periodically measure abdomen during ASU stay		

Independent Nursing Actions:
NAME: Cynthia MacDonald
DATE: 9/9/91
NURSING DIAGNOSIS: Powerlessness R/T inability to control illness process
RESOLVED: ___ Yes ___ No   DATE: _____

Assessment	**Nursing Orders**	**Implementation**	**Evaluation**
1. Tense, stated "My life seems totally out of control since I became ill."	1. Allow patient to participate in decision making in order to regain a sense of control.	1. Ask patient to make decisions about care as often as possible.	

Exhibit 12-3 Preoperative nursing care plan.

Interdependent Nursing Actions:
DATE: 9/12/91
MEDICAL DIAGNOSIS: Cholecystitis with Cholelithiasis
RESOLVED: _X_ Yes ___ No   DATE: 9/12/91

	Medical Orders	Implementation	Evaluation
	1. NPO	1. NPO	1. NPO maintained
	2. Prep abdomen	2. Abdomen prepped	2. Area of skin prep free of razor damage
	3. Demerol, 100mg Atropine, 0.4 mg at 08:15	3. Preop meds given	3. Preop meds given at 08:15
	4. Start at 500cc LR IV	4. IV started	4. IV running; no infiltration.

Independent Nursing Actions:
NAME: Cynthia MacDonald
DATE: 9/9/91
NURSING DIAGNOSIS: Altered nutrition, more than body requirements, R/T eating habits
RESOLVED: ___ Yes ___ No   DATE: _____

Assessment	Nursing Orders	Implementation	Evaluation
1. Ht. 5'5" Wt. 155 20# wt. gain	1. Educate as to diet/exercise for health promotion at time of discharge		

Independent Nursing Actions:
NAME: Cynthia MacDonald
DATE: 9/9/91
NURSING DIAGNOSIS: Knowledge deficit R/T assuming patient role
RESOLVED: _X_ Yes ___ No   DATE: 9/9/91

Assessment	Nursing Orders	Implementation	Evaluation
1. Verbalized "I am totally ignorant about what will happen to me."	1. Educate patient as to perioperative routine and laser procedure	1. Patient will view perioperative video and laser procedure video, booklets sent home with patient	1. Patient asked many questions after viewing videos and thanked the staff for the written materials.

Independent Nursing Actions:
NAME: Cynthia MacDonald
DATE: 9/9/91
NURSING DIAGNOSIS: Anxiety R/T impending procedure
RESOLVED: ___ Yes ___ No   DATE: _____

Assessment	Nursing Orders	Implementation	Evaluation
1. Verbalized anxiety about impending procedure	1. Provide support. Explain the procedure and the perioperative routine.	1. Staff will provide emotional support during all routine procedures and will provide explanations before procedures.	

Exhibit 12-3 (Continued)

Independent Nursing Actions:
NAME: Cynthia MacDonald
DATE: 9/9/91
NURSING DIAGNOSIS: Pain R/T disease process
RESOLVED: _X_ Yes ___ No   DATE: 9/12/91

Assessment	Nursing Orders	Implementation	Evaluation
1. Abdomen tender on palpation. Abdomen distended; circumference 42 in.	1. Position patient for comfort. Periodically measure abdomen during ASU stay.	1. Turned to side with pillow at back.	1. Some relief of pain when on side; pain persists.

Independent Nursing Actions:
NAME: Cynthia MacDonald
DATE: 9/9/91
NURSING DIAGNOSIS: Powerlessness R/T inability to control illness process
RESOLVED: ___ Yes ___ No   DATE: _____

Assessment	Nursing Orders	Implementation	Evaluation
1. Tense, stated "My life seems totally out of control since I became ill."	1. Allow patient to participate in decision making in order to regain a sense of control.	1. Ask patient to make decisions about care as often as possible.	

Exhibit 12-4 Intraoperative nursing care plan.

Interdependent Nursing Actions:
DATE: 9/12/91
MEDICAL DIAGNOSIS: Cholecystitis with cholelithiasis
RESOLVED: _X_ Yes ___ No   DATE: 9/12/91

Medical Orders	**Implementation**	**Evaluation**
1. Supine position	1. Supine position	1. Supine position
2. Cover patient's eyes with saline-soaked pads and eye shields.	2. Eyes protected	2. Eyes protected
3. ND: YAG equipment	3. ND: YAG equipment in room and calibrated	3. ND: YAG equipment in room and calibrated

Independent Nursing Actions:
NAME: Cynthia MacDonald
DATE: 9/9/91
NURSING DIAGNOSIS: Altered nutrition; more than body requirements, R/T eating habits
RESOLVED: ___ Yes ___ No   DATE: _____

Assessment	**Nursing Orders**	**Implementation**	**Evaluation**
1. Ht. 5'5" Wt. 155 20# wt. gain	1. Educate as to diet/exercise for health promotion at time of discharge		

Independent Nursing Actions:
NAME: Cynthia MacDonald
DATE: 9/9/91
NURSING DIAGNOSIS: Knowledge deficit R/T assuming patient role
RESOLVED: _X_ Yes ___ No   DATE: 9/9/91

Assessment	**Nursing Orders**	**Implementation**	**Evaluation**
1. Stated "I am totally ignorant about what will happen to me."	1. Educate patient as to perioperative routine and laser procedure.	1. Patient will view perioperative video and laser procedure video; booklets sent home with patient.	1. Patient asked questions after viewing videos and thanked the staff for the written materials.

Independent Nursing Actions:
NAME: Cynthia MacDonald
DATE: 9/9/91
NURSING DIAGNOSIS: Pain R/T disease process
RESOLVED: _X_ Yes ___ No   DATE: 9/12/91

Assessment	**Nursing Orders**	**Implementation**	**Evaluation**
1. Abdomen tender on palpation Abdomen distended; circumference 42 in.	1. Position patient for comfort. Periodically measure abdomen during ASU stay.	1. Turned to side with pillow at back.	1. Relief of pain when on side, pain persists.

Exhibit 12-4 (Continued)

Independent Nursing Actions:
NAME: Cynthia MacDonald
DATE: 9/9/91
NURSING DIAGNOSIS: Anxiety R/T impending procedure
RESOLVED: ___ Yes ___ No   DATE: _____

Assessment	Nursing Orders	Implementation	Evaluation
1. Verbalized anxiety about impending procedure	1. Provide support. Explain the procedure and the perioperative routine.	1. Staff will provide emotional support during all routine procedures and will provide explanations before procedures.	

Independent Nursing Actions:
NAME: Cynthia MacDonald
DATE: 9/9/91
NURSING DIAGNOSIS: Powerlessness R/T inability to control illness process
RESOLVED: ___ Yes ___ No   DATE: _____

Assessment	Nursing Orders	Implementation	Evaluation
1. Tense, stated "My life seems totally out of control since I became ill."	1. Allow patient to participate in decision making in order to regain a sense of control.	1. Ask patient to make decisions about care as often as possible.	

Independent Nursing Actions:
NAME: Cynthia MacDonald
DATE: 9/12/91
NURSING DIAGNOSIS: Altered skin integrity R/T surgical intervention
RESOLVED: _X_ Yes ___ No   DATE: 9/12/91

Assessment	Nursing Orders	Implementation	Evaluation
1. Skin intact and shave prep done	1. Monitor skin prep.	1. Proper skin prep technique will be maintained.	1. Proper prep done
	2. Monitor aseptic technique of OR team members.	2. Aseptic technique of team members monitored	2. Aseptic technique maintained
	3. Monitor dressing applications.	3. Dressing applications monitored.	3. Dressing technique satisfactory

Independent Nursing Actions:
NAME: Cynthia MacDonald
DATE: 9/12/91
NURSING DIAGNOSIS: High risk for Injury R/T foreign bodies
RESOLVED: _X_ Yes ___ No   DATE: 9/12/91

Assessment	Nursing Orders	Implementation	Evaluation
1. All sponge, needle, and laser tip counts conducted and recorded	1. Monitor sponge, needle, and laser tip counts during procedure.	1. Additional sponges recorded; all counts maintained	1. All counts correct

Exhibit 12-5 Postoperative nursing care plan.

Interdependent Nursing Actions:
DATE: 9/12/91
MEDICAL DIAGNOSIS: Cholecystectomy
RESOLVED: _X_ Yes ___ No   DATE: 9/12/91

Medical Orders	Implementation	Evaluation
1. Monitor vital signs.	1. Vital signs remained stable.	1. Vital signs stable
2. Monitor LOC.	2. Responding	2. LOC stable
3. Check dressing on admission and q1h.	3. Dressing intact and sterile	3. Dressing intact
4. Demerol, 100 mg, IV for pain.	4. Total Demerol given in PACU was 90 mg.	4. Demerol relieved pain.
5. Compazine, 10 mg q4h prn nausea.	5. No nausea	5. No nausea
6. Admit to short stay unit when awake.	6. Orders sent to short-stay unit.	6. Bed available in short-stay unit.

Independent Nursing Actions:
NAME: Cynthia MacDonald
DATE: 9/12/91
NURSING DIAGNOSIS: Pain R/T surgical intervention
RESOLVED: _X_ Yes ___ No   DATE: 9/12/91

Assessment	Nursing Orders	Implementation	Evaluation
1. BP, 132/74; P, 88; R,12	1. Monitor vital signs.	1. Vital signs monitored.	1. Vital signs remained stable.
2. Drowsy, responding		2. Level of consciousness monitored	2. Responding
3. Dressing dry, and intact	3. Check dressing.	3. Dressing dry and intact	3. Dressing intact and sterile
4. C/O incisional pain radiating to back	4. Titrate Demerol as needed per order.	4. Demerol, 100 mg given IV in increments of 15 mg until patient is comfortable	4. Total Demerol given in PACU was 90 mg and pain was relieved.
5. No C/O nausea		5. No nausea	5. No nausea

Independent Nursing Actions:
NAME: Cynthia MacDonald
DATE: 9/12/91
NURSING DIAGNOSIS: Impaired airway clearance R/T anesthesia and sedation
RESOLVED: _X_ Yes ___ No   DATE: 9/12/91

Assessment	Nursing Orders	Implementation	Evaluation
1. Resp. rate 16	1. Monitor resp. and auscultate lungs.	1. Respirations monitored; lung fields clear	1. Airway remained patent; resp. rate 20 on discharge
	2. Check LOC.	2. LOC clearing	2. Responding to name
2. Responding to verbal commands			

Exhibit 12-5 (Continued)

Independent Nursing Actions:
NAME: Cynthia MacDonald
DATE: 9/9/91
NURSING DIAGNOSIS: Altered nutrition; more than body requirements, R/T eating habits
RESOLVED: _X_ Yes ___ No   DATE: 9/12/91

Assessment	Nursing Orders	Implementation	Evaluation
1. Ht. 5'5" Wt. 155 20# wt. gain	1. Educate as to diet/exercise for health promotion at time of discharge.	1. Diet/exercise booklet given to the patient; Health promotion explained and questions answered.	1. Patient understands the need for diet and exercise for health promotion.

Independent Nursing Actions:
NAME: Cynthia MacDonald
DATE: 9/9/91
NURSING DIAGNOSIS: Knowledge deficit R/T assuming patient role
RESOLVED: _X_ Yes ___ No   DATE: 9/12/91

Assessment	Nursing Orders	Implementation	Evaluation
1. Stated "I am totally ignorant about what will happen to me."	1. Educate patient as to perioperative routine and laser procedure.	1. Patient will view perioperative video and laser procedure video, booklets sent home with patient.	1. Patient asked questions after viewing videos and thanked the staff for the written materials.

Independent Nursing Actions:
NAME: Cynthia MacDonald
DATE: 9/9/91
NURSING DIAGNOSIS: Anxiety R/T impending procedure
RESOLVED: _X_ Yes ___ No   DATE: 9/12/91

Assessment	Nursing Orders	Implementation	Evaluation
1. Verbalized anxiety about impending procedure	1. Provide support. Explain the procedure and the perioperative routine.	1. Staff will provide emotional support during all routine procedures and will provide explanations before procedures.	1. Patient stated she was less anxious, and thanked staff for support.

Independent Nursing Actions:
NAME: Cynthia MacDonald
DATE: 9/9/91
NURSING DIAGNOSIS: Powerlessness R/T inability to control illness process
RESOLVED: _X_ Yes ___ No   DATE: 9/12/91

Assessment	Nursing Orders	Implementation	Evaluation
1. Tense, stated "My life seems totally out of control since I became ill."	1. Allow patient to participate in decision making in order to regain a sense of control.	1. Ask patient to make decisions about care as often as possible.	1. Patient advised to discuss with surgeon what to expect during recovery based on surgical findings.

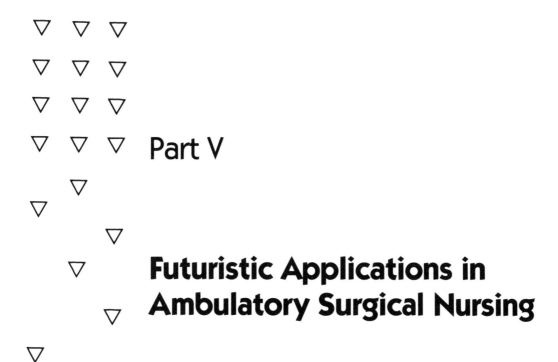

Part V

Futuristic Applications in Ambulatory Surgical Nursing

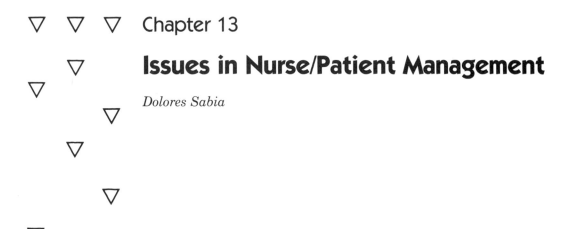

Chapter 13

Issues in Nurse/Patient Management

Dolores Sabia

One of the leading advantages of the ambulatory surgery concept is the ease and simplicity of patient care. The most attractive aspect of this type of patient care is the minimal effect that the experience usually has on the patient's life-style. The variety of patients seen in ambulatory surgical units (ASUs) requires a great deal of flexibility in scheduling and in staffing. As more ASUs are opened, there will be more competition among them for patients. It is important, then, for these units to adapt to patients' needs. The purpose of this chapter is to examine the issues underlying nurse/patient management by answering the following questions:

1. What are the pros and cons of flexible patient scheduling from the perspective of both the nurse and the patient?
2. What pain management techniques are used for the more complex surgical procedures performed in the ambulatory surgical setting?
3. What are the legal issues that arise in relation to signed consent, patient education, documentation of care, and discharge planning as complex procedures are added to the ambulatory surgical schedule?
4. What are the professional issues related to standards of practice and nurse reimbursement in the ambulatory surgical setting?

Flexible Patient Scheduling

One of the most effective marketing tools for ASUs is the flexibility of patient scheduling in this setting. Hospitals and free-standing investor-owned centers that compete for ambulatory services are finding that flexibility and ease of scheduling have a high market value for both physicians and their patients. As patients become more knowledgeable and sophisticated in their choices of health care, the services that are offered must compete with those provided by existing facilities. A free-standing center may have more flexibility in its scheduling practices, as the operating rooms (ORs) are not shared by inpatient services or held open to be ready for emergencies. As society moves at an increasingly faster pace, the expectation of patients is access to surgery with little fuss or bother.

Scheduling preferences may vary according to the patient's age or lifestyle. The pediatric patient is an ideal candidate for procedures in the ASU. These patients should be scheduled for surgery as early in the day as possible. Because pediatric patients are usually kept NPO for general anesthesia, maintenance of their delicate hydration balance is maintained if the anesthetic is administered early in the morning. School-aged patients may want to schedule surgery as late in the week as possible to allow for recovery over the weekend, thereby reducing absenteeism from school. Likewise, adult patients who are taking time off from their work week for surgery may also want to schedule the procedure as late in the week or work day as possible to allow for a weekend recovery and thus reduce the amount of time spent away from work. Female patients who are also mothers may wish to arrange surgery around the schedule of a babysitter. Older adults may have similar constraints if they rely on others for transportation on the day of surgery.

Just as cost containment efforts dictate that nurses must provide services quickly and efficiently, nursing care must also meet safety and professional standards. The future promises ever-increasing financial constraints, especially given a system in which prospective payment mandates high utilization of the services offered. To meet these high utilization requirements, the ASU functions as an intensive work environment. In this intense work environment, the nurse must maintain the patient's safety and well-being. The inherent pressure for accuracy is enhanced by the time factor. Flexible scheduling, although an attractive option for both patients and physicians, must be managed well so that both the staff and the clients may benefit. The system of flexible scheduling in the ASU is an attractive advantage to the consumer; however, it also requires flexibility in the scheduling of staff members.

▽

Flexible Staff Scheduling

Careful attention must be paid to the staff scheduling needs of the surgery center. Flexible staff scheduling throughout the day ensures adequate coverage and helps to minimize overtime. The overall effect of adequate flexible scheduling is that nurses are present at the center when they are needed and the staff is free to give care to the patients in an unrushed manner. As consumers become more knowledgeable about many aspects of the care they receive, the nurse will need to communicate with the patient in a calm and reassuring manner. If the staff feels overworked, the patient may feel that they are being rushed through the surgical experience. Expensive staff training programs in guest relations may be negated if the nursing staff, in their efforts to keep the schedule running on time, end up rushing the patient.

Adequate staff must be employed to meet the needs of flexible scheduling, and sufficient staff resources must be available to reduce overtime, which is a costly alternative to insufficient staffing. Curtailing overtime also reduces the added stressor of irregular hours for the staff. It is important for the nursing staff to stagger work schedules to cover early morning cases, as well as late evening and weekend cases. As mentioned earlier, it is necessary to maintain flexible staff schedules as a unit marketing technique. Just as client marketing is important, so is the marketing of the attributes of the unit important in attracting employees.

An attractive option for prospective nurse employees might be innovative scheduling policies. For instance, a nurse with school-aged children might prefer to work the hours that their children are in school. Another approach would be to accommodate those nurses who want to work only evenings or weekends. Too frequently, the nursing staff is required to work the hours prescribed by the institution, rather than patterning their work hours according to patient scheduling needs.

▽

Pain Management Techniques

One of the greatest concerns patients have is the degree of pain following their surgery. Pain is a complex condition for postoperative patients, and many factors affect the way in which they feel or perceive pain. Often, the preoperative emotional state of patients affects their postoperative pain threshold. Moreover, a complex set of other factors may affect their perception of pain. For instance, if this is the patient's first surgical experience, fear of the unknown, or perhaps the negative surgical experiences of family or friends, may color the patient's perceptions. The patient's ethnic/cultural background may also influence his or her experience of or reaction to pain. The ASU staff can participate in efforts to alleviate or minimize patient discomfort.

An effective method of reducing a patient's pain is through preadmission education. A preoperative telephone call or the availability of printed informational materials prior to admission may help to answer basic questions the patient may have. Even the simplest information can help the patient understand the surgical experience. Alleviating the fear of the unknown can assist the patient in reducing anxiety and understanding instructions. This may have a positive effect on the patient's mental state, which may help the patient to manage pain after surgery.

During the initial preoperative nurse/patient contact, any questions the patient may have should be answered. The nursing staff may point out to the patient that some discomfort is to be expected. A simple strategy, such as using the word discomfort rather than the word pain, may reassure the patient. The patient should also be reassured that pain medication will be available to them if it is needed. It may also be helpful to inform the patient that arrangements can be made with the physician to make prescription analgesics available for home care.

There is a great deal of debate as to the necessity for preoperative medication. Midazolam hydrochloride (Versed) is a new parenteral benzodiazapine that offers a positive alternative to the traditional benzodiazapines which are longer-acting. Physicians were once reluctant to order the traditional benzodiazapines, especially for outpatient use, owing to their prolonged effect and the possible complication of thrombophlebitis. These new medications are appropriate for the relatively healthy patient seen in the ASU because, although they are shorter-acting, they offer a sufficient degree of hypnotic, anticonvulsant, and muscle-relaxing effect. The differences between these agents and diazepam and lorazepam include the higher potency, rapid onset, lipid solubility, and the rapidity with which the former agents cross the blood–brain barrier. For example, systemic elimination of midazolom is rapid, as it has a half-life of 1.8 to 2.5 hours, which is well within the time frame for observation of the patient during an ambulatory surgical visit. Moreover, some are water-soluble agents that reduce pain on injection and reduce the threat of thrombophlebitis.

Attempts to reduce a patient's anxiety before surgery can have a positive effect on the patient's perceptions following surgery. Pain control for the ambulatory surgical patient may be started intraoperatively by anesthesia personnel. Use of a narcotic intraoperatively helps to reduce the patient's pain while in the postanesthesia care unit (PACU). Patients who have received a narcotic must be closely observed by the nursing staff to ensure patency of the airway and adequate oxygen exchange. Most of the inhalation agents currently available for general anesthesia allow patients to awaken quickly.

Because ambulatory surgical procedures and the effect of the medications administered are usually of short duration, these patients awaken quickly in the PACU and may experience pain shortly after their admission to the unit. The appropriate use of intravenous, short-acting narcotics may prevent the patient from experiencing severe pain. Untreated pain will result in nausea and vomiting, and may have other physiological effects, as evidenced by vital sign changes. Fast and effective use of narcotics for pain usually reduces the total amount of medication that is necessary for pain relief. A small intravenous injection of a narcotic may provide enough analgesia for the patient to ambulate and prepare for discharge. Patients will be very reluctant to leave the unit if they are experiencing pain and if they believe that that the pain may increase on arriving home.

Because ambulatory surgical patients are discharged to family or friends rather than to other areas within the hospital, safety precautions must be taken at the time of discharge. A fine line may exist between discharging a patient too soon and sending a patient home who is in pain and apprehensive. Discharge criteria are established by the physician and must be adhered to strictly so that patient safety is assured.

▽

Legal Issues

The legal issues that pertain to the nurse/patient relationship and case management include informed consent. The ambulatory setting offers a very different challenge in this area. In an effort to streamline ASU operations, signed surgical consents can be obtained by a variety of staff. In some instances, the physician or their office staff will obtain signed consent for the surgery; this, however, does not remove the responsibility of the perioperative nurse to ensure that proper consent has been documented. There may be several variations of surgical consent, but certain information is required. Legal counsel familiar with medical practice can provide expert advice on the criteria for proper consent. It is advisable to have ASU standard consent forms either conform to hospital policy (for hospital-based units) or be reviewed by legal counsel to ensure that proper procedure is followed. It is also advisable to reevaluate consent forms as the unit changes or adds procedures or services.

A basic operative consent form will indicate the patient's name, name of the surgeon, the complete and correct name of the procedure to be performed, and the date of surgery. Such phrases as "and other indicated procedures" only provide legal support if the surgeon is required to extend the original scheduled procedure. These phrases are not precise and may be insufficient when opened to legal interpretation. It is the responsibility of the medical staff to make sure that the patient understands the nature of the procedure and the expected outcome. The patient has the right to know both the expected benefits of the procedure and any reasonable, foreseeable potential risks involved. It is advisable to obtain consent before the day of surgery, as fear and apprehension can alter a patient's understanding. At the very least, the patient must have had the surgery, the benefits, and the risks explained by the surgeon, usually during an office visit. If patients are required to sign the surgical consent on the day of surgery, this provides an opportunity for the ASU nurse to restate and reinforce what is already understood by the patient. The explanation to the patient should be simple and straightforward, using terms and language the patient understands.

Patients who are minors—that is, patients who are younger than the legal age as defined by their state's law—must be given special consideration. A minor may be defined in a variety of ways by different states' laws. In some, the age of maturity is 18 years of age; in others, it is 21 years; and in some instances, a patient may be considered to be of legal age if they are emancipated from their parents or guardians. It is vital that the nurse know the criteria established by the state in which the nurse is practicing. Informed consent for a minor patient must be signed by a parent or legal guardian. In some cases, a court official or nursing home administrator will be assigned legal guardianship for very young or elderly patients. A copy of the guardianship papers is required to verify signatures, and is an added safeguard for proper patient documentation.

Liability for patient care is always minimized by patient education. Patients who understand their surgery and its expected effects are unlikely to bring legal action against a staff member or the unit. In ambulatory surgery, the contact with the patient is limited to a very short period of time. The more the nurse can do to educate patients and answer their questions, the more positive the experience will be for patients and their families. Simple measures, such as providing patients with brochures about the unit, can educate the patient about what to expect on the day of surgery. Generic printed postoperative material can minimize the number of questions patients have in regard to their surgery and what to expect during their recovery period.

The short interaction of the staff in the ASU also has an effect on proper documentation. The patients are in the care of nurses for only a short time, and there is no opportunity to observe them over the course of several days. The short-term stay places the nurse at a disadvantage for evaluating care, so nurses must be more vigilant in their documentation.

▽

Standards of Nursing Practice

Evaluation of care is frequently recommended in the standards of practice established by professional nursing organizations. The initial assessment, the surgical experience, the recovery period, and the evaluation of the patient at the time of discharge must be documented. Policies and procedures must reflect the practice of the unit and be tailored to meet the needs of the patients. Health care standards in the community must also be met, and all activities of the patient while at the ASU must be documented. A preoperative note should be written in the patient's chart to provide a description of the preoperative condition of the patient so that a comparison can be made during the recovery period. The nursing documentation of the patient's preoperative status should include vital signs and a short narrative describing the patient's condition before surgery. The operative record should state the surgical and anesthesia time frames, type of surgical procedure, type of anesthesia, persons responsible for patient care while in the OR, positioning of the patient during surgery, preoperative medical diagnosis, and postoperative diagnosis.

Any medication given by the nurse must be documented, as must any ancillary studies, such as x-rays, that are conducted.

The equipment used during the procedure and the amount of blood loss, if appropriate, should also be recorded. It is also advisable to indicate the surgical service and wound classification for quality assurance purposes. Any dressings or casts that are applied, and any appliances (such as drains or catheters) that are to remain with the patient must be documented. The third part of the documentation is completed in the PACU, where vital signs, intake, output, and the PACU scoring criteria for the patient should be recorded.

Documentation of the operative site, dressings, and patient education strategies used should be recorded in the nurses' notes. The documentation may follow a variety of formats, but must adhere to policy for the unit.

The nursing documentation should include an area where the staff can record the type of patient education conducted prior to discharge. It is advisable, and in some instances required, to send the patient home with written instructions, a copy of which is placed in the patient's permanent record. These instructions must direct the patient's home care. Information regarding anesthesia recovery and surgical recovery should be detailed on the instruction sheets. Any special instructions that the surgeon has should also be included. It is also advisable to document any medication the physician may have prescribed for the patient's home use.

Written information is especially helpful should the patient need to contact the unit about a question regarding their home care. A telephone number for patients to call if they have any questions also helps to reassure the patient. It is recommended that patients or responsible parties sign their names to the chart copy of the instructions, indicating that they have been instructed adequately in home care techniques and have had their questions answered.

A preprinted discharge instruction sheet, with both a patient and chart copy, makes discharge teaching more uniform and complete. If a preprinted sheet is to be used, it is recommended that the information given to the patient meet with physician approval and be individualized for the patient. This eliminates any questions that might arise regarding what information was given to the patient at the time of discharge.

▽

Summary

Although there are many issues that pertain to patient care and nursing management in the ASU, nurses must remember that, in today's competitive health care market, the primary goal is to meet patients' needs. Patients' needs may include flexible scheduling and pain management, both of which must be governed by standards of practice. This chapter has discussed some of these issues; other nursing care issues will emerge as more complex procedures are performed in the ambulatory surgical setting.

Bibliography

Atsberger, D. B., & Shrewsburg, P. (1988). Minisymposium: Postoperative pain, postoperative pain management. The PACU nurse's challenge. *Journal of Post Anesthesia Nursing, 3*(6):399–403.

Burden, N. (1988). Nursing care of the patient undergoing laparoscopy in the ambulatory setting. *Journal of Post Anesthesia Nursing, 3*(3), 189–195.

Glandon, G. L., Colbert, K. W., & Thomasma, M. (1989). Nursing delivery models and RN mix: Cost implications. *Nursing Management, 20*(5), 30–33.

Hyna, W., & Gutmann, C. (1984). *Management of surgical facilities.* Rockville, MD: Aspen Publications.

Kitz, D. S., Robinson, D. M., Schiavone, P. A., Walsh, P. R., & Conahan, T. J. (1988). Discharging outpatients. Factors nurses consider to determine readiness (3rd ed.). *AORN Journal, 48*(1), 87–91.

Morath, J. M. (1989). Empathy training: Development of sensitivity and caring in the hospital. *Nursing Management, 20*(3), 60–62.

Squibb, C. B. (1988). Outpatient surgical evaluations. *Nursing Management, 19*(1), 32L, 32N, 32P.

Swehla, M. A. (1988). Nursing diagnosis as a standard: Methodology for identifying validating diagnosis in an ambulatory setting. *Nursing Administration Quarterly, 12*(2), 18–23.

Ver Steeg, D. F. (1988). Computer use and nursing research. A computerized taxonomy of nursing diagnoses for use in ambulatory care nursing education, practice, and research. Part 2: The use of modifiers. *Western Journal of Nursing Research, 10*(6), 778–781.

Welcher, B. V. (1985). *Anesthesia for ambulatory surgery.* Philadelphia: J. B. Lippincott.

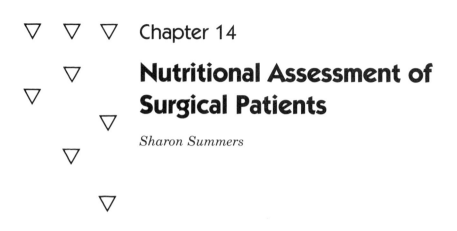

Chapter 14

Nutritional Assessment of Surgical Patients

Sharon Summers

Nutritional status of ambulatory surgical patients is an important part of assessment, yet little attention is given to this factor. It is estimated that more than 50 percent of the patients admitted to hospitals have preexisting malnutrition.[1-3] Preexisting malnutrition is believed to result in a reduced ability to tolerate the stressors of surgery, an increased susceptibility to nosocomial infections, and a longer hospital stay.[4] Other complications related to preexisting malnutrition include muscular deterioration, increased rate of complications, and impaired wound healing.[5-7] With the increased emphasis on ambulatory surgery as a cost containment measure, there may also be an increased incidence of malnutrition in these patients. Thus, nurses in the ambulatory surgical setting need to assess their patients' nutritional status and institute patient education regarding nutrition in order to expedite postoperative recovery. Therefore, the purpose of this chapter is to answer the following questions:

1. What methods can be used to measure nutritional status in ambulatory surgical patients?
2. What are the nutritional needs of ambulatory surgical patients?
3. What nutritional methods can be used to promote quick recovery among ambulatory surgical patients?
4. What computer applications facilitate the assessment of nutritional status in ambulatory surgical patients?

Measurement of Nutritional Status

Little consensus was found in the medical, nursing, or dietetic literature regarding how to measure nutritional status.[8-13] Tricep skinfold thickness, arm muscle circumference, body mass index, creatinine/height ratio, hemoglobin, hematocrit, height, weight, lymphocyte count, total lym-

Exhibits for Chapter 14 are located at the end of the chapter on pages 272–274.

phocyte count (white blood cell count × % lymphocytes × 100), protein, albumin, retinol binding protein, prealbumin, and serum iron levels have all been cited as measures of nutritional status. In addition, the sources just cited classified malnutrition in surgical patients as either marasmus (protein and calorie) malnutrition or as kwashiorkor (protein) malnutrition.

Summers' Nutritional Assessment Profile

Drawing from these literature sources and from physiology texts,[14,15] Summers' Nutritional Assessment Profile (SNAP) was developed to measure nutritional status in hospitalized surgical patients.[16] The SNAP (Exhibit 14-1) consists of two parts: demographic data and nutritional status data. The nutritional status section was further divided into six indices: protein, fat, carbohydrate, hematological indicators, chemistry, and physical parameters. These six indices were selected as they are the routine laboratory tests and admission criteria that are most frequently recorded for hospitalized patients. Financial support from a National Center for Nursing Research grant paid for one additional laboratory test—prealbumin levels—the results of which were also reported to be a very sensitive marker of nutritional status.

After institutional approval, surgical patients were approached, the study was explained, and written informed consent was obtained from the participants.* Data were then collected on 70 surgical patients, who were classified as either ill or well, from a single medical center in the Midwest. Typical ill patients (N = 35) were those who had been ill at home prior to admission, but who did not have cancer, diabetes, life-threatening illness, or hemorrhagic disorders. Typical well patients (N = 35) were those admitted for elective surgery, such as inguinal herniorrhaphy, who had not been ill prior to admission.

Results

The demographic data shown in Table 14-1 profile the subjects. The SNAP was statistically analyzed for instrument reliability; coefficient alpha reliability was 0.7136, which is acceptable for a new instrument. Factor analysis was used to establish construct validity, which determines whether the SNAP actually measured the construct of nutritional status. When data were forced into six factors, as measures of the six dimensions, then the SNAP items accounted for 74 percent of the variance, indicating that only 26 percent of other factors that measure nutritional status remained unexplained.

Analysis of the data indicated that, of all the laboratory tests, total

*This study was funded by an Emphasis Grant Component Study #14, awarded to the University of Kansas Medical Center, School of Nursing by the National Center For Nursing Research, 1988–1989.

Table 14-1 Demographic Data of Surgical Patients
(N = 70)

Average age	50.19 yrs (range 19–65 yrs)
Sex	
Male	39
Female	31
Decrease in energy	
Yes	50
No	20
Decrease in appetite	
Yes	31
No	39
Decrease in food intake	
Yes	33
No	37

Table 14-2 Stepwise Discriminant Analysis of SNAP Laboratory Values
for Ill and Well Subjects

	Average	Values		Significance
Variable	Ill	Well	F Ratio	(p <0.05)
Total protein	6.17	6.70	5.54	0.02*
Blood urea nitrogen	14.73	15.54	0.16	0.68
Albumin	3.36	4.40	21.60	0.00*
Prealbumin	17.37	34.18	3.85	0.05*
Cholesterol	170.95	192.56	4.92	0.02*
Potassium	3.95	4.25	7.39	0.00*
Hemoglobin	12.42	13.61	5.56	0.02*
Red blood cell count	4.17	4.56	6.37	0.01*
Glucose	120.26	111.72	0.94	0.33
Calcium	8.45	8.98	2.24	0.14
Lymphocytes	18.19	22.29	2.37	0.07
Total lymphocytes	1642.00	1720.58	0.13	0.71
Hematocrit	35.85	39.09	3.34	0.07
Leukocytes	10.02	8.61	2.24	0.14

*Significant difference between ill and well subjects

protein, serum albumin, and prealbumin levels (protein indices); cholesterol values (fat indices); potassium levels (mineral indices); and hemoglobin, and red blood cell levels (hematological indices) were the significant (p < 0.05) indicators of nutritional status in the patients studied (Table 14-2). As hemoglobin is routinely measured in ambulatory surgical patients, this may be the best, most cost-effective method for assessing nutritional status.

Table 14-3 Discriminant Function Analysis

Actual Group	Number	Predicted 1	Group 2
Ill subjects	35	25 (70.7%)	10 (29.3%)
Well subjects	35	10 (29.3%)	25 (70.7%)

Percent correctly classified = 70.65

Further data analysis, using discriminant function analysis, sorted the patients by ill and well categories for the purpose of analyzing and classifying the patients by nutritional status. As seen in Table 14-3, 70.65% of the patients were correctly classified into categories of ill and well based on the laboratory test results listed on the SNAP.

Conclusions

The literature cited earlier categorized malnutrition as either marasmus and kwashiorkor; however, these terms have usually been used to describe extreme protein/calorie deprivation. The results of this study found significant differences in ill and well surgical patients based on protein indices, but the values did not indicate severe malnutrition. It is suggested, then, that *nutritional deficit* may be a better term than malnutrition to describe what happens to surgical patients when they are deprived of their usual intake of oral food and fluids. It was noted that one patient in the well group had a decrease in serum albumin level from 4.2 gm/100 ml to 2.8 gm/100 ml during hospitalization. The decrease in serum albumin level indicated that the nutritional needs of "routine" or well patients may be ignored, whereas ill patients tend to receive nutritional support. (The nutritional needs of ambulatory surgical patients are assumed to be those of the well patient group in this study.)

Although body weight is a standard measure whereby judgments are made as to nutritional status, some overweight individuals may be malnourished. Height/weight tables are based on averages and do not always "fit" when describing individual patient's nutritional status—hence, the need for the SNAP. Nutritional needs of the ambulatory surgical patient are a function of the metabolic demands made in response to the stressors of surgery. Thus, regardless of the patient's ill or well status, the surgical experience is a stressor that leads to an increased need for nutrients.

▽

Nutritional Needs of Ambulatory Surgical Patients

As seen in Figure 14-1, the nutritional needs of surgical patients are a function of the percentage of energy requirements for postoperative recovery, which ranges from approximately minus 2 to plus 5, and activates the stress response. Selye defined stress as the "nonspecific response of

Figure 14-1 Energy requirements of critically ill patients. (From Wilmore, D. W. [1977]. *The metabolic management of the critically ill* (p.36). New York: Plenum Publishing Corporation, with permission.)

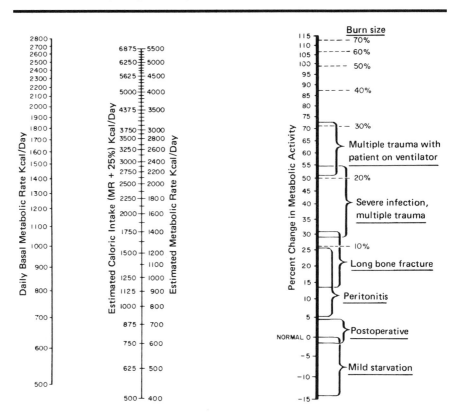

the body to any demand (p. 32)."[17] The stress theory consists of two forms of adaptation—general adaptation syndrome and local adaptation syndrome. The general adaptation syndrome is further defined by the alarm reaction, the resistance stage, and the exhaustion stage. Selye states that the general adaptation stages occur in addition to the normal, life-sustaining physiological processes. Events that evoke the general adaptation syndrome are known as stressors, and these stressors may be either pleasant or unpleasant, physical or psychological. In contrast to the general adaptation syndrome, the local adaptation syndrome pertains to a local tissue response that includes inflammation, proliferation of fibrous connective tissue to prevent the spread of pathogens, granulation of new tissue to replace damaged tissue, and chemotaxis to neutralize waste and toxins and to kill pathogens.

The stress response is a series of events that may be precipitated by psychological or physiological mechanisms (Figure 14-2). Psychological stress may be precipitated by admission to the unit and fear of the un-

Figure 14-2 Stress response.

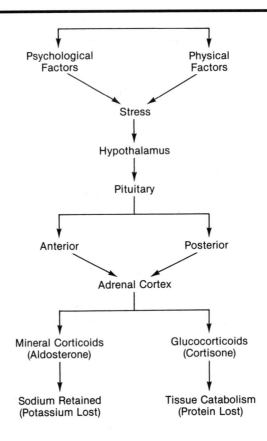

known related to unit routines. Physiological stress may be precipitated by general anesthesia and the trauma of surgery. The anesthetized patient, although not perceiving stressors, has physiological stressors that evoke the stress mechanism at the hypothalamic level.[18,19] Hypothalamic stress results in a rapid response and a slow response. The rapid response is mediated through the sympathetic-adrenal medulla mechanism. The sympathetic-adrenal medulla mechanism results in the release of catecholamines that may have a deleterious effect on the cardiovascular system,[20] whereby tachycardia and hypertension may occur and myocardial oxygen consumption may be compromised. The slow response is mediated through the pituitary-adrenal cortex mechanism. Delayed responses of the pituitary-adrenal cortex mechanism may elicit changes in such parameters as antidiuretic hormone (ADH) levels. ADH is believed to be elevated by circulating catecholamines, which elevation results in fluid retention.

Increased fluid retention is believed to cause an increase in cardiac workload and hypertension. Blitt indicated that surgery and general anesthesia evoke the acute sympathoadrenal catecholamine response.[20] The effects of general anesthesia may mask the physiological responses; however, the stress response may be evidenced by tachycardia, hypertension, compromised myocardial oxygenation, and dysrhythmia, especially in the presence of halothane.[20] Boucher and Witt[21] found that all inhalation anesthetics are myocardial depressants that precipitate dysrhythmias and premature ventricular contractions. In addition, "all general anesthesia agents temporarily decrease renal blood flow and glomerular filtration rate as a direct consequence of hemodynamic changes induced by myocardial depressant effects and venous and arterial dilatation" (p. 66).[21]

Other stressors include the pain response, which promotes the release of catecholamines; inadequate ventilation, which promotes catecholamine release; hypothermia and subsequent shivering; a distended bladder or catheterization, which are associated with an autonomic nervous system response; and preoperative anxiety.[22] It was assumed that the surgical experience elicited the general adaptation syndrome. Blitt indicated that the negative effects of stress may include altered wound healing and inhibition of the immune response to infection.[20] Stressors that stimulate the release of pituitary and adrenal hormones also increase the body's need for energy and nutrients.

Guyton stated that the principle substrates to produce cellular energy are carbohydrates, proteins, and fats in the presence of oxygen.[14] Carbohydrates, proteins, and fats are nutrient precursors needed by cells to produce adenosine triphosphate (ATP), which is an energy source for cellular function; whereas water and carbon dioxide are by-products of cellular metabolism. The stress theory describes and explains how the catabolic impact of stressors could affect recovery of the ambulatory surgical patient.

In order to explain further the impact of surgical stress on the patient, ten propositions, or assumptions, were developed:

1. Adequate cellular access to the universal requisites of air, food, water, and elimination is necessary to produce ATP for energy.
2. Inadequate cellular access to the universal requisites of air, food, water, and elimination will alter cellular production of ATP for energy.
3. Adequate human access to the universal requisites of air, food, water, and elimination is necessary to promote cellular life, ATP production, and local and general adaptation responses.
4. Inadequate human access to the universal requisites of air, food, water, and elimination will alter cellular life, ATP production, and local and general adaptation responses.
5. Universal requisites of air, food, water, and elimination are frequently combined in food products known as proteins, fats, carbohydrates, oxygen, and by-products of water and carbon

dioxide for the purpose of maintaining cellular life, ATP production, and local and general adaptation.

6. When protein, fat, carbohydrate, oxygen, and by-products of water and carbon dioxide are sufficient to maintain normal human cellular life, ATP production, and local and general adaptation, then the state is known as adequate nutrition.

7. When protein, fat, carbohydrate, oxygen, and by-products of water and carbon dioxide are insufficient to maintain normal human cellular life, ATP production, and local and general adaptation, then the state is known as nutritional deficit.

8. Stressors may disrupt cellular and human access to adequate nutrition and to local and general adaptation.

9. Impending surgery and hospitalization are stressors that may lead to a nutritional deficit and to disruption of cellular life, ATP production, and local and general adaptation.

10. When the stressors of impending surgery and hospitalization are superimposed on preexisting nutritional deficits, then disruption of local and general adaptation responses may threaten human cellular survival.

Patients who are candidates for surgery in the ambulatory setting are assumed to be well, and nutritional deficits are assumed to be related to the routine withholding of food and water instigated by the policy of nothing *per os* (NPO) after midnight before scheduled surgery. It is interesting to note that NPO after midnight became traditional policy when general anesthesia consisted predominantly of drip ether and resulted in violent episodes of postanesthesia nausea and vomiting.[23] Today, the anesthetics used result in less toxic effects, facilitating a smooth postanesthesia recovery. As seen in Table 14-4, not all general or combination anesthetics result in postanesthesia nausea and vomiting. It is suggested that protocols be established so that ambulatory surgical patients do not receive general anesthetics that result in nausea and vomiting during recovery. Hill recommended that the general anesthetics used for ambulatory surgical patients be restricted to nitrous oxide, halothane, enflurane, and isoflurane.[23]

If current practice would restrict the use of general anesthetics to those agents that do not precipitate nausea and vomiting, then it might be possible to allow patients to eat and drink commercially prepared products that are easily digested and quickly absorbed from the stomach. A review of the literature revealed virtually no research studies that systematically evaluated whether or when patients could eat and drink before surgery without a risk of postanesthesia vomiting or aspiration. The rationale for NPO status has been associated with the need to decrease gastrointestinal residue or to decrease abdominal distention. This policy was developed for inpatients who were usually ill. Few research studies have documented that the protocol of NPO after midnight prior to surgery

Table 14-4 Selected Actions of General and Combination Anesthetic Agents

Agent	Selected Side Effects (Nausea and Vomiting)
Cyclopropane	Common
Droperidol (Inapsine)	Uncommon
Diazepam (Valium)	Uncommon
Droperidol and fentanyl citrate (Innovar)	Uncommon
Ether	Common
Enflurane (Ethrane)	Rare
Fentanyl citrate (Sublimaze)	Uncommon
Halothane (Fluothane)	Uncommon
Isothane (Forane)	?
Ketamine hydrochloride (Ketalar)	Common
Methohexital sodium (Brevital)	?
Methoxyflurane (Penthrane)	Common
Nitrous oxide	Moderate
Thiamylal sodium (Surital)	Uncommon
Thiopental sodium (Pentothal)	Uncommon

is necessary with the newer anesthetic agents, suggesting that this procedure remains an unscientific ritual that may interfere with patient recovery.

▽

Nutritional Methods to Promote Quick Recovery

In order to implement nutritional protocols for quick recovery, the ambulatory surgical nurse needs to have an understanding of normal gastrointestinal function. According to Vick, the time for gastric emptying is based on the composition of the intake delivered to the stomach.[15] For example, isotonic saline is transferred from the stomach to the duodenum at a rate of 50 to 100 ml/min, whereas solid food usually leaves at a rate of 3 to 10 ml/min. This time difference for digestion and transfer is related to the time required for secretion of digestive enzymes and the churning motion needed for the breakdown of fibrous particles. Because liquids do not contain fibrous particles, less time is needed for digestion.

There are several products available for supplemental feedings that are usually prescribed for patients who need nutritional support. As seen in Table 14-5, various manufacturers have developed products to supplement patients' nutritional intake. These products are frequently utilized only after patients are stressed from illness or surgery, and are given as tube feedings. Little research has been conducted regarding "preventive" nutritional programs designed to meet metabolic stressors in outpatients.

Table 14-5 Nutritional Supplements*

Formula	Caloric Density (Kcal/ml)	Protein (gm)/	Fat (gm)/ (% Kcal)	Carbohydrate (gm)/ (% Kcal)
Criticare HN (Mead-Johnson)	1.06	37.5/(14%)	3.3/(3%)	222/(83%)
Travasorb HN (Travenol)	1.0	45/(18%)	13/(12%)	175/(70%)
Travasorb STD (Travenol)	1.0	30/(12%)	13/(12%)	190/(76%)
Vivonex (Norwich-Eaton)	1.0	20/(8%)	1.4/(1%)	230/(91%)
Vivonex HN (Norwich-Eaton)	1.0	46/(18%)	0.9/(1%)	210/(81%)
Vivonex TEN (Norwich-Eaton)	1.0	38/(15%)	3.0/(2.5%)	206/(82%)
Vital HN (Ross)	1.0	42/(17%)	11/(9%)	185/(74%)

*These are elemental products that are low-residue and require little digestion; they are usually instilled as tube feedings.

However, the available inpatient research will be discussed and suggestions for the ambulatory surgical setting will be offered.

Some research studies have examined methods of feeding inpatients who undergo major abdominal surgery. Moss conducted experimental studies, with both animal models and human subjects, on the effect of early postoperative feeding on recovery from bowel resection and cholecystectomy.[24,25] Although it is not known whether these studies were conducted with the shift in health care from traditional hospitalization to ambulatory surgery in mind, the findings are pertinent for nurses in these units.

Moss conducted a study of 18 patients, aged 18 to 71 years, who underwent colectomy and who had a multiple lumen nasogastric (MLNG) tube inserted during the surgical procedure.[24] (Shea and McCreary refer to the MLNG tube as the "Moss nasogastric duodenal tube."[26]) The MLNG tube is designed to aspirate swallowed air trapped in the esophagus and aspirate stomach contents while delivering an elemental formula into the duodenum. For the purposes of the study, feeding was begun approximately five hours postoperatively, usually while the patient was still in the postanesthesia care unit. Results of this study, and those of similar ones also conducted by Moss, indicate that early resumption of feeding using the MLNG tube resulted in a marked improvement in wound healing.

In a similar study of 37 patients who underwent cholecystectomy, Moss reported results that are pertinent for nurses in the ambulatory surgery unit (ASU).[25] Use of the MLNG tube and early postoperative feeding resulted in a shortened length of stay for patients having cholecystectomy, with the longest hospital stay being 48 hours. Patients ranged in age from 21 to 80 years, and cholecystectomy was performed in the usual manner except that Moss injected the midline incisional tissue (rather than the Kocher incisional site) with 1/2% Marcaine. The MLNG tube was inserted during surgery, esophageal and gastric aspiration was instituted, and elemental feeding was begun in the postanesthesia care unit. The MLNG tube was removed the morning following surgery, after instillation of a saline cathartic, and a "general diet" was resumed. Wound management included replacing skin clips with sterile tape. All patients were discharged within *48 hours* after cholecystectomy; 34 were discharged within the first 24 hours. Also of note in this study was that less pain medication was needed by the patients receiving supplemental MLNG tube feeding than by those who received no supplemental feeding. Meperidine use averaged 50 mg in a 24-hour period, and 25% of the patients (9 patients) did not require any narcotics for pain.

These studies conducted by Moss, as well as the preliminary studies conducted from the 1960s through the 1980s, have exciting implications for health care providers related to shortened length of stay while maintaining quality of care.[27-41] In particular, a question arises for nurses who have cared for patients in both traditional and short-stay settings. How can patients care for themselves at home when, as nurses, we know how much care (injections for pain, assistance with ambulation and wound management, including T-tube drainage) they required in the inpatient setting? As Moss[25] stated, "Paralytic ileus is an avoidable complication. . . . swallowed air and adverse effects of anesthetics, peritoneal irritation, narcotics, [and] intestinal gas become the *coup de grace*" (pp. 69–70).

Moss also reported that esophageal and gastric aspiration, combined with early feeding and saline cathartic, restored gastric function.[24,25] Early feeding also promoted wound healing (albumin and globulin levels were triple compared to those in unfed dogs), and more new collagen was observed in the wounds of animals that were fed than in those that remained unfed. It is concluded from these studies that early feeding provides patients with the energy necessary to care for themselves, and that fewer gastrointestinal side effects result. Moss reported early feeding of patients with an elemental diet supplying 3,600 Kcal plus 133 gm of amino acids; however, concerns have been raised with regard to renal overload from the increase in amino acids,[14] and other considerations need to be given to patient self-care when feeding is instituted prior to admission.[24,25]

A research study is in the developmental stage in which results of nutritional research from sports medicine will be applied to ambulatory surgical patients.[38] The nutritional needs of athletes have been studied extensively regarding the best means of preparing for marathon events. The basis of marathon nutrition is determining how to provide sustained energy to meet an athlete's metabolic needs during high-energy, stressful athletic events. It is assumed that, like the athlete, surgical patients face a high-energy marathon when undergoing surgery, except that little is done to prepare them metabolically.

A study will be conducted in which a group of elective ambulatory surgical patients (with inguinal hernias) will be fed high-carbohydrate athlete supplements, in addition to their usual diets, for 72 hours prior to admission. A control group of matched patients (of the same ages and undergoing the same procedure) will eat their usual diet prior to surgery. The two groups will then be compared on the basis of differences in recovery using the SNAP. Thus, prefeeding prior to surgery is intended to be a nutritional method for promoting quick recovery in ambulatory surgical patients.

In today's health care arena, with the prevailing concerns about shortened length of stay, "customer satisfaction," quality of care, and the legal implications of early discharge, nutritional preparation should be a priority concern. Undernutrition or disregard for nutritional preparation prior to surgery is analogous to not putting enough gas in the gas tank of a car and yet expecting the car to run. Surgical patients will not "run" if they do not have sufficient energy stores prior to surgical stress.

▽

Computerized Methods for Assessing Nutritional Status

Computer applications were discussed indepth in Chapter 3; however, the applications presented were aimed at general use in the ambulatory surgical setting. Just as computers can be used for general use, so, too, can they be used for specific applications, as with assessment of nutritional status. A variety of software packages is available to assess the nutritional needs of patients,[39,40] and these range in cost from $100 to $5,000. The content of these programs ranges from the assessment of individual critically ill patients to maintenance of wellness in other patients. Most programs contain data on thousands of types of foods, allowing detailed analysis or profiles of patients.

The results of the SNAP study, as discussed earlier, indicated that total protein, prealbumin, cholesterol, potassium, and hemoglobin levels, together with red blood cell count, were the best measures of nutritional status. In the ASU, potassium levels and hemoglobin are frequently measured upon admission of a patient. If these values are lower than acceptable norms, the nurse could then alert the surgeon as to possible nutritional deficits.

One method for evaluating a patient's nutritional status is to use a computerized spreadsheet, constructing items and writing formulas that will calculate a patient's recovery risk when laboratory values are below acceptable norms. For example, Exhibit 14-2 shows a typical computer screen where patient data are entered onto a spreadsheet and the recovery risk is calculated. When a patient example is inserted into the spreadsheet, this risk can quickly be calculated (Exhibit 14-3). For example, low risk implies no anticipated problems, moderate risk implies that some problems may occur, and high risk implies that the patient is at risk for surgical complications.

If institutional computers are unavailable to the ambulatory surgical nurse, then the patient's nutritional status may be monitored with a pocket computer. Thompson[41] reported the use of the TRS-80 model computer, with a program written in BASIC, to monitor patients receiving total parenteral nutrition. The data entered included intake during the past 24 hours, current caloric requirements, and projected nutrient needs for the current period. An advantage of using computers to assist in monitoring recovery risk and calculating nutrient needs is that they permit nursing assessment of a patient's nutritional status. In busy practice settings, laboratory data frequently are placed in charts, and few nurses integrate the available laboratory study results into a risk evaluation.

▽

Summary

This chapter has presented the importance of nutritional assessment as part of the ambulatory surgical nurses' patient evaluation. Emphasis has been placed on the importance of patient assessment and nursing intervention should the patient be at risk during recovery from surgery. The research presented reviewed methods for measuring nutritional status, methods for instituting early postoperative feeding, and the means by which computers can assist nurses in meeting the nutritional needs of ambulatory surgical patients.

References

1. Mullen, J. L. (1981). Consequences of malnutrition in surgical patients. *Surgical Clinics of North America, 61*(3), 465–487.
2. Palmer, P. N. (1984). Malnutrition: Reversing the trend in the surgical patient. *AORN Journal, 40*(3), 347–352.
3. Kamath, S. K., Lawler, M., Smith, A. E., Kalat, T., & Olson, R. (1986). Hospital malnutrition: A 33-hospital screening study. *Journal of the American Dietetic Association, 86,* 203–206.
4. Seltzer, M. H., Bastidas, J. A., Cooper, D. N., Engler, P., Slocum, B., & Fletchers, H. S. (1979). Instant nutritional assessment. *Journal of Parenteral and Enteral Nutrition, 3,* 157.
5. Edwards, H., Rose, E. A., & King, T. C. (1982). Postoperative deterioration in muscular function. *Archives of Surgery, 177,* 899–901.
6. Warnold, I., & Lundholm, K. (1983). Clinical significances of preoperative nutritional status in 215 noncancer patients. *Annals of Surgery, 199*(3), 299–305.
7. Haydock, D. A., & Hill, G. L. (1986). Impaired wound healing in surgical patients with varying degrees of malnutrition. *Journal of Parenteral and Enteral Nutrition, 10,* 550–554.
8. Blackburn, G. L., & Thornton, P. A. (1979). Nutritional assessment of the hospitalized adult. *Medical Clinics of North America,* Vol. 63, No. 5 1103–1115.
9. Baker, G. P., Detsky, A. S., Wesson, D. E., Wolman, S. L., Stewart, S., Whitewell, J., Langer, B., & Jeejeebhoy, K. N. (1982). Nutritional assessment: A comparison of clinical judgment and objective measures. *New England Journal of Medicine, 306*(16), 969–972.
10. Krey, S. H., & Murray, R. L. (1986). *Dynamics of nutrition support.* Norwalk, CT: Appleton-Century-Crofts.

11. Grant, J. P., Custer, P. B., & Thurlow, J. (1981). Current techniques of nutritional assessment. *Surgical Clinics of North America, 61*(3), 437–463.
12. Williams, C. S. (1986). Laboratory values and their interpretation. In S. H. Krey, & R. L. Murray (Eds.), *Dynamics of Nutritional Support.* Norwalk, CT: Appleton-Century-Crofts.
13. Roy, L. B., Edwards, P. A., & Barr, L. H. (1985). The value of nutritional assessment in the surgical patient. *Journal of Parenteral and Enteral Nutrition, 9*(2), 170–172.
14. Guyton, A. C. (1986). *Textbook of medical physiology.* Philadelphia: W. B. Saunders Company.
15. Vick, R. L. *Contemporary medical physiology.* Menlo Park, CA: Addison-Wesley Publishing.
16. Summers, S. L. (1989). *Nutritional assessment of surgical patients.* Unpublished manuscript.
17. Selye, H. (1978). *The stress of life.* St. Louis: McGraw-Hill.
18. Levy, C. J. (1982). Changes in plasma chemistry associated with stress. In J. Watkins, & M. Salo (Eds.), *Trauma, stress, and immunity in anesthesia and surgery.* (p. 141). London: Butterworth Scientific.
19. Salo, M. (1982). Endocrine response to anaesthesia and surgery. In J. Watkins, & M. Salo (Eds.), *Trauma, stress, and immunity in anesthesia and surgery.* (pp. 158–173). London: Butterworth Scientific.
20. Blitt, C. D. (1985). *Monitoring in anesthesia and critical care medicine.* New York: Churchill Livingstone.
21. Boucher, B. A., & Witt, W. O. (1986). The postoperative adverse effects of inhalation anesthetics. *Heart & Lung 15,*(1), 63–69.
22. Glass, P. M. (1982). Postoperative hypertension. *Breathline 2,*(4), 63–64.
23. Hill, G. J. (1984). *Outpatient surgery.* Philadelphia: W. B. Saunders.
24. Moss, G. (1981). Maintenance of gastrointestinal function after bowel surgery and immediate enteral full nutrition. II. Clinical experience, with objective demonstration of intestinal absorption and mortality. *Journal of Parenteral and Enteral Nutrition, 5*(3), 215–220.
25. Moss, G. (1983). Mini-trauma cholecystectomy. *Journal of Abdominal Surgery, 25*(7,8), 66–74.
26. Shea, M., & McCreary, M. J. (1984). Early postop feeding. *American Journal of Nursing, 84*(10), 1230–1231.
27. Scovill, W. A., Saba, T. M., Kaplan, J. E., Bernard, H. R., & Powers, S. R., Jr. (1977). Disturbances in circulating opsonic activity in man after operative and blunt trauma. *Journal of Surgical Research, 22,* 709–716.
28. Moss, G., & Friedman, R. C. (1977). Abdominal decompression: Increased efficiency by esophageal aspiration utilizing a new nasogastric tube. *American Journal of Surgery, 133,* 225–228.
29. Moss, G. (1979). Postoperative ileus in an avoidable complication [editorial]. *Surgery, Gynecology, and Obstetrics, 148,* 81–82.
30. Greenstein, A., Rogers, P., & Moss, G. (1978). Doubled fourth day colorectal anastomotic strength with complete retention of wound mature collagen and accelerated deposition following immediate full enteral nutrition. *Surgical Forum, 29,* 78–81.
31. Zikria, B. A., & King, T. C. (1979). Gastrointestinal function and nutrition in surgical patients. *Contemporary Surgery, 14,* 37–41.
32. Moss, G., Greenstein, A., Levy, S., & Bierenbaum, A. (1980). Maintenance of gastrointestinal function after bowel surgery and immediate enteral full nutrition. I. Doubling of canine colorectal anastomotic bursting pressure and intestinal wound mature collagen content. *Journal of Parenteral and Enteral Nutrition, 4,* 535–538.
33. Jain, K. M., Rush, B. F., Jr., Seelig, R. F., Cheung, N. K., & Dikdan, G. (1981).

Changes in plasma amino acid profiles following abdominal operations. *Surgery, Gynecology, and Obstetrics, 152*, 302–306.

34. Moss, G., & Wells, J. (1981). Rapid return to normal of postoperative plasma amino acid concentrations by immediate full enteral nutrition [abstract]. *Federal Proceedings, 40*, 851.

35. Moss, G. (1982). Full enteral nutrition aborts postoperative plasma amino acid depression [abstract]. *Federal Proceedings, 41*, 274.

36. Robinson, G., & Moss, G. (1982). Accelerated leucine turnover for protein synthesis following experimental bowel resection and immediate postoperative full enteral nutrition [abstract]. *Federal Proceedings, 41*, 274.

37. Moss, G. (1983). Postcolectomy plasma amino acid levels maintained above basal by immediate full enteral nutrition [abstract]. *Federal Proceedings of Federation of American Societies for Experimental Biology, 42(4)*, 1071.

38. Summers, S. L. (1991). *Effect of feeding on wound healing in humans*. Proposal development in progress.

39. Williams, S. R. (1985). *Nutrition and diet therapy*. St. Louis: C. V. Mosby Co.

40. Polacseu, R. A. (1987). The fourth annual medical software buyers' guide. [Special Issue]. *M. D. Computing, 4(6)*, 23–139.

41. Thompson, D. A. (1984). Monitoring total parenteral nutrition with the pocket calculator. *Computers in Nursing, 2(5)*, 183–188.

Exhibit 14-1 Summers' nutritional assessment profile.

CODE #_____

PART 1 DEMOGRAPHIC DATA

1. Age _____   2. Sex _____   3. Body Temperature at Time of Data
                                    Collection _____

4. Does the Patient have enough energy for daily activities?

                        Yes _____   No _____

5. Has the Patient had a change in appetite?   Yes _____   No _____

6. Has the Patient had a decrease in food intake?   Yes _____   No _____

7. Primary Diagnosis

   _____
   _____
   __

8. Secondary Diagnosis

   _____
   _____
   __

PART 2 NUTRITIONAL STATUS

PROTEIN INDICES   ELECTIVE _____   GENERAL _____
1.   Total Protein _____
2.   Albumin _____
3.   Blood Urea Nitrogen _____
4.   Prealbumin _____

FAT INDICES
5.   Cholesterol _____

CARBOHYDRATE INDICES
6.   Glucose _____

MINERAL INDICES
7.   Potassium _____
8.   Calcium _____
9.   Zinc _____
10. Magnesium _____

HEMATOLOGIC INDICES
11. Hemoglobin _____
12. Hematocrit _____
13. RBC _____
14. WBC _____
15. Lymphocytes _____
16. Total lymphocyte count _____
     (lymph x wbc/100)

Exhibit 14-2 Computerized spreadsheet for measuring nutritional status.

```
AGE:_____

SEX:_____
                              UNDER | NORMAL | OVER

                              _____|_____|_____

HEMOGLOBIN:___GMS____

RED CELL COUNT:___CU CM___

POTASSIUM:___MEQ/L___

CHOLESTEROL:____MG/100ML____

HEMATOCRIT:_____%

TOTAL PROTEIN:____GMS____

ALBUMIN:___GM/100ML___

WEIGHT:___LB__
                              LOW | MODERATE | HIGH

RECOVERY RISK:                ____|_____|_____
```

Exhibit 14-3 Computerized spreadsheet for assessing recovery risk: An example.

```
AGE:  44

SEX:  F
                         UNDER | NORMAL | OVER
                         _____|_____|_____

HEMOGLOBIN: 10.2 GMS

RED CELL COUNT: 3.5CU CM

POTASSIUM: 4.0 MEQ/L

CHOLESTEROL: 247 MG/100ML

HEMATOCRIT: 32 %

TOTAL PROTEIN: 5 GMS

ALBUMIN: 2.9 GM/100ML

WEIGHT: 115 LB
                         LOW | MODERATE | HIGH
RECOVERY RISK:           ____|_____|__X___

     LOW = NO ANTICIPATED
       PROBLEMS

     MODERATE = SOME
       PROBLEMS MAY
       OCCUR

     HIGH = HIGH RISK
       OF RECOVERY PROBLEMS
```

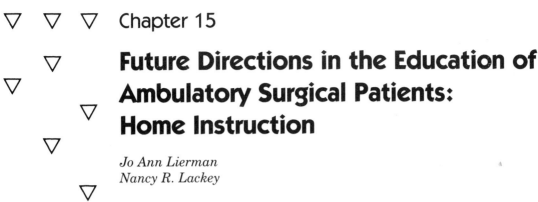

Chapter 15

Future Directions in the Education of Ambulatory Surgical Patients: Home Instruction

Jo Ann Lierman
Nancy R. Lackey

As a result of economic and regulatory forces restructuring the health care system, the ambulatory surgery unit (ASU) has become one of the most recognized and encouraged strategies for reducing health care costs. The current decade has seen a dramatic shift in the number and types of surgical procedures performed on an ambulatory basis. Increasingly, more complex surgeries are being performed on an outpatient basis. Ambulatory surgery centers, whether free-standing or operating within an institution, are beginning to feel the strain of the burgeoning number of surgeries. Nurses who work in these centers may experience role conflict, knowing that they should be spending more time with patients to allay fears, to answer questions, and to teach. As the number of surgical cases increases, the amount of time the nurse spends with the patient, both preoperatively and postoperatively, may decrease. Although the benefit of ambulatory surgery for the patient is minimal interruption of personal and family functioning, the psychological and physiological needs of these patients likely remain unchanged from those of inpatients. Nurses need to be prepared to meet the challenge of patient education in this health care setting to ensure that ambulatory surgical patients experience minimal discomfort and side effects from their surgical experience. The key questions to be answered in this chapter include:

1. What are the appropriate methods of assessing levels of preoperative patient anxiety?
2. What methods may be used to decrease anxiety and promote preoperative relaxation in the ambulatory surgery patient?
3. What is the role of the nurse in decreasing intraoperative anxiety through patient education?
4. What are some innovative teaching techniques that can be developed that are cost-effective and meet patient informational needs?

Exhibits for Chapter 15 are located at the end of the chapter on pages 288–290.

▽

Methods of Assessing Preoperative Anxiety

Many definitions of anxiety and many points of view on the subject of anxiety may be found in the literature.[1,2] Anxiety can be a mood, a feeling, an emotional response, a symptom, a syndrome, or an illness. Anxiety can be a diffused apprehension. It may generate feelings of uncertainty and helplessness in the face of danger.[2]

Anxiety is a normal human phenomenon. "At lower levels, anxiety is a useful state associated with mastery of the environment" (p. 2).[3] Anxiety is regarded as pathological when it interferes with general well-being or efficiency.

Lader also stated that:

A person experiencing anxiety responds with an increase in central nervous and peripheral sympathetic activity, such as increased muscle tone, which may be especially marked in the scalp muscles, and is manifested as tension headaches. The anxious person may be restless, unsettled, and fidgety. Tendon jerks and tic movements may often occur. The person may twist a lock of hair or bite fingernails. Respirations may be deeper and more frequent. Sighing is noticeable. Cardiovascular function may be disturbed, [with] tachycardia occurring. The person may perceive this disturbance as pounding in the chest or head. Peripheral vasoconstriction may be assessed as coldness in the extremities with an increased pulse pressure. In stressful situations, glandular activity changes may be noted in the form of decreased salivary output and increased palmar sweat. Hollow organ activity is noticed with an increased frequency of micturition and defecation, looseness of bowel movements, increased eructation, and borborygmi. The appetite and sleep patterns are disturbed. There may be a weight loss due to a poor appetite; although eating often is found to relieve anxiety and a weight gain may occur. The anxious person may have an inability to fall asleep followed by fitful and unrefreshing sleep (p. 56).[4]

Hospitalization frequently is psychologically threatening and can be conducive to the occurrence of anxiety in patients.[1,5] It is widely accepted that most people respond to anxiety-producing situations with increased anxiety, and that anxiety reactions are characterized by feelings of apprehension, tension, and activation of the autonomic nervous system.[6,7] The level of anxiety—mild, moderate, or severe—has implications for the planning and delivery of nursing care.[1,8]

Because surgical intervention and the ASU may be threatening, and anxiety may reach a level which could be detrimental to patient adaptation, nurses need to be able to assess and relieve anxiety in patients. High levels of anxiety have been shown to correlate with poor physical recovery.[9,10] Early significant nursing studies have shown that psychologically prepared patients have a better postsurgical recovery, based on one or more indices of recovery, than do those who are psychologically unprepared.[11-14]

When ill, a patient may be overwhelmed by anxiety about such factors as the perceived threat to life, the complexity of the disease and its attendant treatment modalities, and an unfamiliar environment. A sense of powerlessness may result because of an inability to control events. The extent of feelings of loss of control may influence the individual's ability to make short- and long-term adjustments to illness.[1,8]

The nurse must be able to recognize whether a patient is anxious. Subjective and objective anxiety data that the nurse should assess are outlined in Table 15-1. During a preoperative visit, the perioperative nurse has an ideal opportunity to assess anxiety in the patient and perhaps in the significant other. The nurse should be aware of physiological, emotional, and behavioral clues that would indicate the patient is anxious. At the time of the preoperative visit, the nurse should verbally encourage the patient or significant other to express any feelings of anxiety. On the day of surgery, the perioperative nurse has another opportunity for assessment of emotional status. While preparing the patient for the operation to be performed, the perioperative nurse can assess and intervene to reduce anxiety.

In the immediate postoperative period, assessment of the patient's anxiety level is also necessary. The patient's anxiety level may again increase as a result of factors such as concern regarding home care, family/significant others, what outcomes might result from surgery, type of dis-

Table 15-1 Signs of Anxiety

Subjective Data	Objective Data
Report of apprehension	Stuttering, voice quivering
Report of nervousness or worry	Hand tremors
Report of anxiety or symptom of anxiety (e.g., headache, low back pain, gastrointestinal distress)	Repetitive, purposeless movement
	Muscle tension, increased muscle tone
	Increased blood pressure and pulse
	Increased respirations
	Pupillary dilation
	Increased rate, volume, and pitch of voice
	Increased palmar sweating
	Increased bowel sounds
	Difficulty concentrating, self-focusing
	Narrowed perceptual field
	Inappropriate anger, guilt, fear, or regression
	Withdrawal, denial
	Increased wariness
	Excessive or repetitive questioning
	Avoidance of topics related to feelings

comfort to be expected at home, or the handling of potential complications at home. The nurse needs to remember that the postoperative period can be as anxiety-provoking as the preoperative period.

There may be occasions when the perioperative nurse makes initial contact with the patient by phone; anxiety can be assessed at this time as well. The nurse should be aware of the patient's communication patterns, voice tone, speech patterns, ability to focus on the conversation, general affect, any sign of unusual self-focusing or excessive questioning, or other signs that might indicate a highly anxious state.

▽

Methods to Decrease Preoperative Anxiety and Promote Relaxation

Illness frequently interrupts the typical day-to-day patterns that patients may have established to feel safe and secure. Surgical intervention involves many anxiety-producing situations for the patient, and may require various devices to assist in anxiety reduction. Basic to anxiety reduction is the need for the patient to attach some meaning to the event. It is important for the nurse to know how the anxiety of a patient can best be reduced and what factors need to be considered to divert the patient's energies most effectively. Since the perioperative nurse will certainly affect how patients respond to their environment, the nurse needs to provide patients with methods of coping with the anxiety-producing situations that arise.

Perioperative nursing practice is patient-centered. Preoperative and postoperative meetings with the patient can promote continuity of care and reduce anxiety. Reduction of the patient's anxiety level is important, and may enhance postoperative recovery.[15-18]

Many classic studies can be found in the literature which document, as early as the 1960s, that perioperative nursing interventions affect patients' psychological and physiological responses to the surgical experience. Meyers conducted a study involving 72 medical-surgical patients in which three different nursing approaches to patient communication—structured, irrelevant, and no communication—were examined.[19] The study revealed that the group of patients who received structured communication showed the greatest reduction in anxiety.

Groah conducted a survey of surgical patients and found that preoperative visits with the perioperative nurse were valued, and that the patient would be willing to pay for these visits.[20] Preoperative visits to the ASU could provide the patient with a tour, with information, and with the opportunity for the nurse to establish rapport with the patient. When the patient sees a familiar face the day of surgery, then the patient's anxiety may be reduced. Other studies found that preoperative nurse-patient interaction benefited the patient's surgical recovery, as measured by such factors as decreased use of narcotics, compliance with instruction, and decreased anxiety levels.[11,14,20-26]

Nurses need to be able to recognize anxiety in patients. It is first important to understand that illness, or the threat of it, usually generates anxiety. One of the roles of the nurse is to minimize patient anxiety by helping the patient channel energies into anxiety-reducing activities; the nursing literature has continually supported this idea.[1–5,26–27] An important point to remember is that the patient's perception or interpretation of the situation as a threat will determine the degree of anxiety present. If an event is not perceived as a threat, then the anxiety response may not be observed.

To understand patients, the nurse must encourage verbal disclosure of what patients are experiencing—their worries, fears, joys, and just how their world seems to them. Patients will act on the basis of their perception and the meaning it has for them. Nurse-patient interaction is fundamental to the concept of patient-centered care. One of the goals of this interaction is the fulfillment of emotional needs.[28]

The nurse-patient interaction involves communication. Communication is defined as a process that is continuous and involves change.[27] It includes all the processes by which people influence one another. Interpersonal communication attempts to understand other people's points of view from their frame of reference, which includes their feelings about the situation.[27] It is the transmission of messages from one person to another. Communication is most accurate when there is free feedback between persons. When patients feel free to ask questions, they arrive at a better understanding of what the nurse is trying to communicate.[27] Communication is also most effective when nonverbal messages are recognized, acknowledged, and accurately interpreted. Communication that is nonthreatening aids the flow of information and conveys a sincere interest toward others, facilitating positive interactions. The real value of effective communication lies in its ability to increase understanding.[27]

It is important for the nurse to be concerned with the patient's level of distress, because prevention and treatment of disease proceeds best when health care management does not cause the patient additional suffering. The pathological process and treatment may deplete the patient's inner resources. The success of preventive measures or treatments ultimately rests on the patient's own capacity to use them.[27] Any observation that is shared and explored with the patient is immediately useful in assessing and meeting their needs.[27]

Patient teaching that is individualized according to perceived patient needs may assist the patient in maintaining or regaining a sense of control.[16] Patient teaching has been recognized as an independent nursing role. Peplau describes nursing as a maturing force, an educative instrument.[15]

Redman defined teaching as "communication especially structured and sequenced to produce learning" (p. 9).[29] Redman stressed that the anxieties of hospitalization and surgery can be relieved by teaching. Wheeler believes the nurse must help patients cope with upcoming surgery.[28] By helping them to look at the situation realistically, by providing information, and by helping the patient resolve the stressful situation, a crisis situation secondary to excessive anxiety can be avoided.[28] The patient of the 1990s desires factual information. Anxiety can be a common reaction to the surgical experience when the patient lacks information, and this, in turn, can lead to ineffective coping. It is desirable to minimize the factors creating anxiety. Accurate expectations about physical sensations that are likely to be experienced will reduce anxiety attributable to threatening events. Johnson, Morrisey, and Leventhal conducted a study involving 48 subjects who were undergoing gastrointestinal endoscopic examinations.[30] Results of the study indicated that the group receiving information about the test, prior to its taking place, exhibited less anticipatory anxiety and required less tranquilizer sedation than the group that did not receive that information. The literature reviewed supports the idea that, regardless of the type of surgical intervention, psychoeducational interventions and therapeutic communication can be useful approaches in relieving anxiety and in influencing the outcome of day surgery.[16]

Teaching requires that the nurse listen and have respect for the patient's right to choose the type of information they want to hear. Based on the premise that patients are rational people who can understand all but perhaps the most technical aspects of their care, teaching must be varied according to each patient's need (see Chapter 7). It is unlikely that a patient will ask for more information than they are ready to assimilate, or for an answer they cannot bear to hear. Patients frequently worry about the present, and probably will reject teaching that is not relevant to the present. Teaching is an integral part of nursing for, through teaching, the patient is encouraged to talk about personal apprehensions and fears. Teaching, even if most of it is giving information, will foster an atmosphere of caring. Information enables patients to think about alternatives and express, mull over, or fight back at alternatives facing them. This nurse-patient interaction allows the patient to be an active partner in health care.[31] Numerous studies in the literature indicate that planned, interpersonal communication and the presentation of structured information reduce patient anxiety.[9,16,31]

Several behavioral strategies can be taught to patients preoperatively which may help the patient to control their own anxiety and cope more effectively. Various techniques of systematic muscle relaxation may be helpful in reducing sympathetic arousal symptoms of anxiety. The perioperative nurse can easily teach patients during a preoperative visit how to manage their anxiety effectively. Patients can be guided through a relaxation routine involving deep breathing and induced relaxation through guided imagery. Once relaxed, the patient can be taught some additional, progressive muscle relaxation techniques for long-term use. Diaphragmatic breathing routines and progressive muscle relaxation techniques provide the patient with a focal point and elicit control over body functions, leading to a decrease in anxiety levels. Muscle relaxation and breathing techniques are interventions that are easily implemented by the nurse to help patients cope effectively with the experience of surgery.[32]

It is commonly assumed that surgical intervention and the ASU environment are anxiety-provoking. Therapeutic communication, patient teaching, and the use of behavioral strategies can lead to a satisfying surgical experience for the patient and one in which the patient can cope effectively with anxiety. Exhibit 15-1 lists some nursing interventions and expected patient outcomes that are appropriate for patients with a nursing diagnosis of anxiety related to (R / T) the surgical experience.

▽

Intraoperative Anxiety Reduction

Intraoperative anxiety reduction for the ASU patient begins when the patient's case is scheduled. Perioperative nurses, however, report that patients frequently arrive in the operative room in a state of anxiety. Patients may exhibit anxiety by talking excessively, by body tremors, by crying, by facial expressions, and by increased heart rate and blood pressure. Preoperatively, some patients may conceptualize ideas about the procedure and what will happen during the surgical experience. The anxiety state may be the result of fear of the unknown or lack of information concerning what will happen in the operative area.

Anxiety and apprehension can be intensified in patients who have local rather than general anesthesia. The patient may be fearful of impending sights and pain. If the patient is undergoing facial surgery, for example, surgical drapes over the head, as well as the overhead lights that generate heat, and the pressure exerted on the face may combine to potentiate a feeling of suffocation. Grating, rasping, or suction noises may increase the patient's anxiety level.

Perioperative nurses may have responsibility for physiological monitoring during a surgical procedure undertaken with local anesthesia, but they must also remember to monitor the patient's anxiety level constantly. Anxiety can be assessed by monitoring vital signs, color changes, and perspiration levels. The nurse must validate what the patient is feeling, as some perioperative medications produce some of the same symptoms as anxiety. A list of physiological and psychological signs the nurse should assess as indicators of increased anxiety are listed in Table 15-2.

Defense mechanisms function to protect the individual from feelings of anxiety. These defense mechanisms may take the form of behavioral responses, like anger, denial, somatic complaints, and withdrawal, all of which may be used to reduce or avoid anxiety awareness. Regardless of the signs and symptoms that the patient exhibits, the perioperative nurse must be prepared to intervene when anxiety becomes too great.

A caring nurse-patient relationship is the first step in dealing with a

Table 15-2 Signs of Anxiety in the Patient Undergoing Local Anesthesia

Muscle cramps	Excessive questioning
Muscle tenseness or twitching	Clenching of fist
Muscle tremors	Jaw setting
Facial and body rigidity	Anxious, apprehensive look
Increased pulse and blood pressure	Inappropriate laughing
Rapid, shallow respirations; dyspnea	Excessive joking
Increased self-awareness	Scattered thoughts
Increased self-consciousness	Stuttering; blocking; rapid, pressured speech
Heightened perception of surroundings	Increased perspiration
Crying, tearfulness, sobbing	Flushing or pallor of face
Facial grimace	Darting eyes
Inappropriate anger, irritability	Quivering voice

patient's anxiety level. If the patient's anxiety level becomes excessive, the nurse may need to report the patient response to the surgeon and suggest that medication, such as a tranquilizer, be administered. Maladaptive anxiety occurs when an exaggerated response results in inappropriate behavioral patterns and decreased levels of performance.

The perioperative nurse must be an accepting listener and create opportunities for the patient to talk and express concerns. Therapeutic interactive communication is extremely important. The nurse's actions, voice tone, and eye expression should convey interest and concern for the patient as a person. As activity in the room and noises can heighten the patient's anxiety level, traffic in the room should be limited, and noise should be kept to a minimum. A sign on the outside of the operating room (OR) door helps to alert others that the patient is awake. Conversations in the room should include the patient in an effort to decrease anxiety.

Empathy on the part of the perioperative nurse can be enhanced if the nurse is educated to view the operative experience through the eyes of the patient. Attention to patient comfort and ventilatory ability greatly helps to reduce anxiety. Every effort should be made to meet patient requests, thereby allowing the patient to gain a sense of control and thus further reducing anxiety. The nurse needs to remember to keep the patient informed of the progress of the surgical experience. Information and knowledge regarding the surgical experience help to alleviate anxiety. A frequently overlooked anxiety intervention is touch. A gentle pat on the shoulder or holding the patient's hand can help to reduce anxiety in the awake patient. The awake patient presents a challenge to the perioperative nurse. The patient's anxiety level greatly affects postoperative recovery. Early recognition of anxiety and responsive intervention can provide a successful, satisfying surgical experience for the patient.

▽

Innovative Teaching Techniques to Meet
Patient Informational Needs

Patients who are admitted to ambulatory surgical centers vary as much as do their individual surgeries, ranging from the very young to the frail elderly; from the highly educated to the illiterate; from the upwardly mobile young career executive to the mentally retarded and physically handicapped individual. Professional nurses are taught that, before effective teaching/learning can occur, the learning needs of the patient should be assessed and a plan made for each patient. This method, devised for the inpatient, must be modified for the ambulatory surgery patient, primarily because of the decrease in contact time with the patient.

Currently, most patient teaching is done in the ASU one to two hours before the actual surgery begins. The nurse may well question how much of what is taught at this time is comprehended and retained by the patient. Immediately preoperatively, the patient may be focused only on their imminent surgery and its outcome. In the postoperative phase, prior to discharge, their focus changes to concerns about their activity level at home, as well as when they can return to work and their normal activities. Little thought is given to the possible complications that may arise as they recover at home without medical supervision. At this time, anxieties and fears may arise. If ambulatory surgical nurses are going to deal with these patient fears and reduce potential anxiety, they need to abandon traditional patient teaching techniques and develop new, innovative ones. These techniques must meet the patient's needs, be effective, and be both cost- and time-efficient. Both the content of patient teaching and the method of delivery must be changed to meet ASU patient demands and the numerous changes in the ambulatory setting that will be commonplace in the next century.

Research needs to be conducted before implementing any teaching techniques on a wide scale. The ASU nurse must first determine what patients need to know to make their experience a positive one. Too often, nurses assume that they know what patients need to know, without asking them, and then proceed to teach that content. Some of the questions that nurses need to ask include: What do ambulatory surgery patients perceive as their learning needs? How do ASU patients deal with their fears and anxieties? What causes ASU patient anxiety? What kind of information do ASU patients need to facilitate their postoperative recovery? When would be the best time to present information to the ASU patient, and by what method? Teaching strategies and content based on the results of a study designed around the answer to these questions would be an ideal approach to the development of innovative patient teaching techniques (see the section on Comparison of the Perceived Learning Needs of Patients and Nurses in Chapter 7).

There is basic information that is needed by all patients having ambulatory surgery, regardless of the type of procedure (see Chapters 3 and 7). In addition, information that might decrease patient anxiety could easily be included in a booklet that could be sent to the patient at the time the surgery is scheduled.

Some ASUs have established various teaching/learning protocols that require the patient to come to the unit a few days before the scheduled surgery for instruction. At this time, a nurse does one-on-one teaching in a session that lasts 30 to 90 minutes. Any member of the health care team deemed appropriate may be involved in these preadmission sessions, which are designed to teach the patient about the impending surgery and recovery phase. Nurses have prepared slide-tape presentations or closed circuit television programs that can be used for either individual or group instruction.[33,34] Ideally, after viewing such a program, there would be a follow-up session with the nurse that would allow an opportunity for patients to ask questions and to receive further information specific to their impending surgery. The main disadvantage to this type of learning is that patients scheduled for surgery have to take time off from work or family obligations and come to the ASU for instruction at a time that may not be convenient for them. One solution might be to develop cost-effective, preoperative teaching programs that could be utilized by patients in their home environment at their leisure, yet still be effective in providing the patient with information needed for surgery and recovery.

In a study completed by Lierman and Lackey, a videotape was produced that taught anxiety reduction techniques to patients who were scheduled for arthroscopy in the ambulatory surgery setting.[35] A two-group experimental design was used (N = 50 for each group). Patients in the experimental group completed a questionnaire and were required to view the videotape with the investigator, and practice the relaxation methods as they viewed the tape. Patients were then loaned the tape and told that they could view the tape and practice the relaxation techniques as many times as they wished preoperatively and postoperatively. The tape and a post-test with a questionnaire were picked up by the investigators three to four days after surgery. Patients in the control group did not receive a videotape or any instruction in relaxation techniques. They were required to complete a post-test questionnaire only. Patients reported that they liked being able to view the tape as needed to relax.[35] Similarly, it may be possible to produce videotapes containing information on specific surgical procedures. When patients were scheduled for a specific procedure, they could then be sent the appropriate tape and could view it as many times as they desired preoperatively and postoperatively. Hotlines could also be established that would allow the patient to call for answers to questions not covered by the tape.

Alternatively, the ASU could establish a dial-a-surgery information service. When the prospective patient was scheduled for surgery, they could call the service at their convenience and as many times as needed for specific instructions about admission procedures, the recovery phase, and general information about their particular impending surgery. At the end of the message, an additional telephone number could be given that would allow the ASU patient to call and talk to a nurse regarding answers to specific questions that were not covered in the recorded message.

Many prospective surgical patients now have access to computers, either at home or in their place of employment. Computer-structured packages could be developed and given to the prospective patient at the time their surgery was scheduled. Again, the patient could work through the tutorial package at their convenience, and as many times as they desired. Prospective patients having computers with modems could access a hospital tutorial program designed to give them general instructions, as well as specific instructions regarding their surgery and postoperative recovery.

Patient teaching by means of videotapes, telephone, and computer programs are, indeed, innovative methods. Nursing research is needed to explore these methods further and to determine their degree of usefulness.

Programmed learning packages have been utilized with success in some learning environments. Wong and Wong developed five learning activity packages (LAP) that were designed to teach patients who were scheduled for total hip replacements.[36] These packages contained information about surgery, admission, preoperative procedures, (deep breathing, leg exercises and logrolling), possible postoperative complications, immediate postoperative procedures, and long-term rehabilitation. Patients receiving this type of preoperative instruction expressed a high level of satisfaction with this teaching approach.[36] Similar learning packages could be developed for the ASU patient and distributed, along with instructions for their use, at the time surgery was scheduled.

Learning packages can also be developed for those prospective patients who have special needs. For the segment of the patient population that is illiterate, booklets similar to comic books have been developed for patient teaching. These booklets, which include numerous pictures that demonstrate various procedures, contain a minimum amount of written instructions (Exhibit 15-2). Patients who have been given these booklets have expressed a high level of satisfaction regarding the material covered and the method of presentation.

Audiotapes covering specific preoperative and postoperative instructions could be developed for the visually impaired. Closed-caption videotapes containing similar instructions could be used for the hearing impaired.

▽

Summary

Perhaps the most effective teaching/learning techniques for ASU patients involve a combination of audiovisual methods. Preoperative teaching techniques and materials need to be developed that allow patients to utilize them at their own pace and within their own home. Before any type of teaching/learning techniques are developed, more research must be conducted that describes the ambulatory surgery population and identifies their specific learning needs. Once appropriate teaching/learning techniques have been developed, they need to be subjected to additional testing to determine their effectiveness. The ASU is becoming a permanent part of the health care setting. Professional nurses can play a vital role in the development of methods to decrease patient anxiety. It is an opportune time to move from traditional patient teaching methods to new ones that enhance the ASU experience for patients by decreasing their anxiety.

References

1. Nyamathi, A., & Kashiwabara, A. (1988). Preoperative anxiety: Its effect on cognitive thinking. *AORN Journal, 47,* 164–170.
2. May, R. (1950). *The meaning of anxiety.* New York: The Ronald Press Company.
3. Lader, M. & Marks, I. (1971). *Clinical Anxiety.* New York: Grune & Stratton.
4. Lader, M. H. (1970). Physical and psychological aspects of anxiety and depression. *The British Journal of Clinical Practice, 24,* 55–59.
5. Alberts, M. S., Lyons, J. S., & Moretti, R. J. (1989). Psychological interventions in the pre-surgical period. *International Journal of Psychiatry in Medicine, 19,* 91–106.
6. Freud, S. (1936). *The problem of anxiety.* New York: W.W. Norton.
7. Spielberger, C. D., & Sarason, I. G. (1975). *Stress and anxiety.* New York: John Wiley & Sons.
8. Scott, I. O. (1983). Anxiety, critical thinking and information processing during and after breast biopsy. *Nursing Research, 32,* 24–28.
9. Jamison, R. N., Parris, W. C. V., & Maxson, W. S. (1987). Psychological factors influencing recovery from outpatient surgery. *Behavior Research and Theory, 25,* 31–37.
10. Mathews, A., & Ridgeway, V. (1981). Personality and surgical recovery: A review. *British Journal of Clinical Psychology, 20,* 243–260.
11. Johnson, J. E. (1972). Effects of structuring patients' expectations on their reactions to threatening events. *Nursing Research, 21,* 499–504.
12. Johnson, J. E., Dabbs, J. M., & Leventhal, H. (1970). Psychosocial factors in the welfare of surgical patients. *Nursing Research, 19,* 18–29.
13. Hartfield, M., Cason, C., & Cason, G. (1982). Effects of information about a threatening procedure on patient's expectations and emotional distress. *Nursing Research, 31,* 202–206.
14. Schmitt, F. E., & Wooldridge, P. J. (1973). Psychological preparation of surgical patients. *Nursing Research, 22,* 108–116.
15. Peplau, H. E. (1952). *Interpersonal relations in nursing.* New York: G. P. Putnam's Sons.
16. Rothrock, J. C. (1989). Perioperative nursing research: Preoperative psychoeducational intervention. *AORN Journal, 49,* 597–619.
17. Icenhour, M. L. (1988). Quality interpersonal care: A study of ambulatory surgery patients' perspectives. *AORN Journal, 47,* 1415–1418.
18. Kempe, A. R. (1987). Patient education for the ambulatory patient. *AORN Journal, 45,* 500–507.
19. Meyers, M. E. (1964). The effects of types of communication on patients' reactions to stress. *Nursing Research, 13,* 126–131.

20. Groah, L. (1979). Do patients value preoperative assessment? *AORN Journal, 29,* 1250–1256.
21. Dumas, R. G., & Leonard, R. C. (1963). The effects of nursing on the incidence of postoperative vomiting. *Nursing Research, 12,* 12–15.
22. Egbert, L. D., Battit, G. E., Welch, C. E., & Bartlett, M. K. (1964). Reduction of postoperative pain by encouragement and instruction of patients. *New England Journal of Medicine, 270,* 825–827.
23. Kinney, M. R. (1977). Effects of preoperative teaching upon patients with differing modes of response to threatening stimuli. *International Journal of Nursing, 14,* 49–59.
24. Wallis, R. (1971). Preoperative visits—A challenge for O.R. nurses. *AORN Journal, 14,* 53–56.
25. Lindeman, C. A., & Van Aernam, B. (1971). Nursing intervention with the presurgical patient—Effects of structured and unstructured preoperative teaching. *Nursing Research, 20,* 319–331.
26. Wolfer, J. A., & Davis, C. E. (1970). Assessment of surgical patients' preoperative emotional condition and postoperative welfare. *Nursing Research, 19,* 402–414.
27. Beare, P. G., & Myers, J. L. (1990). *Principles and practice of adult health nursing* (pp. 416–421). St. Louis: C.V. Mosby.
28. Wheeler, B. R. (1988). Crisis intervention: Recognizing and helping patients overcome anxiety. *AORN Journal, 47,* 1242–1248.
29. Redman, B. (1988). *The process of patient teaching in nursing.* St. Louis: C. V. Mosby.
30. Johnson, J. E., Morrisey, J. F., & Leventhal, H. (1973). Psychological preparation for an endoscopic examination. *Gastrointestinal Endoscopy, 19,* 180–182.
31. DeMuth, J. S. (1989). Patient teaching in the ambulatory setting. *Nursing Clinics of North America, 24,* 645–654.
32. Wilson, J. F. (1981). Behavioral preparation for surgery: Benefit or harm? *Journal of Behavioral Medicine, 4,* 79–102.
33. Colton, M., Lowi, M., & McCann, M. (1986). Preoperative patient program lightens nurses' teaching load. *Dimensions in Health Services 63,* 21,37.
34. Worobey, J. (1985, May). *Using closed-circuit television as a teaching tool: Implications for health communication educators.* Paper presented at the Eastern Communication Association, Instructional Practices Interest Group, Providence, RI.
35. Lierman, J. A., & Lackey, N. R. (1989). *The effect of relaxation on reduction of anxiety and pain.* Unpublished manuscript, University of Kansas, School of Nursing, Kansas City, Kansas.
36. Wong, J., & Wong, S. (1985). A randomized controlled trial of a new approach to preoperative teaching and patient compliance. *International Journal of Nursing Studies, 22,* 105–115.

Exhibit 15-1 Nursing care plan.

Nursing Diagnosis	Patient Goal	Nursing Orders	Evaluation
Preoperative			
Anxiety R/T unfamiliar surroundings and surgical procedure	Patient will express understanding of surgical procedure, preparatory actions, and surroundings.	Review sequence of and rationale for perioperative events.	Patient expressed an understanding of the sequence and purpose of events.
		Encourage verbalization of questions and concerns.	
		Provide noninvasive relaxation techniques.	
		Give emotional support.	
		Review anticipated effects/ sensations of preparatory medications.	
		Assure patient of constant care and monitoring.	
Sensory-perceptual alteration R/T loss of vision after block and postoperatively	Patient will verbalize expectation of temporary vision loss and alteration in depth perception	Describe blocking procedure and the resulting loss of vision in the operative eye.	Patient anticipated loss of vision after block and expressed understanding of monocular vision.
		Review the doctor's routine for postoperative patching.	
		Discuss the perceptual alteration resulting from monocular vision (lack of depth perception, decrease in field).	
		Approach patient from non affected side.	
High risk for injury R/T sedation and impaired sensory/perceptual functioning	Patient will remain injury free.	Continuously orient patient to environment.	Patient was free from injury related to transfers or positioning.
		Keep side rails up and safety strap on.	
		Assess patient's ROM and position for comfort throughout perioperative stay.	
		Supervise patient during all transfers.	
High risk for injury R/T infection	Patient will remain free of infection.	Monitor aseptic technique throughout perioperative period.	Patent was free of signs and symptoms of infection postoperatively.
		Educate patient postoperatively regarding signs and symptoms of infection (fever, drainage).	
High risk for ineffective breathing pattern R/T sedation, draping	Patient will maintain adequate oxygen exchange.	Review rationale for administering oxygen while applying patient's cannula.	Adequate respiratory exchange was maintained throughout procedure.
		Explain purpose of oxygen monitor.	
		Check drape position to ensure proper cannula positioning and patient comfort.	

Exhibit 15-1 (Continued)

Nursing Diagnosis	Patient Goal	Nursing Orders	Evaluation
High risk for injury R/T positioning, prepping solution, alterations in skin integrity	Patient will remain free from injury related to positioning or physical hazards.	Encourage patient to provide feedback to ensure comfortable positioning; position according to policy and procedure. Assess skin integrity and pressure points. Cleanse patient's skin of residual prepping solution prior to discharge from OR.	Patient remained injury-free and comfortable in relation to alterations in skin integrity and reactions to prepping solutions.
Altered communication, R/T sensory deprivation secondary to draping	Patient will continue to express needs and concerns intra-operatively.	Discuss the need to remain quiet with minimal movement during procedure. Implement a communication system (e.g. patient will move exposed hand, not head, when needing to speak).	Patient squeezed nurse's hand before speaking.
Altered oral mucus membranes (dryness), R/T NPO status and use of diuretics, hyperosmotics.	Patient will remain comfortable.	Explain the drying effects of NPO and medications. Moisten patient's lips with water or lemon glycerin swab prior to procedure	Patient verified increased comfort after nursing intervention.

Postoperative

Nursing Diagnosis	Patient Goal	Nursing Orders	Evaluation
Altered health maintenance R/T postoperative care regimen	Patient will express an understanding of postoperative regimen.	Review postoperative activity restrictions and medication instructions Provide large print written instruction sheet. Provide time for and encourage patient questions. Demonstrate eye drop instillation and bandaging technique. Discuss pain management. Explain importance of protecting operative eye (shield, glasses). Review normal and abnormal signs and symptoms. Make follow-up call to patient two days after surgery.	Patient expressed an understanding of instructions and expectations prior to discharge from unit. Patient repeated eye drop instructions.
Altered home maintenance management R/T change in vision and activity levels	An effective plan for patient's home management will be in place prior to discharge.	Review importance of compliance with activity restrictions. Emphasize the perceptual impact of monocular vision. Facilitate involvement of patient's support system.	Patient and support system had an understanding of the need for assistance and participated in formation of plan for dealing with alteration in visual acuity and activity levels. Follow-up phone call was made to evaluate effectiveness of plan.

HOME RECOVERY EXERCISES

Rebuilding the muscles that support your knee—your quadriceps, hamstrings, and calf muscles—is one of the best ways to help your knee recover fully. The sooner you start these exercises, the better. Your goal is to avoid both overuse of these muscles (this causes inflammation, pain, and swelling) and underuse (this causes stiffness and

☐ For Strength

☐ **Quadriceps sets** help rebuild your front thigh muscles, which give your knee its greatest stability. "Quad sets" can be done anywhere, anytime, lying down or sitting. Simply tighten your quadriceps to press your knee toward the floor or bed. Hold for 5–10 seconds, then relax. It may help to rest your hand on your kneecap and feel it move upward slightly as you tighten your muscles.

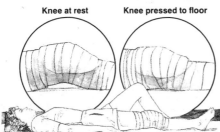

Knee at rest   Knee pressed to floor

Starting date	Repetitions	Sets per day

☐ **Toe presses** help rebuild your calf muscles. Simply press up on your toes with both feet, hold for 5–10 seconds, and slowly lower your heels. Use a support for balance.

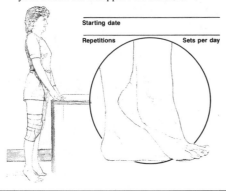

Starting date		
Repetitions		Sets per day

☐ **Straight leg raises** help rebuild all of the muscles that support your knee.

To the front. Lie on your back and do a "quad set." Lift your leg 8"–12". Hold 4–6 seconds, then slowly lower and repeat.

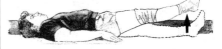

To the back. Lie on your stomach and lift your leg straight behind you 8"–12". Hold 4–6 seconds, then slowly lower and repeat.

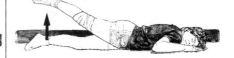

To the outside. Lie on your side, and lift your bandaged leg 12"–24". Hold 4–6 seconds, then slowly lower and repeat.

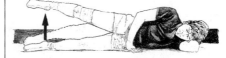

To the inside. Rest your leg on a low support as shown. Lift your bandaged leg up to touch ankles. Hold 4–6 seconds, lower, and repeat.

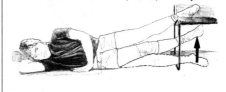

Starting date	Repetitions	Sets per day

▽ ▽ ▽ Chapter 16

Nursing Education Strategies: Ambulatory Surgery to Home Care

Elizabeth Monninger

Unprecedented changes are occurring in health care every day that not only affect the nursing care given and the structure of the nurse/client relationship, but also the economics, ethical decisions, accountability, and learning processes underlying health care delivery. Naisbitt describes many societal transformations in his book, *Megatrends*. His charge to all of us fits well with the goals of nursing care: "We must learn to balance the material wonders of technology with the spiritual demands of our human nature" (p. 40).[1] Further, Naisbitt notes important trends that impact our lives and our professions; among these are the movements from an industrial to an informational society, and from a purely technological focus to a high tech/high touch society.[1] Technology, as well as the acuity of illnesses and new patterns of providing care also have an impact on nursing education. Nursing educators must find ways to prepare graduates of nursing programs to be effective in future systems. Nursing's body of knowledge, categories of phenomena, and relationship with other disciplines and clients must be examined; the scope of nursing care, as well as nursing process and focus, must change, or professional stagnation will be rampant. Such was the case in one country long ago.

> Once upon a time, in a country far away, the sabertooth tiger curriculum was the most famous in all the land. Sabertooth tigers were feared by all the citizens because they were so ferocious and they killed many people. Leaders of the land formed a committee and demanded that an effective curriculum be developed to teach all men and women to rid the country of the dreaded animals. Educators responded and designed an excellent course of study, teaching students to stalk and kill sabertooth tigers. In fact, the courses were so good that soon, no sabertooth tigers were to be found in the whole country. However, since the curriculum was judged to be so outstanding, the educators continued to teach sabertooth tiger hunting long after those tigers existed.[2]

This analogy is applicable to the education of nurses. Early in the twentieth century, most health care took place outside the hospital. Few sophisticated treatment regimens were available, so palliative measures

Exhibits for Chapter 16 are located at the end of the chapter on pages 306–313.

were the preferred mode of care until technology, antibiotics, and other drug treatments were developed. In order to accommodate implementation of scientific health care measures, hospitals expanded rapidly. Nursing care shifted from the home care setting of earlier times to hospitals, which became nurses' principal place of employment. Therefore, the culture of nursing reflected the bureaucratic nature of hospitals, and nursing care was shaped to respond to large inpatient populations. The hospitalized clients' incumbency extended as long as was needed to recover from hospital-instituted treatments. A team nursing approach was formulated to organize the provision of care for large groups of patients by multiple levels of providers. Intensive care and cardiac care teams of nurses became technically proficient. Patients entered the hospital for treatment, only to lose their identity and to be required to adhere to the "hospital routine." Hospitals and the hospitalized patient population continued to grow for more than 30 years.

During the 1980s, prospective payment plans for insurance and governmental reimbursement became the driving force that reshaped the focus of health care and determined the amount of care available, as well as where that care was delivered. As a result of burgeoning costs, hospital stays were abruptly reduced. Innovative outpatient treatments were found to be effective. The focus of health care again shifted to the community outside the hospital. Health care is now on the fast track; clients frequently receive highly technical care, including surgical treatment, in ambulatory care facilities, and return home in less than 24 hours. The number of occupied hospital beds has decreased daily, whereas ambulatory treatments and home care follow-up programs are expanding rapidly. The recipients of care are informed consumers who are now learning self-care and preventive measures that will reduce their health care expenditures.

Now, in the 1990s, nurses need to prepare for predicted changes in health care. In a recent publication, *Ten Trends To Watch,* the next decade was described as an "era of opportunity for nursing."[3] Nursing is projected to be the link between the client and quality health care, with an increasing focus on the total person. Cost-containment pressures will result in greater and more frequent ethical dilemmas. Independent nursing decision making and advances in health care technology mandate refocused educational preparation, as do an increasing consumer health awareness and the shift of health care from the hospital to the community. These emerging trends should be reflected in nursing curricula if nursing is to be a viable and effective profession.

Will nursing education respond to these new trends and prepare health care providers who collaborate with clients to reduce health care needs and improve health? Or will nurses continue to teach "sabertooth tiger hunting" long after those tigers cease to exist? A new educational perspective reflecting the projected health care changes is proposed.

The purpose of this chapter is to present a framework for preparing nursing students to provide holistic patient care in the future, using the emerging model of short-stay or ambulatory surgery-to-home clients. The following questions are addressed:

1. What educational strategies and clinical experiences are needed for placing the ambulatory surgical nurse role in the undergraduate curriculum?
2. What are the curricular needs to educate the master's-prepared perioperative clinical specialist?
3. What are the future directions in nursing education that may meet nurse/patient needs in ambulatory surgery settings?

▽

Strategies for Placing the Ambulatory Surgical Nurse Role in the Undergraduate Curriculum

Undergraduate nursing education provides preparation for nurse generalist practice. Undergraduate students learn theory and practice in all areas of nursing in order to acquire a context for the needs of all clients, and also to be able to practice nursing in any setting, at least at a beginning level. In baccalaureate nursing (BSN) programs, students are taught decision-making processes, which include assessment, prioritizing needs, use of data from clients, families, communities, and other sources for diagnosing client needs; planning; implementing and evaluating nursing care.

Bevis has suggested that the following criteria be used for guiding BSN curriculum planning:[4]

1. Implement a conceptual framework that supports rendering nursing care for real community health needs.
2. Employ the knowledge explosion and rapid change in scientific knowledge.
3. Provide student learning in reality situations.
4. Graduate nurses who are capable of delivering creative nursing care for the next 15 to 20 years.

Traditionally, BSN curricula have merely expanded the historical precedent of the hospital/pathology-based patient care model. Even though students study health-oriented content and provide some care for individuals and families in the community, the nursing culture defines acute, institutional care as the benchmark in nursing. One often hears of the standard which indicates that the nurse needs a substantial amount of hospital experience, before and after graduation, in order to be an effective nurse in the area of community/out-of-hospital patient care. It is interesting that the hospital is still the focal point of a profession whose goal is optimal health and high-level functioning.

Nursing education programs must respond to the health needs of society and provide clinical practice for students in reality situations. Even though out-of-hospital clinical placements may create problems with student supervision, these are the settings that offer contemporary nursing practice opportunities. In ambulatory care settings, students may be placed with preceptors who are experienced role models. A contractual arrangement between the school of nursing and agencies may involve financial reimbursement for preceptor supervision. Although this requires an investment on the part of both the school and the agency, unless student nurses become comfortable with practice in ambulatory settings, nursing's role in out-of-hospital settings will not develop to the extent that intensive and cardiac nursing care and other inpatient roles have matured. Nursing students must master discharge planning; patient teaching; advocacy and support of self-care; assessment of the contextual parameters of care in homes; administration of highly technical care in out-of-hospital environments; consultation with lay health care providers, such as family members; accessing community resources; and case management. Independent functioning and decision making, as well as interdisciplinary collaboration, are necessary in less structured settings, and must be incorporated into the goals of educational programs. These behaviors are learned through teaching methods and by providing settings for student practice that accommodate and provide support for autonomy and role modeling by faculty, preceptors, and other professionals. Ambulatory surgical units (ASUs) are excellent examples of practice settings in which student learning takes place in reality situations, and in which provisions are made for appropriate role models and patient care practices essential for mastery of the behaviors needed for futuristic roles.

The goal of patient care in ASUs is to achieve optimal functioning, comfort, and effective self-care. Ambulatory surgical clients need high tech/high touch care. In this setting, the novice student can gain experience in wellness and self-care practices. In fact, this setting may offer a wide and varied perspective for beginning students: interviewing and other communication skills practice; holistic assessment, with emphasis on health histories; observation and beginning participation in high tech care in operating rooms (OR) and recovery units; family dynamics; discharge planning; client and family teaching; anticipatory guidance; marketing; health care economics; and nursing care planning, with functional health patterns as the focus.

Advanced students may benefit from investigating and practicing in more complex situations in ASUs, with more indepth study of change, adaptation to stress, bioinstrumentation (e.g., the use of ventilators), and client/family education for those requiring technological devices, such as pacemakers, computerized drug delivery systems, or multiple devices. These advanced students may also assist with discharge decisions based on computerized acuity indexing, and may consult with members of other disciplines, including social workers, physical therapists, and speech therapists.

These patterns of undergraduate education synthesize Carnaveli's concepts of the domains or categories of phenomena that are of central concern to nursing[5] and the Dreyfus model of levels of proficiency.[6] They also incorporate major trends influencing health care.[5]

Carnaveli's Nursing Model

Carnaveli described the essence of the discipline of nursing according to major categories of concern and the relationships that exist among those phenomena. She categorized the essence or central concern of nursing as activities of daily living and functional health status.[5] The relationships, according to Carnaveli, are "concerned with the interaction and inter-dependence between these two groups of phenomena, daily living as it affects functional health status and conversely, functional health status as it affects participation in daily living" (p. 16).[5]

This model focuses on a person's resources and requirements for daily living, and may be viewed as a framework for providing wellness care. Further, Carnaveli suggested that nurses assess, diagnose, and treat those occurrences, issues, or phenomena that affect daily living, and assist with incorporating those circumstances or their consequences (whether they be crises, technology, or other treatment regimens) into their life-styles.[5]

Dreyfus Model

The Dreyfus model of proficiency served as the basis for Benner's hall-mark work, *From Novice to Expert: Excellence and Power in Clinical Nursing Practice,*[6] in which levels of competency in nursing practice were delineated. This model characterizes the various levels of proficiency:[6]

Novice—One who has little or no experience and therefore must use rules to guide practice;

Advanced beginner—One who performs adequately, but continues to rely on directions or preformulations to guide practice and is beginning to be able to prioritize;

Competent—That practitioner who is able to envision long-term goals of care and to organize that care;

Proficient—One who is able to perceive a situation and its context as a systematic process, and uses experience as well as knowledge to evaluate data and make decisions; and

Expert—One who is quickly able to assess situations, make effective decisions in an expeditious manner, and identify broad solutions, taking into consideration the context and dynamics of a particular circumstance.

These definitions of levels of competency in nursing may be used in planning clinical experiences in BSN and master's degree in nursing educational programs, with the BSN students performing at the novice and advanced beginner levels and the graduate student performing at the competent and proficient levels.

New Perspectives for BSN Student Learning

If ASUs are defined as emerging examples of community-based care, the perspective of nursing education strategies in those settings must reflect that notion. The ambulatory surgical client is a family and community member who is seeking assistance for a defined problem and returns to the family and community immediately after the surgical intervention. Therefore, the phenomena of concern must include the patient's functional health status and activities of daily living in the context of the client's family and community. Too often, the client is viewed from the perspective of the medical diagnosis, or only the individual's health status, ignoring contextual factors—the realism of where the person functions, the support systems that affect that functioning, the legal constraints, and the economic factors that impact the activities of daily living. Ambulatory surgical clients can provide learning opportunities for students to gain this holistic nursing care experience.

The novice student should study the less complex and more predictable client example, such as an individual anticipating repair of a simple hernia in the ASU. The student may have first contact with such a client in the presurgical assessment unit. A health assessment may be completed which would include not only the client's health history, but information about support systems in the family and community and economic perspectives (such as sick leave from the job and health insurance coverage and the need for child care during and after the surgical intervention). The novice student may use a structured approach to assessment, utilizing preestablished history forms, such as the "Perioperative Assessment Tool" shown in Exhibit 16-1. This form assists the novice student in synthesizing family, cultural, economic, and community perspectives, and relates clients' problems to functional health patterns, activities of daily living, and nursing diagnoses. The student may also assess the client in preoperative, intraoperative, and postoperative phases. The student should participate in discharge planning and family teaching. Follow-up home visits are essential in order for the student to assess the context of care in the family and community. This view of the client as one who comes from the community and then returns to the community provides experience for students that establishes a contemporary and broad concept of the scope of nursing practice. Exhibit 16-2 shows a course outline that illustrates this perspective and places the novice student in the ambulatory surgical setting.

Advanced beginners (junior or senior students) may assume responsibility for more complex client care. Teams of more advanced students may study multiple modes and sites for providing nursing care in the community, using a broad body of knowledge to plan a more inclusive scope of nursing care. For example, this team of students might study a designated community. Contextual data may be collected that describes the spectrum of sociocultural and economic characteristics, community resources, employment situations, housing descriptions, and legal constraints of that community. Health risks would be identified, as would exemplary patient care situations.

Each student could assess, plan, and provide care for a client or a group of clients, each with differing care needs than other students' clients. For instance, one student may identify a client with hypertension through participation in an industrial health screening experience in the designated community. In a community clinic, another student may identify a client who has a high-risk pregnancy. Other students could identify prototype clients through study of a variety of community organizations, such as physician groups, home health agencies, schools, emergency rooms, ASUs, and other community-based health care organizations. The family and community data base thus forms the common context and organizational structure for all the clients being cared for by the student group. The purpose of this group client-care experience is to conceptualize the scope of nursing practice in a specified community by asking: "What nursing care is needed by this community?" Concepts involved in the practice of nursing may be studied, such as quality of care assessment, total patient care, cost containment, consumer health awareness, abuse problems, epidemiology, interdisciplinary communications in health care, and case management. The resulting perception of nursing care will be that of professional practice, and a community-based, rather than an institution-based job.

The ASU is a rich setting for studying exemplary clients who may provide case management experiences for students. The case manager assumes responsibility for coordinating all care provided by a variety of health care team members, such as the physician, physical therapist, pharmacist, and others. The case manager plans with the client to identify stressors, as well as strategies for continuity of care. For example, the initial contact with the client may be in an industrial setting, where severe pain in the right hand of the client is diagnosed as carpal tunnel syndrome and surgical treatment is prescribed by a surgeon. The student nurse may work with the industrial nurse, who serves as both a resource and a preceptor regarding health care in the work place. Home visits reveal support resources, as well as potential stressors, in the family. The student, as case manager, may oversee the client's preparation for surgery, examine health insurance coverage, participate with a surgical nurse preceptor in the ASU, and provide surgical ambulatory care under the direct supervision of a preceptor and the instructor. Assessment of family support, formulation of a teaching plan regarding residual muscle weakness, and coordination among the patient and physical therapy and supervising daily regimes of exercise, may be case management responsibilities. Follow-up by the student case manager of the client's recovery from surgery to regained muscle strength, as well as assessment of any disability and coordination with the industrial nurse are all measures of continuity of care and case management.

Study of the community and case management of a variety of clients in ambulatory care units by a group of students provides an understanding of the spectrum of community nursing care needs and a survey of case management experiences. The most important outcomes of such an arrangement are the assumption of responsibilities and the recognition of the scope of nursing function which include not only acute care needs (such as surgical intervention and immediate recovery care), but the community to acute care and return to the community spectrum of nursing care. Too often we segregate client care to isolated settings and time periods. If ASUs and other prevailing health care settings are specified as the fulcrum for continuity of care and student experiences, the field of nursing practice may begin to extend. Clients may begin to expect that nurses are the professionals who have the unique ability to strengthen their coping with illness and direct their way to recovery. If student experiences continue to be isolated to a specified setting, nursing practice will continue to be fragmented and establishment-oriented, instead of client-centered.

▽

Curricular Strategies for Educating the Master's-Prepared Perioperative Clinical Specialist

Clinical nurse specialists are prepared through graduate study and advanced levels of patient care. These nurses deliver advanced nursing care based on indepth theoretical study and application of theory to practice. Clinical specialist preparation also focuses on the development of beginning research skills. According to the Dreyfus model of practice, clinical specialists' competency level is "competent to proficient"; that is, they are able to envision long-term goals of care and assume organizational responsibilities. Some clinical specialists may well be at the level of "proficient"; that is, they are able to perceive a situation as a systematic process, using their experience to evaluate data and to make decisions.[6]

The perioperative clinical specialist curriculum focuses on the following components: theoretical approaches to practice; beginning research process; evaluation of the use of biotechnology; management and marketing; health care and community systems; and perioperative case management.

Theoretical approaches in perioperative practice may apply systems theory and models of nursing practice. For example, Sister Callista Roy's model explains adaptation of the person and his environment. Other theoretical concepts are described by Orem, Rogers, Stevens, Neuman, and Johnson.[7] A survey of nursing theories is useful to analyze the processes and goals of nursing practice, and to provide direction for planning, providing, and evaluating nursing care. Marriner proposes that "nurses' power is increased through theoretical knowledge because systematically developed methods are more likely to be successful."[8] Further, Chinn and Jacobs contend that the study of theory develops analytical skills and links concepts guiding professional practice.[9]

Research or scientific inquiry is essential for any profession in order to improve the practice of its members and to develop the body of knowledge that is fundamental to practice.[10] Clinical specialists are called upon to identify clinical problems and to work with doctorally prepared nurses to investigate these problems. A continual and cooperative process of inquiry is needed in order for the nursing service that is provided for clients to be effective. Therefore, the clinical specialist program must provide preparation in beginning research skills, as well as in the application of theory.

As the discipline of nursing develops through practice, theory development, and scientific inquiry, master's-prepared clinical specialists have increasing responsibilities to assist in refining and testing the nursing diagnoses and functional health patterns now being formulated. The challenge is to translate theory into practice in a variety of settings.[11–14] According to Benner:[6]

> A [nursing] theory is needed that describes, interprets, and explains not an imagined ideal of nursing, but actual expert nursing as it is practiced day to day. This type of theory could be used to develop curricula in which practice informs nursing education in a way that nursing education has always influenced practice.

The interaction of theory, practice, and education begins at the undergraduate level, is studied in more depth and tested in master's education, and new theories emerge through doctoral preparation. It is only through the interaction of practice, research, and education that nursing practice and its taxonomy (nursing diagnoses and functional health patterns) will develop and be refined.

The ASU may emerge as the prototype for nursing practice because it spans institutional and community nursing responsibilities. Perioperative nursing as a specialty practice in ambulatory settings involves marketing[15] and management skills,[16] as well as direct care of clients and families involving caring,[17,18] continuity of care,[19,20] and biotechnology.[21] Study of these concepts is integral to graduate clinical specialist preparation.

Gamotis and associates have noted that "the pendulum has swung from the patient as a docile, passive recipient of health care to the well-informed consumer who questions health care and evaluates health care providers."[15] These authors call our attention to the importance of patient satisfaction and a professional portrait that depicts competence and quality. Customer satisfaction is the goal of all marketing ventures. The consumer's voice and the perceptions of the well-informed client are primary concerns of health care organizations as well as of nurses themselves. Further, clients who respond most positively to therapeutic regimens are those who believe that the nurse providing their care is knowledgeable; engages in answering questions, explanations, and demonstration; and shows interest and listens.[15] Outpatient clients were shown to be most satisfied with teaching efforts on the part of nurses.[15]

Health care has become a competitive market. Therefore, those professions that can provide the best quality care with the most positive outcomes will be the professions that gain reimbursement and recognition as desirable providers.[15] Nursing knowledge is broad and caring. Nurses must become proactive in the marketplace, demonstrate effectiveness, respond to consumer needs, and disclose their competence.

The proliferation of the use of technology and specialized devices in health care sometimes diverts the focus from caring and patient interaction to the application and servicing of machinery. Recently, Watson,[22] Leininger,[23] and Benner[24] published works describing caring in nursing. Benner alleges that "a caring relationship is central to most nursing interventions," and that caring is an "enabling condition of caring and concern . . . [that] sets up the possibility of giving help and receiving help."[24] Caring, together with sensitive, informed use of technology, is imperative to quality nursing care in this age of technology and information. Educational programs must establish links between providing support and utilizing devices.

Reed, in a conference studying the importance of education in the use of technology in nursing care, said:

> As the largest health professional group in the nation and often the primary link between the patient and the vast array of health care technology, nurses are vital to this endeavor. Nurses have long established responsibilities for the safe and effective administration of drugs to the patient and the challenge to them in the medical device area may be even greater. . . . Because development of the technology often originates with the scientific community that may be somewhat removed from the realities of patient care, the role of nurses in adapting it to the needs of patients—perhaps even in helping with its design before it reaches the bedside—is critical to its effective and safe use.[25]

Further, Reed describes the nurse's responsibility as encompassing not only the use of technology, but also the promotion of clients' and families' understanding of the role of devices in their treatment. The patient who is subjected to innumerable tubes, probes, electronic monitors, or infusion pumps undoubtedly feels overwhelmed, fearful, and quite helpless. According to Reed and Dressler,[25,26] such patients need assurance that the equipment is being used safely and effectively.

Graduate preparation in nursing seldom focuses on bioinstrumentation, according to a 1986 survey of programs accredited by the National League for Nursing (NLN).[27] Only 34% reported courses on bioinstrumentation, or even support courses, such as physics. A survey of nurses in agencies in a large metropolitan area revealed that 97% believed that a clinical instrumentation course was needed. Home health nurses expressed the greatest need for such a course.[27] Abbey and Shephard have proposed a device education model that shows the components needed for preparation of nurses for expert use of bioinstrumentation. Their model is shown in Figure 16-1, and may be used as a framework for a graduate course in the use of technology.

Dressler[26] suggests that educational programs may integrate learning of technological skills into models of care, such as Carnaveli's depiction of nursing's role in helping clients maintain activities of daily living. Nurses need to be prepared to assess comprehensively "all dimensions of patient health status,"[26] keeping abreast of rapidly changing conditions, detecting impending problems, and interpreting indicators of change in health status. Graduate programs that prepare nurse specialists, includ-

Figure 16-1 Nursing knowledge and skills for device use. (From The Abbey-Shepherd device educational model. In *Nursing and Technology: Moving into the 21st century: Conference proceedings of May 16–18, 1988, Annapolis, MD,* 1989, Washington, D.C.: Department of Health and Human Services. Reproduced with permission of the authors.)

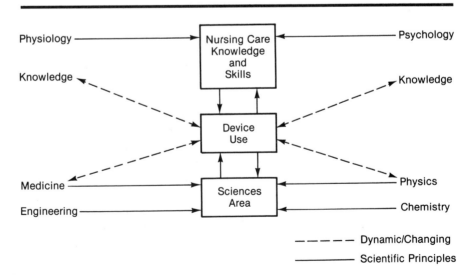

ing perioperative nurse clinicians, must offer coursework in bioinstrumentation in order to provide preparation for futuristic practice.

The perioperative nurse specialist may be cited as a unique futurist
role that combines technological expertise, continuity of care (community
to institution to community), marketing strategies, and caring. The role
is emerging, but must be developed through new directions in graduate
education and research.

▽

Future Directions in Nursing Education That May Meet Nurse/ Patient Needs in Ambulatory Surgery Settings

Nursing education must be open to changing modes of practice, new reimbursement patterns, new technologies and sites of care, and competitive
markets. Just as the focus of the curriculum must be progressive, so, too,
must the methods of teaching, the organization of learning experiences,
the use of educational technology to enrich learning, and the relationship
between schools of nursing and clinicians be open to examination and
collaborative planning.

The evolution of ambulatory surgery settings has underscored the
need for preparation of nurses for broader roles. Undergraduate curricula
should be based on concepts that may be applied in any setting, not just
inpatient acute care or community care. Continuity of care is one of the
foremost concepts that must thread throughout the curriculum. Thor-
ough assessment skills must be taught so that graduates may assume
decision-making responsibilities. Also, the interaction of contextual data
with assessment parameters must be integrated throughout the course
of study. The expectation in the future will be that nursing practice will
be able to adapt to any setting, with the nurse assuming the role of primary nurse or case manager.

With these impending or continued changes, what will nursing education programs be like? Computers will provide technical support in a
variety of ways: textbooks may be available on computer disks; course
syllabi, student assignments, papers, and patient data may be accessed
from students' homes via computer networking; and clients may be able
to record their own health history using computer networks, with the
history and physical assessment data subsequently being analyzed using
specialized computer software. Computerized discharge planning will be
managed by ambulatory care nurses. With the mass of information available, data will require skillful analysis by nurses. Computer proficiency
will be required for all nurses.

As technology and new surgery techniques are perfected, the role of
ambulatory surgery and the policy of early discharge will expand. Highly
skilled self-care teaching and planning with clients will be in increasing
demand. Nurses will need to be involved in the production of health care
technology because they have a unique knowledge of reactions to disease

and the problems with which clients cope 24 hours a day. Nursing education must provide preparation in physics, computer applications, client teaching, and communication with health team members, as well as with clients.

Teaching methods will need to be adapted so that new technology can be used to advantage. Specifically, independent learning will become an expectation so that faculty can spend their time with students, focusing on critical analysis, planning, and application of knowledge. Faculty must have time available to develop computer simulations, in consultation with practitioners.

Video simulations and "nursing Nintendo" programs (interactive video learning packages) will be available for independent study. Many classes will be taught using telecommunication networks and computer-aided instruction. Faculty and clinical preceptors will cooperatively plan clinical conferences, as well as client care experiences. Because of this atmosphere of continuous change, it will become increasingly important for clinical agencies and educators to collaborate in order to keep nursing preparation current, and to enhance nursing practice through faculty research. Graduate programs preparing ambulatory surgical specialists will offer interdisciplinary preparation in nursing and business or marketing. Other programs will prepare nurses in the sciences, such as computer science, physics, or engineering, in order to involve nursing in highly specialized client care management. Ambulatory surgical clinical specialists who are knowledgeable about legal and ethical dilemmas will also be needed, and nurses with dual preparation in law will be in increasing demand.

Watson, in her discussion of nursing and nursing education of the future, contends:

> This comprehensive delivery, coordination, and management of expert human caring, healing, and health will occur in the midst of biotechnology and computer technology, but within the context of the individual patients' and families' personal human caring and health needs . . . the nurse of the future is an expert in human caring who is directly accountable to society—one prepared as a full health professional who works collaboratively across settings within a continuous care model, as an equal member of the interdisciplinary team.[28]

Nurses in ambulatory care settings are the new breed in the professional practice of nursing. Through collaboration among educators and practitioners in these new settings, significant contributions to future health care will be made.

References

1. Naisbitt, J. (1982). *Megatrends* (pp. 11–53). New York: Warner Books Inc.
2. Benjamin, H. (1939). *Saber-tooth curriculum.* New York: McGraw-Hill Book Company.
3. Ten trends to watch. (1986). *Nursing and Health Care 7,* 17.

4. Bevis, E. M. (1982). *Curriculum building in nursing* (p. 179). St. Louis: C.V. Mosby.
5. Carnaveli, D. L. (1982). Nursing perspectives in health care technology. *Nursing Administration Quarterly 9,* 12, 16, 17.
6. Benner, P. *From novice to expert: Excellence and power in clinical nursing practice.* (1980). Menlo Park, CA: Addison-Wesley Publishing Company.
7. Riehl, J. P., & Roy, C. (1980). *Conceptual models for nursing practice.* New York: Appleton-Century-Crofts.
8. Marriner, A. (1986). *Nursing theorists and their work.* St. Louis: C. V. Mosby.
9. Chinn, P. L., & Jacobs, M. K. (1983). *Theory and nursing.* St. Louis: C. V. Mosby.
10. Polit, D., & Hungler, B. (1987). *Nursing research: Principles and methods.* Philadelphia: J. B. Lippincott.
11. Ver Steeg, D. F., (Guest Ed). (1988). Computer use and nursing research: A computerized taxonomy of nursing diagnosis for use in ambulatory care nursing education, practice, and research. Part 1: Development and major headings. *Western Journal of Nursing Research, 10,* 506–509.
12. Hamilton, P., (1983). Community nursing diagnosis. *Advances in Nursing Science, 6,* 21–36.
13. Guzzetta, C. E., Bunton, S. D., Prinkley, L. A., Sherer, A. P., & Seifert, D. C. (1989). *Clinical assessment tools for use with nursing diagnosis.* St. Louis: C. V. Mosby.
14. Dela Cruz, F. A. (1989). *Measuring clinical nursing judgment in home health nursing.* Paper presented at Society for Research in Nursing Education 7th Annual Research in Nursing Education Conference, San Francisco.
15. Gamotis, P. B., Dearmon, V. C., Doolittle, N. O., & Price, S. C. (1987). Inpatient vs. outpatient satisfaction. *AORN Journal, 46,* 5.
16. Ward, S. F., & Kazokowski, J. L. (1987). The nurse as the knowledge worker. *AORN Journal, 46,* 896–901.
17. Wolf, Z. R. (1986). The caring concept and nurse identified caring behaviors. *Topics in Clinical Nursing, 8,* 84–93.
18. Icenhour, M. L. (1988). Quality interpersonal care. *AORN Journal, 47,* 1414–1419.
19. Stephenson, M. (1988). The case for day care surgery. *Nursing Times, 84,* 37–38.
20. Mortonsen, M., & McMullin C. (1986). Discharge score for surgical outpatients. *American Journal of Nursing, 86,* 1347–1349.
21. Department of Health and Human Services. (1988). *Nursing and technology: Moving into the 21st century.* (Conference Proceedings, Annapolis, MD, May 16–18). Washington, DC: Department of Health and Human Services.
22. Watson, J. (1979). *The philosophy and science of caring.* Boston: Little, Brown & Co.
23. Leininger, M. M. (1981). *Caring: An essential human need.* Thorofare, NJ: Charles B. Slack.
24. Benner, P. (1988). *The primacy of caring.* Menlo Park, CA: Addison-Wesley Publishing Company.
25. Reed, R. (1988). Response to a challenge. In Department of Health and Human Services: *Nursing and technology: Moving into the 21st century.* (Conference Proceedings, Annapolis, MD, May 16–18). Washington DC: Department of Health and Human Services.
26. Dressler, D. K. (1988). Nursing and technology: The Carnaveli nursing education model. In Department of Health and Human Services: *Nursing and technology: Moving into the 21st century.* (Conference Proceedings, Annapolis, MD, May 16–18). Washington DC: Deparment of Health and Human Services.

27. Abbey J., & Shephard, M. D. (1988). The Abbey-Shephard device educational model. In Department of Health and Human Services: *Nursing and technology: Moving into the 21st century.* (Conference Proceedings, Annapolis, MD, May 16–18). Washington DC: Department of Health and Human Services.
28. Watson, J. (1989). The future-in-the-making: Creating the new age. In E. M. Bevis & J. Watson (Eds.), *Toward a caring curriculum: A new pedagogy for nursing.* New York: National League For Nursing.

Figure 16-1 Nursing knowledge and skills for device use. (From The Abbey-Shepherd device educational model. In *Nursing and Technology: Moving into the 21st century: Conference proceedings of May 16–18, 1988, Annapolis, MD, 1989,* Washington, D.C.: Department of Health and Human Services. Reproduced with permission of the authors.)

PERIOPERATIVE ASSESSMENT TOOL

Name _____ Age _____ Sex _____
Address _____ Telephone _____
Significant other _____ Telephone _____
Date of admission _____
Allergies _____ Medical diagnosis _____
Planned surgical intervention _____
Anticipated length of surgery _____
Wound classification _____
Informed consent _____

Preoperative Phase

Nursing Diagnosis
(Potential or Altered)

COMMUNICATING ■ A pattern involving sending messages
Read, write, understand English (circle) — Communication
Other languages _____ — Verbal
Intubated _____ Speech impaired _____ — Nonverbal
Physical deformities (jaws wired, cleft palate) _____
Alternate form of communication _____
Perioperative implications _____

VALUING ■ A pattern involving the assigning of relative worth
Religious preference _____ — Spiritual state
Name of minister, priest, rabbi _____ — Distress
Cultural practices _____ — Despair
Perioperative implications _____

RELATING ■ A pattern involving establishing bonds
Role
Marital status _____ — Role performance
Age & health of significant other _____ — Parenting
_____ — Sexual dysfunction
Number of children _____ Ages _____
Role in home _____
Financial support _____ — Family processes
Occupation _____
Job satisfaction/concerns _____

Socialization
Social relationships: functional/dysfunctional (circle) — Impaired social interaction
Prefers to be alone/with family/with friends (circle)
Perioperative implications _____

KNOWING ■ A pattern involving the meaning associated with information
Current health problems _____

Are you or could you be pregnant? _____
Current medications _____
Previous illnesses/hospitalizations/surgeries (list dates) _____

Previous transfusion/transfusion reaction: _____

History of the following problems (specify self or family):
Heart _____ Rheumatic fever _____
Peripheral vascular _____ Cerebrovascular _____
Lung _____ Kidney _____ Hepatitis _____
Liver _____
Thyroid _____ Cancer _____
Human immunodeficiency virus _____
Other _____ — Knowledge deficit

Risk factors — Present — Perceptions/knowledge of
1. Hypertension _____
2. Hyperlipidemia _____
3. Smoking _____
4. Obesity _____
5. Diabetes _____
6. Sedentary living _____
7. Stress _____
8. Alcohol use _____
9. Oral contraceptives _____
10. Bleeding _____
11. Family history _____

Perceptions/expectations of surgery _____

Misconceptions _____
Readiness to learn _____
Educational level _____ — Thought processes
Learning impeded by _____
Surgical consent signed: Yes _____ No _____
Blood/blood products ordered: Yes _____ No _____ Number of units _____

Orientation
Level of alertness _____ — Orientation
Orientation: Person _____ Place _____ Time _____ — Confusion
Appropriate behavior/communication _____

Memory
Memory intact: Yes _____ No _____ Recent _____ Remote _____ — Memory
Perioperative implications _____

FEELING ■ A pattern involving the subjective awareness of information
Comfort
Pain/discomfort: Yes _____ No _____ — Comfort
Onset _____ Duration _____ — Pain/chronic
Location _____ Quality _____ Radiation _____ — Pain/acute
Associated factors _____ — Discomfort
Aggravating factors _____
Alleviating factors _____

Emotional Integrity/States
Recent stressful life events _____ — Grieving
— Anxiety
Verbalizes feelings of _____ — Fear
Source _____ — Anger
Physical manifestations _____ — Guilt
Perioperative implications _____ — Shame
— Sadness

Exhibit 16-1 (Continued)

Pupils
Reaction: Brisk _____
Sluggish _____ Nonreactive _____

Eye Opening
No response (1)
To pain (2)
To speech (3)
Spontaneous (4)

Best Verbal
No response (1)
Incomprehensible sound (2)
Inappropriate words (3)
Confused conversation (4)
Oriented (5)

Best Motor
Flaccid (1)
Extensor response (2)
Flexor response (3)
Semipurposeful (4)
Localized to pain (5)
Obeys commands (6)

Glasgow Coma Scale total _____

Cerebral tissue perfusion

Cardiac
Apical rate & rhythm _____
Heart sounds/murmurs _____
Pacemaker: Yes _____ No _____ Type _____
BP: Reading _____ Location _____
IV fluids/medications _____
Invasive monitoring: CVP _____ Swan-Ganz _____
A-line _____ Other _____

Cardiopulmonary tissue perfusion
Fluid volume
  Deficit
  Excess

Peripheral
Pulses: A = absent   B = bruits   D = doppler
+3 = bounding   +2 = palpable   +1 = faintly palpable
Location _____ Side _____
Skin temp _____ Color _____
Edema _____ Capillary refill _____

Peripheral tissue perfusion
Fluid volume
  Deficit
  Excess
Cardiac output

Physical Integrity
Skin Integrity
Petechiae _____ Rashes _____ Lesions _____
Abrasions _____ Bruises _____
_____ Scars _____
Proposed incision site _____

Impaired skin integrity
Impaired tissue integrity
Injury
Infection

Oxygenation
Complaints of dyspnea _____ Precipitated by _____ Depth _____
Respiratory rate _____ Rhythm _____
Labored/unlabored (circle)
Use of accessory muscles _____
Cough: productive/nonproductive _____
Breath sounds _____
Pulmonary function studies _____
Last chest x-ray study _____
Tracheostomy/endotracheal tube _____
Ventilator _____

Impaired gas exchange
Ineffective airway clearance
Ineffective breathing patterns

Physical Regulation
Immune Status
Lymph nodes enlarged _____ Location _____
Compromised immune system _____
WBC count _____ Differential _____
HCT _____ Hb _____
Consent for HIV testing _____ Results _____
Chemotherapy _____ Steroid therapy _____
Prophylactic antibiotic therapy _____
Temperature _____ Route _____

Infection
Hypothermia
Hyperthermia
Body temperature
Ineffective thermoregulation

Nutrition
Eating patterns: Changed _____ Unchanged _____
Number of meals per day _____

Nutrition

(Continued)

MOVING ■ A pattern involving activity
Activity
Limitations in daily activities
Related to: Arthritis _____ Back pain _____
Prosthetic devices _____ Muscle weakness _____
Fatigue _____ Other _____
Exercise habits _____

Activity intolerance
Impaired physical mobility

Self-Care
Ability to perform ADLs independently: Yes _____ No _____
Specify deficits _____
Discharge planning needs _____

Self-care
Feeding
Bathing/hygiene
Dressing/grooming
Toileting

Rest
Hours slept/night _____ Feels rested: yes/no _____
Difficulty falling/remaining asleep _____
Sleep aids (pillows, meds, food) _____

Sleep pattern disturbance
Insomnia
Hypersomnia
Nightmares

Recreation
Leisure activities _____
Social activities _____

Deficit in diversional activity

Health Maintenance
Health insurance _____
Regular physical checkups _____

Health maintenance

Environmental Maintenance
Home maintenance management
Size & arrangement of home (stairs, bathroom) _____
Safety needs _____
Housekeeping responsibilities _____
Perioperative implications _____

Impaired home maintenance management
Safety hazards

PERCEIVING ■ A pattern involving the reception of information
Self-Concept
Verbalizes change in feeling about self due to: Diagnosis _____
Illness _____ Surgery _____ Other _____

Body image
Self-esteem
Personal identity

Sensory/Perception
Vision impaired _____ Glasses _____
Auditory impaired _____ Hearing aid _____
Kinesthetics impaired _____
Gustatory impaired _____
Tactile impaired _____
Olfactory impaired _____
Reflexes: grossly intact _____

Visual
Auditory
Kinesthetic
Gustatory
Tactile
Olfactory

Meaningfulness
Verbalizes hopelessness/powerlessness (circle) _____
Perioperative implications _____

Hopelessness
Powerlessness

EXCHANGING ■ A pattern involving mutual giving and receiving
Circulation
Cerebral (circle appropriate response)
Neurologic changes/symptoms (headaches/seizures/convulsions/blackouts) _____

Cerebral tissue perfusion

Exhibit 16-1 (Continued)

Special diet
Caffeine intake (coffee, tea, soft drinks, chocolate)

Nausea/vomiting
Condition of mouth/throat
Teeth (chipped, loose)
Dentures (upper, lower, full mouth)
   Disposition of dentures
Height _____ Weight _____
Current therapy
   NPO _____ NG suction _____ TPN _____
Labs (indicate abnormal values with *)
   Na _____ K _____ PT _____ CL _____ Glucose _____
   Serum albumin _____ PTT _____ BUN _____
   Other _____

Oral mucous membrane
More than body
   requirements
Less than body requirements

Elimination
Gastrointestinal/bowel
Usual bowel habits
Alterations from normal

Bowel elimination
   Constipation
   Diarrhea
   Incontinence

Renal/urinary
Usual urinary pattern _____ Output q.d. _____
Alteration from normal
Urinary catheter _____ **Bladder distention** _____
Hemodialysis
Perioperative implications

Urinary elimination
   Incontinence
   Retention
Renal tissue perfusion

CHOOSING ▪ A pattern involving the selection of alternatives
Coping
Patient's usual problem-solving/coping methods

Ineffective individual coping
Ineffective family coping

Family's usual problem-solving/coping methods

Patient's affect
Physical manifestations

Participation
Compliance with past/current health care regimens

Noncompliance
Ineffective participation

Willingness to comply with future health care regimen

Judgment
Decision-making ability
   Patient's perspective
   Others' perspectives
   Perioperative implications

Judgment
   Indecisiveness

Prioritized nursing diagnosis/problem list: PREOPERATIVE
1.
2.
3.
4.
5.

Signature _____ Date & time _____

Exhibit 16-1 (Continued)

Intraoperative Phase

GENERAL INFORMATION
Name _____ Room _____ Age _____ Sex _____
Allergies
Patient in _____ Patient out _____
OR # _____ Anesthesia start _____ Anesthesia stop _____
Surgery start _____ Surgery stop _____
Surgeon _____ Assistant(s) _____
Circulator _____ Relief _____
Scrub _____ Relief _____
Anesthesiologist _____ CRNA _____
Other/students
Type of procedure: Scheduled _____ Emergency _____ Urgent _____
Wound class: Clean _____ Clean-contaminated _____ Contaminated _____ Dirty/infected _____
Informed consent

Nursing Diagnosis
(Potential or Altered)

KNOWING ▪ A pattern involving meaning associated with information
Preoperative diagnosis
Procedure
Postoperative diagnosis

Orientation
Level of alertness

Orientation
Confusion

FEELING ▪ A pattern involving the subjective awareness of information
Comfort
Anesthesia: General _____ Mask _____ Intubated _____
   Regional _____ Local/monitor _____
   Local _____
Pain/discomfort: Yes _____ No _____
Location
Aggravating factors
Alleviating factors
Comfort measures offered (warm blanket, pillow)

Comfort
Pain/acute
Discomfort

Emotional Integrity/States
Verbalizes feelings of

Anxiety
Fear
Shame

MOVING ▪ A pattern involving activity
Positioning: Supine _____ Prone _____ Lithotomy _____
Right side up _____ Left side up _____ Jack-knife _____
Other
Padding/supports/restraints

Impaired physical mobility

Transfer to OR bed: Self _____ Assisted _____
Presence/disposition of prosthesis

PERCEIVING ▪ A pattern involving the reception of information
Sensory/Perception
Disposition of sensory aids (glasses, hearing aid)

Sensory/perception
   Visual
   Auditory

Exhibit 16-1 (Continued)

EXCHANGING ■ A pattern involving mutual giving and receiving

Circulation
Blood/blood products administered _____   Tissue perfusion
Estimated blood loss _____   Fluid volume
Pulse checks performed: Time _____ Location _____   Deficit
Rate _____   Excess
Monitoring: ECG _____ Rhythm _____   Cardiac output
BP: _____ Time _____ BP: _____ Time _____

Physical Integrity
Invasive lines: Peripheral _____ A-line _____   Impaired skin integrity
CVP _____ Swan-Ganz _____   Impaired tissue integrity
Skin Integrity: electrosurgery unit # _____
Settings _____ Ground pad site _____   Injury
Skin condition _____   Infection
Skin Prep: Iodophor _____ Hibiclens _____ Other _____
Tourniquet # _____ Location _____ Pressure _____
Padding _____ Time up _____ Time down _____
Implants/Prostheses: Mfr _____ Model _____
Lot _____ Serial # _____ Size _____
Site _____

Counts: Initial   1st   2nd   3rd
Sponge _____
Needle _____
Instrument _____
Other _____   Initials _____
Drains/Catheters: Type _____ Size _____ Location _____
Packing: Type _____ Location _____
Dressings: type _____

Oxygenation
O₂ administered by RN: Yes _____ No _____ Rate _____ Route _____   Impaired gas exchange
Ineffective airway clearance
Ineffective breathing patterns

Physical Regulation
Temperature _____ Route _____ Time _____   Body temperature
Specimens: Pathology _____ Bacteriology _____   Hypothermia
Cytology _____ Other _____   Hyperthermia
   Infection

Nutrition
Disposition of dentures _____

Elimination
Urinary catheter _____ Inserted by _____   Renal tissue perfusion
Size _____ Output _____   Urinary elimination

Medications

Drug	Route	Time	Prepared by	Administered by

Fluid volume
Deficit
Excess
Injury

Exhibit 16-1 (Continued)

Discharged to _____ Via _____ Report given: Yes _____ No _____
By _____
Patient status _____

Prioritized nursing diagnosis/problem list: INTRAOPERATIVE
1
2
3
4
5

Signature _____   Date & Time _____

Postoperative Phase

                   Nursing Diagnosis
                   (Potential or Altered)

KNOWING ■ A pattern involving the meaning associated with information
Orientation
Level of alertness _____   Orientation
Orientation: Person _____ Place _____ Time _____   Confusion
Perception/expectation of surgery performed _____   Memory
   Thought processes
Misconceptions _____   Knowledge deficit
Knowledge of:
   Care of incision site
   Potential complications
   Symptoms to report
Need for referral to home health agency: Yes _____ No _____

FEELING ■ A pattern involving the subjective awareness of information
Comfort
Pain/discomfort: Yes _____ No _____ Duration _____   Comfort
Onset _____ Location _____ Radiation _____   Pain/acute
Quality _____
Associated factors _____
Aggravating factors _____
Alleviating factors _____

MOVING ■ A pattern involving activity
Ability to perform ADLs independently: Yes _____ No _____   Impaired physical mobility
Specify deficits _____   Self-care
Discharge planning needs _____

PERCEIVING ■ A pattern involving the reception of information
Self-Concept
Effects of surgery on self-concept _____   Body image
   Self-esteem
   Personal identity

EXCHANGING ■ A pattern involving mutual giving and receiving
Circulation
Neurologic changes _____   Tissue perfusion
Cardiovascular changes _____   Cerebral
   Cardiopulmonary
   Peripheral

(Continued)

Exhibit 16-1 (Continued)

Physical Integrity
Skin integrity: Incision site _____ Color _____
  Temperature _____ Drainage _____
  Electrosurgery grounding site _____
  Other _____

Oxygenation
Ability to deep breathe and cough
  Mechanical ventilation: Yes _____ No _____

Physical Regulation
  Temperature _____ Route _____
  WBC count _____ Other labs _____

Nutrition
  Current therapy: NPO _____ NG suction _____
  TPN _____ Diet: Fluid _____ Solid _____

Elimination
  Bowel function _____
  Urinary function _____

CHOOSING • A pattern involving the selection of alternatives
Coping
  Patient's affect _____
  Patient's coping mechanisms _____
  Family's coping mechanisms _____

Participation
  Willingness to comply with health care regimen _____

Infection
Injury
Impaired tissue integrity
Impaired skin integrity

Impaired gas exchange
Ineffective airway clearance
Ineffective breathing patterns

Hypothermia
Hyperthermia
Infection

Nutrition

Bowel elimination
Urinary elimination

Ineffective individual coping
Ineffective family coping

Noncompliance
Ineffective participation

Prioritized nursing diagnosis/problem list: POSTOPERATIVE
1. _____
2. _____
3. _____
4. _____
5. _____

Inpatient: Discussed with primary nurse   Yes _____ No _____

Outpatient: Discharged to: _____ Via _____
Accompanied by _____

Signature _____ Date & Time _____

Exhibit 16-1 (Continued)

Patterns	Emphasis areas to determine
PREOPERATIVE	
Communicating	Ability to read, write, and understand English
	Physical deformities
Valuing	Religious or cultural preferences
Relating	Preference for being alone or with family or with friends
Knowing	Current health problems
	Transfusion and transfusion reaction
	History of bleeding problems, hepatitis, or HIV
	Risk factors
	Surgical consent
	Blood ordered
	Level of alertness
Feeling	Pain or discomfort
	Verbalized feelings such as anxiety, fear, or shame
Moving	Arthritis, back pain, prosthetic devices, or muscle weakness
Perceiving	Sensory/perceptual status
Exchanging	Neurologic and cardiac status
	Skin integrity
	Proposed incision site
	Immune system: WBC, Hct, Hgb, and steroid therapy
	Nausea or vomiting
	Condition of mouth and teeth, dentures, bridges, or plates
	Laboratory information: electrolyte levels and coagulation studies
	Renal perfusion, bladder distension, or hemodialysis
	Patient's affect
Choosing	Compliance with health care regimen
INTRAOPERATIVE	
(General information)	
Knowing	Wound classification
	Preoperative and postoperative diagnosis
	Procedure
Feeling	Comfort
Moving	Positioning
Exchanging	Circulation
	Physical integrity
	Implants
	Counts: sponges, needles, and instruments
	Oxygenation
	Medications
	Patient status
POSTOPERATIVE	
Knowing	Knowledge of incisional care, complications, and symptoms to report
	Need for referral
Feeling	Pain or discomfort
Moving	Discharge planning needs
Perceiving	Effects of surgery on self-concept
Exchanging	Skin integrity
	Deep breathing and coughing
	Physical regulation
Choosing	Coping
	Participation and compliance

Exhibit 16-1 (Continued)

Variables	Focus questions and parameters
EXCHANGING—cont'd	
Proposed incision site	Assess the condition of the proposed incision site. Is the patient at risk for infection?
Immune status	Does the patient have a cold or symptoms of a cold?
Nausea/vomiting	Does the patient complain of nausea or indicate that nausea or vomiting occurred after a previous surgery?
Condition of mouth/throat and teeth	Does the patient wear dentures? Have they been placed in a safe location? Missing teeth? Loose or chipped teeth?
Labs	Are the patient's electrolyte levels within normal limits? Are coagulation studies normal?
Renal/urinary	Has the patient voided recently? Is a urinary catheter ordered? Is the patient on renal dialysis? Where is the shunt or fistula?
CHOOSING	
Patient's affect	What is the patient's affect? Is it appropriate or inappropriate (i.e. extreme anger or euphoria) to the situation?
Compliance with past/ current health care regimens	Will the surgery impose physical or emotional limits on the patient's ability to comply with the anticipated therapeutic regimen? Will the patient or family require referral to a home health agency? Will the patient under local anesthesia be able to comply with intraoperative instructions? (Assess patient's need to retain glasses or hearing aid.)
Intraoperative **(GENERAL INFORMATION)**	
Wound class	Does the wound class predispose the patient to a postoperative infection?
KNOWING	
Preoperative and postoperative diagnoses	What is the patient's understanding of the problem? Is it confirmed by the diagnosis and informed consent?
Procedure	Does the patient confirm the procedure posted?
FEELING	
Comfort	Is the patient uncomfortable before induction? For cases using local anesthetic: Is the patient in pain? What comfort measures (pillows, warm blankets, imagery techniques, or religious items) can be provided? Is more local anesthetic indicated? Does the patient verbalize pain at the incision site?
MOVING	
Positioning	Is the position appropriate for the procedure? Is adequate padding provided to prevent nerve injury? Are pressure areas protected?
EXCHANGING	
Circulation	Assess the patient's circulatory status, including BP, intraarterial pressure, capillary refill, skin color, temperature, ECG, and heart rate. Assess blood loss in suction cannisters, on sponges, and in drapes. What was the preoperative hematocrit?
Physical integrity	Assess skin integrity at site of the grounding pad, ECG leads, invasive lines, tourniquet site, and incision site. "Do you have any allergies to medications or (irrigating or cleansing) solutions?"
Implants/prostheses	Note the manufacturer, model, lot, serial number, size, and implant site is appropriate paperwork completed to ensure follow up?
Counts	Account for all surgical items to avoid the possibility of a retained foreign object or infection.

Exhibit 16-1 (Continued)

Variables	Focus questions and parameters
Preoperative **COMMUNICATING**	
Read, write, understand English	Assess the patient's ability to communicate. If needed, is a translator available (before and after surgery)?
Physical deformity	Does the patient have a physical deformity that impairs communication?
VALUING	
Religious preference and cultural practices	Has a specific spiritual leader been requested? Has the patient requested to keep certain religious items (rosary)? Is it a cultural practice to have family and friends nearby? Are important cultural meanings attached to limbs or to the disposition of body parts?
RELATING	
Prefers to be alone/with family/with friends	Does the patient prefer to be alone, or with a family member or friend? Where will the family and significant other be during surgery?
KNOWING	
Current health problems	"Tell me why you are having surgery. Where?"
Previous transfusion/ transfusion reaction	"Have you ever had a blood transfusion? Any reactions?"
History of the following problems	Do you have a history of HIV, hepatitis, malignant hyperthermia, anesthetic reaction or prolonged recovery time?
Risk factors	Is the patient obese or diabetic or have a coagulapathic condition?
Surgical consent signed	"What has your surgeon told you about your surgery? Do you have any questions?"
Blood/blood products ordered	Determine the blood or blood products available.
Level of alertness	Is the patient alert, lethargic, or comatose?
FEELING	
Pain/discomfort	"Are you in pain? Where?" Are there nonverbal indicators of pain such as shallow breathing, guarding, or grimacing?
Verbalizes feelings of anxiety/fear	Does the patient demonstrate muscle tension, pallor, or increased pulse or respiration? Does the patient verbalize anxiety or fear regarding the surgery or outcome?
MOVING	
Limitations in daily activities	Does the patient have arthritis, back pain, prosthetic devices, or muscle weakness that will affect positioning or transferring to the OR bed?
PERCEIVING	
Sensory/perception	Are any of the patient's senses impaired? Have eye glasses, hearing aids, or other items been placed in a safe location?
EXCHANGING	
Neurologic and cardiac changes/symptoms	Are there any neurologic deficits that may affect positioning, or increase the potential for nerve or pressure injury? Does the patient have cardiovascular disease that might pose a risk under anesthesia?
Skin integrity	Assess the skin for scars, cuts, bruises, cysts, pimples, and abrasions; note color and warmth. What is the condition of the skin at the pressure sites of the planned surgical position? At the site of the electrocautery grounding pad? What invasive lines have been or will be inserted? "Are you allergic to any cleansing agents?"

(Continued)

Exhibit 16-1 (Continued)

312

Variables	Focus questions and parameters
EXCHANGING—cont'd	
Oxygenation	Is the patient's airway patent? Are laboratory results within normal limits? Does positioning allow for optimum oxygenation?
Medications	Are there any allergies to medications used during surgery?
Patient status	Is the patient's status stable or unstable on entering and leaving the OR? Are there special concerns such as history of nausea and vomiting, laryngospasm, or malignant hyperthermia related to recovery?
Postoperative	
KNOWING	
Knowledge of	
Care of incision site	Assess patient's knowledge and understanding of incision care.
Potential complications	Assess patient's knowledge and understanding of complications.
	"Can you tell me what you should look for to be sure you're healing properly?"
Symptoms to report	"Can you describe what changes (in your incision and in how you feel) that you should report?"
Need for referral	Is there a need for follow-up wound care or dressing change?
FEELING	
Pain/discomfort	Does pain interfere with deep breathing and coughing, ambulation, or exercises?
	Does the patient know how to splint the incision site?
MOVING	
Discharge planning needs	"Is there someone to help you at home?"
	Assess the need for transportation, special devices, and home health referrals.
PERCEIVING	
Effects of surgery on self-concept	"How do you feel about yourself now that your surgery is over? How do you think you'll feel 6 months from now?"
EXCHANGING	
Skin integrity	Is there evidence of tenderness, redness, swelling, or drainage at the incision site?
	What is the appearance of the skin at the site of grounding pad, ECG leads, and pressure areas?
	Is there evidence of nerve injury?
Ability to deep breathe and cough	Is the patient able to deep breathe and cough?
	Are breath sounds clear?
	What are the results of pulmonary function studies?
Physical regulation	Is the patient's temperature elevated? WBC elevated?
	Is there evidence of infection?
CHOOSING	
Coping	What is the patient's affect?
	Do family members and significant others verbalize or demonstrate concern or anxiety over their ability to care for the patient? What assistance is available?
Participation	Does the patient verbalize a willingness to comply with the prescribed regimen?
	Does the patient understand the discharge instructions?
	Does the patient have telephone numbers for health care professionals?

Exhibit 16-2 Nursing Therapeutics II: Course description and objectives.

Course description: A practicum which provides the opportunity to examine nursing concepts, practice nursing behaviors, participate in an interdisciplinary health care team, and evaluate nursing care outcomes in a variety of settings.

Objectives: At the completion of this level the student will effectively and appropriately be able to:

1. Demonstrate knowledge of selected concepts, principles, and theories from the physical and behavioral sciences, humanities and nursing which serve as the foundation for baccalaureate nursing practice and professional role development.

2. Apply the problem solving process in providing care for individual client systems.

3. Utilize nursing process with emphasis on assessment and diagnosis of adaptive responses to stressors.

4. Apply basic communication principles in establishing and maintaining relationships with clients.

5. Identify characteristics of clients from diverse, multicultural populations across the life span in selected settings.

6. Function as a member of an interdisciplinary health care team in providing nursing care to clients.

7. Identify principles of the teaching-learning process that are an integral part of professional nursing practice.

8. Use beginning management skills to organize and provide client care.

9. Demonstrate awareness of the value of research in nursing.

Exhibit 16-2 (Continued)

Nursing Therapeutics II

10. Demonstrate accountability and responsibility for professional nursing practice through the communication of pertinent information to health care providers both verbally and through written documents.

11. Identify concepts and principles (of change) which promote system integrity.

12. Demonstrate self awareness and professional development based on assessment of strengths and limitations.

Learning Activities:

1. Plan, provide and evaluate continuity of care in ambulatory surgery/short stay units and home visits and outpatient clinics and offices.

2. Prepare, complete and evaluate self care teaching plan.

3. Analyze coping strategies of caregivers for clients with high technology treatments in the home.

4. Participate in interdisciplinary team patient care planning and/or participate with a preceptor in case management.

▽ ▽ ▽ Chapter 17

▽ ▽ **Ambulatory Surgical Nursing**
▽ **Education Strategies: College Credit**
▽ **or Continuing Nursing Education in a**
▽ **Two-Week Course**

▽ *Sharon Summers*

▽ A common concern among nurses is where and how they can learn to practice in the ambulatory surgical setting. As has been discussed previously, there is limited general or ambulatory surgical nursing content or experiences in any of the various professional nursing education programs, and yet these special skills are needed.[1–13] The current trends toward shortened length of stay and increased patient care in ambulatory settings support the need to prepare nurses for this new practice arena. Currently, when students have experiences in ambulatory surgical units (ASUs), the goals are usually to learn to care for surgical patients, rather than to become proficient in ambulatory surgical nursing. The purpose of this chapter is to discuss a method whereby student nurses enrolled in professional nursing education programs, or practicing professional nurses, could gain ambulatory surgical experience, either for college credit or for continuing education. To meet this goal, this chapter addresses the following four questions:

1. How can students gain knowledge and experience in integrating the nursing process into perioperative ambulatory surgical nursing course?
2. How could a two-week perioperative course applicable to ASUs be included in nursing education programs?
3. What clinical content would introduce beginning perioperative clinical skills applicable for the ASU students in a two-week course?
4. What strategies can be used to teach the student about the patient's total perioperative experience?

▽

Nursing Process in Perioperative Ambulatory Surgical Nursing

As described in Chapter 4, nursing process is an important framework with which to organize nursing practice. As the pivotal point in nursing

Exhibits for Chapter 17 are located at the end of the chapter on pages 324–330.

process, nursing diagnosis can be used as the central theme when planning the goals and objectives of a perioperative ambulatory surgical nursing course. Perioperative nursing diagnoses that are pertinent for student learning (also discussed in Chapters 4 and 12) can then be used to make student assignments.

In the past, perioperative or operating room (OR) assignments have been structured around the medical model of body system, diseases, and disorders. In early diploma nursing education, students were required to scrub on a required number of major and minor surgical cases. Major and minor cases were differentiated by the level of time involved, and the extent of the procedures (i.e., gastric resection was considered a major case and tonsillectomy was deemed a minor case). Courses in OR nursing were structured around the available textbooks, which were organized around surgical procedures, thus promoting the medical model for nursing practice. The major content of these texts described anatomy, physiology, and surgical procedures, including instruments, positioning, and dressings, organized by body systems. Little attention was given to nursing care; rather, emphasis was placed on step-by-step surgical procedure. Although it is important to learn surgical technique to work as a surgical team member, nurses need to learn to practice as nurses, not as surgeons.

Current OR nursing texts include the nursing process; however, nursing diagnosis is either not included or not elaborated on sufficiently. Current medical-surgical nursing texts contain content on perioperative nursing; however, little attention is given to the incorporation of nursing process and nursing diagnosis.[14] Nursing diagnosis can be used to guide assignments and can be an effective method for learning both the nursing and surgical aspects of patient care.[15] For example, a nursing diagnosis of "body image disturbance" can be used as a criterion for student clinical assignments, with students selecting patients admitted for surgical procedures such as burn scar revision, breast biopsy, or reconstructive surgery. Because ambulatory surgical nursing is relatively new, at least from a curriculum perspective, components can be adapted from traditional OR nursing courses and added to the curriculum goals and objectives for ambulatory surgical nursing practice.

▽

Perioperative Ambulatory Surgical Nursing Course Content

Ambulatory surgical nursing course content can be integrated into a nursing education program which typically is arranged around a given theoretical or conceptual framework.[16] Goals and objectives are usually written for the curriculum, for the courses, and for the specific lesson plans, all of which flow from the overall conceptual framework. Goals are defined as desired achievements. For example, a goal might be teaching a perioperative ambulatory surgical nursing course. Objectives are defined as the behaviors the student is to demonstrate when the goals are achieved. Learning is usually measured by testing how well the student met the objectives of the course. Therefore, objectives are a very important first step in planning the specific content of any course so that learning can be measured through the testing process.

A perioperative ambulatory surgical nursing course would provide didactic and clinical experiences in the perioperative role of the nurse (objectives) so that the student acquires the beginning level skills needed to practice in the ambulatory surgical setting (goals). The goals and objectives for this ambulatory surgical nursing course flow from the nursing process and, in particular, from nursing diagnoses or the nine patterns established by the North American Nursing Diagnosis Association (NANDA). With this framework in mind, it would be relatively easy to implement the following course within any educational program's theoretical or conceptual framework, as it describes nursing.

The goal to be achieved through a perioperative ambulatory surgical nursing course is to provide the student/nurse with entry-level skills to practice in an ambulatory surgical setting. This includes the development of:

1. Knowledge and skills of the preoperative role of the nurse.
2. Knowledge and skills of the intraoperative role of the nurse.
3. Knowledge and skills of the postoperative role of the nurse.

These goals are broad, which reinforces the need for course objectives that add the specificity of the content.

Perioperative course objectives guide the didactic content and clinical experiences that are to be included in the course. Objectives are established in order to identify desired student behaviors during and upon completion of the course; they may be classified as psychomotor, cognitive, or affective.[17-19]

Psychomotor behaviors, involving hand-eye coordination and manual dexterity, are pertinent for perioperative nursing practice. Nursing, as a practice profession, has historically placed a great deal of emphasis on psychomotor skills. Coordination and manual dexterity are important behaviors to include in perioperative nursing course objectives, and usually consist of practice skills.

Cognitive behaviors, involving knowledge acquisition and utilization, are also important for perioperative nursing practice. These behaviors include comprehension, application, analysis, synthesis, and evaluation of information.

Affective behaviors consist of how the student accepts, values, or appreciates learned concepts for patient care. Affective behaviors are not always defined in course objectives; however, they are important components in shaping positive behaviors that are ultimately conveyed to patients.

These three behavioral classifications can be structured in concert with the five steps of nursing process, thus developing a 3 × 5 course blueprint (Fig. 17-1). Positive affective and cognitive behaviors are desired in all five steps of nursing process, whereas psychomotor behaviors are particularly important during the assessment and implementation steps. The 3 × 5 blueprint of behaviors and nursing process steps can be used to organize specific course content. As seen in Figures 17-2 through 17-4, preoperative, intraoperative, and postoperative nursing activities can be integrated into these blueprints. The blueprints can be used to implement a semester long or two-week perioperative course; only the two-week course will be discussed.

▽

Two-Week Ambulatory Surgical Nursing Perioperative Course Content

Using the nursing process and behavioral objective blueprint just described, perioperative course content could then be developed for a two-week ambulatory surgery clinical experience. The course could be offered for either one credit hour or for continuing education units. A one-credit course would require one hour of classroom contact and three hours of clinical experience per week on a regular semester schedule. When con-

Figure 17-1 Nursing process and behavioral patterns.

NURSING PROCESS	BEHAVIORS		
	PSYCHOMOTOR	COGNITIVE	AFFECTIVE
ASSESSMENT			
NURSING DIAGNOSIS			
NURSING ORDERS			
IMPLEMENTATION			
EVALUATION			

Figure 17-2 Preoperative nursing process and behavioral objectives.

NURSING PROCESS	BEHAVIORS		
	PSYCHOMOTOR	COGNITIVE	AFFECTIVE
ASSESSMENT	Admission Baseline Data Lab Data	Adm.Procedure Informed consent	Empathy
NURSING DIAGNOSIS/ PATTERNS	Transport to OR	Choosing Understanding Relating Communicating Perceiving Feeling	
NURSING ORDERS		Patient Education	Emotional Support
IMPLEMENTATION	Patient Education Give ordered preoperative medication		Under- standing
EVALUATION		Effectiveness of nursing care	

densed into a two-week course, these hours are translate to a total of 16 hours of classroom contact and 44 hours of clinical experience. Preclinical and postclinical conferences are incorporated into the clinical experiences, providing time for special instruction and discussion. Such a concentrated block of time could accommodate many students; however, for the purposes of this discussion, the groups will include a total of 18 students, divided in groups of six, with three faculty members responsible for the course content and clinical experiences. If more than 18 students were to be rotated through such a course, then additional faculty could manage the students in multiple clinical sites.

As seen in Exhibit 17-1, the two-week course schedule is planned so as to include intensive content related to the "Role of the Perioperative Nurse" and "Introduction to Perioperative Nursing," which encompasses preoperative, intraoperative, and postoperative nursing in ambulatory surgical settings. The course is designed so that lectures/discussion,

Figure 17-3 Intraoperative nursing process and behavioral objectives.

NURSING PROCESS	BEHAVIORS		
	PSYCHOMOTOR	COGNITIVE	AFFECTIVE
ASSESSMENT	Move from cart to OR table	Congruence between scheduled procedure and informed consent Monitor patient's welfare	Value patient welfare
NURSING DIAGNOSIS/ PATTERNS		Exchanging Communicating Moving Feeling	
NURSING ORDERS	Assist with procedure Monitor patient	Analyze care Protect patient	
IMPLEMENTATION	Assist with procedure Monitor positioning	Analyze Care	
EVALUATION		Procedure was performed safely Patient stabilized	

audiovisual resources, and computer-assisted instruction are followed by intensive clinical experiences in perioperative ambulatory surgical nursing.

Objectives for the course consist of behaviors to be demonstrated by the students, both daily and upon completion of the course. Using the blueprint for preoperative course content presented in Figure 17-2, objectives can then be written for the first two days of class. The objectives for day 1 include:

Upon completion of the classroom activities, the student will be able to:

1. Define perioperative nursing in ambulatory surgical settings.
2. Define the role of the nurse in preoperative, intraoperative, and postoperative activities.

Figure 17-4 Postoperative nursing process and behavioral objectives.

NURSING PROCESS	BEHAVIORS		
	PSYCHOMOTOR	COGNITIVE	AFFECTIVE
ASSESSMENT	Total body assessment	Analyze patient data for problems	Empathy Protect from harm
NURSING DIAGNOSIS/ PATTERNS		Exchanging Communicating Relating Moving Feeling Perceiving	
NURSING ORDERS	Assess patient Orders related to specific patient problem	Meaning of the patient data	
IMPLEMENTATION	Medications Implement orders implemented Stabilize patient	Patient education Discharge instruct- ions	
EVALUATION	Patient stable	Recovered and discharged	

3. Apply the steps of the nursing process in the perioperative setting.
4. Formulate nursing diagnoses appropriate for perioperative patients.
5. Evaluate perioperative patient education materials for appropriateness to levels of patient education.
6. Comprehend the legal aspects of a signed operative permit.
7. Comprehend the role of the nurse as patient advocate, protector, and counselor.

Day 1 objectives are then tested by measuring students' comprehension of course content. Day 1 objectives are also used to guide the development of lectures and demonstrations, and to select computer-assisted instruction and audiovisual materials. Sample lesson plans for day 1 are presented in Exhibits 17-2 and 17-3. As can be noted, the lesson plans allow for the organization of course content by specific objective (cognitive) and could be developed for all categories for day 1 listed in Figure 17-5. Clinical assignments are a vital step in course planning.

Table 17-1 Clinical Rotations by Groups

| | Groups | | |
Rotations	Day 4	Day 5	Day 6
Preoperative	I	II	III
Intraoperative	II	III	I
Postoperative	III	I	II

▽

Two-Week Ambulatory Surgical Nursing Clinical Content

Clinical assignments the first week would begin with an observation of and orientation to clinical facilities. Next, after successfully completing the clinical laboratory return demonstrations, students would be assigned to one of three groups. Table 17-1 demonstrates a means by which all groups could be rotated for equal experience in perioperative nursing, participating by assisting the circulating nurse or as a second scrub nurse, or caring for patients in the postanesthesia care unit. A sample lesson plan for perioperative clinical experiences is presented in Exhibits 17-4 through 17-6. As seen in Exhibit 17-4, assignments based on cognitive, psychomotor, and affective behavioral objectives and nursing process are included in the preoperative clinical experiences. It is suggested that testing for clinical competency be based on criterion-referenced measurement.[16] Criterion-referenced measurement is used to compare the student to the criterion of clinical safety, rather than comparing one student to another student.

The three groups of students would rotate through the three areas: preoperative, intraoperative, and postoperative. After students have participated in three days of perioperative ambulatory surgical nursing, their next assignment would be in total patient perioperative clinical nursing experience.

▽

Total Patient Perioperative Clinical Experience

The total perioperative clinical assignment allows students to make their own assignments and to care for selected patients from admission through discharge home. Students select two patients per day, morning and afternoon admissions, for total patient care. Students are responsible for admitting those patients, implementing patient teaching, and implementing other preoperative nursing care activities. Students then continue caring for their patients during the intraoperative phase by taking them to surgery and scrubbing on the case. Students then accompany the patients to the postanesthesia area and provide postoperative care, including the planning and implementation of discharge planning and teaching. This allows students to apply all the learned course content and previous clinical experiences for total patient care. Evaluation of student behaviors could be derived from the clinical experience forms. The two days of total patient care with four patients, in combination with the previous structured perioperative clinical experiences, should be sufficient to meet the course objectives.

Continuing education courses for practicing nurses could also follow the same schedule. Some institutions offer courses ranging from one to eight weeks; however, few nurses or employers can afford these extended periods of absence. A two-week course seems more feasible, and allows for indepth content and experience to facilitate learning and retention of information.

▽

Summary

This chapter has presented various methods for providing students with didactic and clinical instruction and experience in ambulatory surgical nursing. Methods were presented to develop course blueprints and to base perioperative course instructions on behavioral objectives and nursing process. Methods were also presented for goal- and behavior-based clinical experiences. Course and clinical content should be adequate to provide student nurses and practicing nurses with the beginning level skills needed to practice perioperative nursing in ambulatory surgical settings.

References

1. Ammon, K. B. (1986). OR experience for BSN students helping educators overcome barriers. *AORN Journal, 43*(1), 266–272.
2. Gruendemann, B. J., & Meeker, M. H. (1987). *Alexander's care of the patient in surgery.* St. Louis: C. V. Mosby.
3. Gutierrez, K., McCormack, C., & Villaverde, M. (1989). Perioperative nursing in the college curriculum. *AORN Journal, 49*(4), 1052–1064.
4. Marta, M. R. (1987). Surgical rotations: A must for nursing education. *AORN Journal, 45*(3), 668–673.
5. Miner, D., & Schueler, H. (1987). Students to perioperative nurses. *AORN Journal, 45*(4), 993–998.
6. Reynolds, A., & Sizemore, M. H. (1986). Perioperative clinical experiences: Opportunities for baccalaureate nursing students. *AORN Journal, 43*(4), 901–906.
7. Roth, R. A., & Gruendemann, B. J. (1986). Use of AORN-recommended practices: Applications in ambulatory surgery. *AORN Journal, 43*(5), 991–999.
8. Rothrock, J. C., & Baldwin, C. A. (1986). Perioperative study for nurses: An onsight, independent study program. *AORN Journal, 43*(3), 490–497.
9. Thiele, J. E., Pendarvis, J. H., Stuky, M. K., Holloway, J. R., & Murphy, D. A. (1989). Perioperative clinical simulations: Development and use in nursing education. *AORN Journal, 50*(2), 370–378.
10. Young, R., Takahashi, J., & Cheney, A. (1981). Project alpha goes into action. *AORN Journal, 34*(5), 920–939.

11. Lowenstein, L., & Rehtz, C. A. (1984). Project alpha. *AORN Journal, 39*(7), 1196–1204.
12. Jones, J. M., & Sorrell, J. M. (1989). Undergraduate OR experience: Are we meeting students' needs? *AORN Journal, 50*(2), 316–325.
13. Fletcher, J., Tighe, S. M., & Vorderstrasse, P. (1985). Perioperative nursing: A survey of schools. *AORN Journal, 42*(4), 548–564.
14. Long, B. C., & Phipps, W. J. (1989). *Medical-surgical nursing: A nursing process approach.* St. Louis: C. V. Mosby.
15. Malen, A. L. (1986). Perioperative nursing diagnosis. *AORN Journal, 44*(5), 829–839.
16. Bevis, E. M. (1982). *Curriculum building in nursing.* St. Louis: C. V. Mosby.
17. Ely, D. P., Urbach, F., Singer, R. N., Simpson, E. J., Fleishman, E. A., Greer, G. D., Hitt, J. D., Sitterley, T. E., & Slebodnick, E. B. (1972). The psychomotor domain. Washington, DC: Gryphon House.
18. Bloom, B. S. (Ed). (1956). *Taxonomy of educational objectives. Handbook I: Cognitive domain.* New York: David McKay Company, Inc.
19. Krathwohl, D. R., Bloom, B. S., & Masia, B. B. (1956). *Taxonomy of educational objectives. Handbook II: Affective domain.* New York: David McKay Company, Inc.

Bibliography

McConnell, E. A. (1987). *Clinical considerations in perioperative nursing.* Philadelphia: J. B. Lippincott.

Kneedler, J. A., & Dodge, G. H. (1988). *Perioperative patient care: The nursing perspective.* Boston: Blackwell Scientific Publications.

Exhibit 17-1 A two-week course schedule for perioperative ambulatory surgical nursing experience.

Exhibit 17-1 (Continued)

WEEK 1   PERIOPERATIVE AMBULATORY SURGICAL NURSING COURSE

DAY 1–   SIX HOURS OF CLASSROOM ACTIVITY

        ROLE OF THE NURSE IN PERIOPERATIVE NURSING
        NURSING PROCESS IN PREOPERATIVE,
        INTRAOPERATIVE, AND POSTOPERATIVE PHASES:
        PATIENT ASSESSMENT, NURSING DIAGNOSIS,
        PLAN, IMPLEMENTATION, AND EVALUATION OF CARE
        PATIENT EDUCATION
        PATIENT ADVOCATE
        PROFESSIONAL/LEGAL RESPONSIBILITIES
        PATIENT COUNSELOR

DAY 2–   SIX HOURS OF CLASSROOM ACTIVITY

        TECHNIQUES AND TECHNOLOGY IN PERIOPERATIVE
        NURSING
        PREOPERATIVE:
            SURGICAL PREPS
            INFORMED CONSENT
            PRIORITY PATIENT EDUCATION
        INTRAOPERATIVE:
            DEMONSTRATION OF ASEPTIC TECHNIQUE
            BASIC PACKS
            STANDARD INSTRUMENTS
            GOWNING & GLOVING
            MONITORS AND EQUIPMENT
            SKIN PREPS AND POSITIONING FOR
            PROCEDURES
        POSTOPERATIVE:
            POST ANESTHESIA CARE UNIT
            EQUIPMENT AND PROCEDURES

DAY 3–   EIGHT HOURS OF LABORATORY ACTIVITY

        RETURN DEMONSTRATION OF SCRUBBING, GOWNING,
        GLOVING, ASEPTIC TECHNIQUE
        TOUR OF CLINICAL FACILITIES
        ORIENTATION AND OBSERVATION IN CLINICAL
        FACILITY
        DAY 4 ASSIGNMENTS

DAY 4–   EIGHT HOURS OF CLINICAL ACTIVITY

        CLINICAL–PRE-CONFERENCE
        PREOPERATIVE PATIENT ASSIGNMENT
        INTRAOPERATIVE PATIENT ASSIGNMENT
            ASSISTING CIRCULATING NURSE
            PARTICIPATE AS SECOND SCRUB NURSE
        POSTOPERATIVE PATIENT ASSIGNMENT
            POST ANESTHESIA CARE UNIT
        POST-CONFERENCE

WEEK 2

DAY 5–   EIGHT HOURS OF CLINICAL ACTIVITY

        CLINICAL–PRE-CONFERENCE
        PREOPERATIVE PATIENT ASSIGNMENT
            TOTAL PATIENT CARE
        INTRAOPERATIVE ASSIGNMENT
            ASSISTING CIRCULATING NURSE
            PARTICIPATE AS SECOND SCRUB NURSE
        POSTOPERATIVE ASSIGNMENT
            POST ANESTHESIA CARE UNIT
        POST-CONFERENCE

DAY 6–   EIGHT HOURS OF CLINICAL ACTIVITY

        CLINICAL PRE-CONFERENCE
        PREOPERATIVE PATIENT ASSIGNMENT
            TOTAL PATIENT CARE
        INTRAOPERATIVE ASSIGNMENT
            ASSISTING CIRCULATING NURSE
            PARTICIPATE AS SECOND SCRUB NURSE
        POSTOPERATIVE ASSIGNMENT
            POST ANESTHESIA CARE UNIT
        POST-CONFERENCE

DAY 7–   EIGHT HOURS OF CLINICAL ACTIVITY

All Groups   CLINICAL–PRE-CONFERENCE
        PERIOPERATIVE PATIENT ASSIGNMENT
            TOTAL PATIENT CARE
            ADMISSION, PATIENT EDUCATION,
            INTRAOPERATIVE,
            POSTOPERATIVE CARE, DISCHARGE
            PLANNING
        POST-CONFERENCE

(Continued)

Exhibit 17-1 (Continued)

WEEK 2 continued

DAY 8—   EIGHT HOURS OF CLINICAL ACTIVITY

    CLINICAL–PRE–CONFERENCE
    PERIOPERATIVE PATIENT ASSIGNMENT
       TOTAL PATIENT CARE
       ADMISSION, PATIENT EDUCATION, INTRAOPERATIVE,
       POSTOPERATIVE CARE, DISCHARGE PLANNING

POST–CONFERENCE

Exhibit 17-2 A sample lesson plan for a perioperative ambulatory surgical nursing course.

Day 1, Class 1
OBJECTIVES: Cognitive

1. Define Perioperative Nursing in Ambulatory Surgical Setting.

2. Define the role of the nurse in preoperative, intraoperative, and postoperative phases of patient care.

3. Reinforce the need for empathy, advocacy, and counseling activities of the nurse.

Student Assignments

1. Read articles #1 through 4 on reference list

2. View video tapes # 1 & 2

STUDENT TESTING

1. Student will be able to write the correct definitions of perioperative nursing and preoperative, intraoperative, and postoperative phases.

2. Students will demonstrate they read article 1 as evidenced by participation in group discussion.

3. Student will be able to write the correct definition of the role of the nurse in the preoperative, intraoperative, and postoperative phases.

4. Students will demonstrate they read assignments as evidenced by participation in class discussion.

5. Students will participate in discussion of video tape.

A-V Materials

1. Perioperative nursing videotapes 1 and 2 are reserved. Content of tape 1: 15 minute overview of general perioperative nursing. Discussion will need to emphasize adapting to the ambulatory setting. Content of tape 2: 45 minute overview of preoperative, intraoperative, and postoperative nursing. Discussion will need to emphasize adapting the nursing process to the three phases.

Exhibit 17-2 (Continued)

Class Lecture Discussion Notes*

1. Define perioperative nursing:

   Perioperative nursing is defined as "nursing activities performed during preoperative, intraoperative, and postoperative phases of patient's experiences (Long & Phipps, 1989, p. 348)." It is also defined as practice focusing on the "individual experiencing surgical intervention (McConnell, 1987, p. ix)."

   A. Preoperative phase is defined as......

   B. Intraoperative phase is defined as....

   C. Postoperative phase is defined as......

2. Preoperative phase of nursing is defined as Beginning with the need for surgical intervention and ends when the patient is transferred to the operating room (Long & Phipps, 1989).

3. Discuss the need to adapt the definition from medical-surgical nursing text, and general hospital admission, to the ambulatory surgical setting.

4. Discuss the need to incorporate the nursing process and nursing diagnosis into each phase.

* Use as many pages as necessary for lecture/classroom discussion materials.

Exhibit 17-3 Sample lesson plans for a perioperative ambulatory surgical nursing course.

Day 2, Class 1
OBJECTIVES: Cognitive and psychomotor behaviors

1. Define techniques and technology used in perioperative nursing: Surgical prep, informed consent, patient education.

2. Defines intraoperative techniques: aseptic technique, basic packs standard instruments, gowning & gloving, monitors and standard O.R. equipment, skin preps, and positioning.

3. Demonstrates aseptic technique while gowning & gloving.

4. Demonstrates aseptic technique when opening a basic pack.

5. Demonstrates aseptic technique when setting-up a basic mayo table.

6. Demonstrate knowledge of postanesthesia care unit equipment.

Student Assignments

1. Read articles #5 – 10 on reference list.

2. Views video tape #3

3. Return demonstration of gowning, gloving, opening basic packs, setting up basic mayo, and use of postanesthesia equipment in the clinical lab on Day 3 after tour and orientation to clinical facilities.

STUDENT TESTING

1. Student will be able to write the correct definition of surgical prep, informed consent, patient education, aseptic technique, basic packs, standard instruments, gowning & gloving, monitors and standard O.R. equipment, skin preps, and positioning.

2. Student will demonstrate they read assignments as evidenced by participation in class discussion.

3. Student will participate in class discussion of video tape

4. Each student will return demonstrate scrubbing, gowning & gloving, opening a pack, setting up a mayo stand with basic instruments.

5. Each student will return demonstrate basic prep for an abdominal and gynecological procedure.

Exhibit 17-3 (Continued)

6. Each student will return demonstrate correct positioning for abdominal and gynecological cases.

7. Each student will return demonstrate use of equipment in postanesthesia unit.

A–V Materials

1. Perioperative nursing videotape #3 is reserved. Content: 45 minute overview of the nurse caring for a patient from preoperative to postoperative phases. Discussion will need to emphasize adapting the nursing process to the three phases.

2. Lab available with all equipment needed to practice return demonstrations.

Class Lecture/Discussion Notes*

1. Demonstrate all preoperative equipment and forms.

2. Demonstrate all intraoperative equipment and forms.

3. Demonstrate all postoperative equipment and forms.

4. Show video tape

5. Discuss articles.

Exhibit 17-4 Preoperative clinical assignments.

Day 4   Perioperative Ambulatory Surgical Nursing

Preoperative Experience Clinical Experience 1
OBJECTIVES: Psychomotor, Cognitive, and Affective

1. Demonstrates ability to admit patients with minimum
   assistance including completion of chart, informed consent,
   admission lab data, nursing assessment, nursing diagnosis.

2. Demonstrates empathy, understanding, and provides emotional
   support when admitting patients.

3. Demonstrates successful patient education while completing
   admission procedures.

4. Applies previous understanding of preoperative medications
   and techniques when giving preoperative medications.

5. Provides emotional support to patient and/or family as
   patient is transferred to the operating room.

Student Assignment

1. Students will make their own assignments and are expected to
   choose patients to provide experiences with the NANDA
   patterns of Choosing, Relating, Communicating, Feeling, and
   Perceiving.

2. Students will successfully complete admission procedures for
   a minimum of 5 patients that included assessment and the
   formulation of nursing diagnosis.

3. Students will successfully implement patient education for a
   minimum of 5 patients with the nursing diagnosis of lack of
   knowledge.

4. Students will demonstrate empathy and understanding of
   patient need by using therapeutic communication techniques
   with patients and families with nursing diagnosis of fear
   and/or anxiety.

5. Students will demonstrate aseptic technique and knowledge of
   preoperative medications by giving a minimum of 5 injections.

Student Testing

1. Students will complete the 5 above assignments when caring
   for patients during the preoperative phase.

Exhibit 17-5 Intraoperative clinical assignments.

Day 4   Perioperative Ambulatory Surgical Nursing

Intraoperative Clinical Experience 1
OBJECTIVES: Psychomotor, Cognitive, and Affective

1. The student will participate in receiving patients into the
    O.R. and verify the correct patient for the scheduled
    procedure.

2. The student will analyze the preoperative medical diagnosis
    and verifies the patient signed consent for the correct
    procedure.

3. The student will monitor patient's welfare by identifying
    NANDA patterns of Exchanging, Communicating, Relating,
    Moving, and Feeling.

4. The student will assist the circulating nurse in monitoring
    and documenting patient care throughout the surgical
    procedure.

5. The student will assists the scrub nurse by maintaining
    aseptic technique while: gowning & gloving, opening packs,
    setting up mayo with basic instruments, and assisting the
    surgeon.

6. The student will value patient's welfare while carrying out
    intraoperative assignments.

7. The student will analyze patient safety throughout surgical
    procedure.

Student Assignment

1. Participates in receiving patients into the O.R. and verifies
    the correct patient for the scheduled procedure.

2. Analyzes the preoperative medical diagnosis and verifies the
    patient signed consent for the correct procedure.

3. Monitors patient's welfare by identifying NANDA patterns of
    Exchanging, Communicating, Relating, Moving, and Feeling.

4. Assists the circulating nurse in monitoring and documenting
    patient care throughout the surgical procedure.

5. Assists the scrub nurse by maintaining aseptic technique
    while: gowning & gloving, opening packs, setting up mayo with
    basic instruments, and assisting the surgeon.

Exhibit 17-5 (Continued)

Day 4 continued

6. Values patient's welfare while carrying out intraoperative
    assignments.

7. Analyzes patient safety throughout surgical procedure.

Student Testing

1. The student will be expected to perform all assignments, on a
    beginning level, during the intraoperative experience.

Exhibit 17-6 Postoperative clinical assignments.

Exhibit 17-6 (Continued)

Day 4   Perioperative Ambulatory Surgical Nursing

Postoperative Clinical Experience 1
OBJECTIVES: Psychomotor, Cognitive, and Affective

1. Perform ongoing assessments until the patient is awake and physiologically stable.

2. Analyze assessment data to promote homeostasis.

3. Formulate nursing diagnosis from the NANDA patterns including Exchanging, Communicating, Relating, Moving, Feeling, and Perceiving.

4. Implement medical orders to promote patient recovery, safety, and welfare.

5. Give ordered medications correctly based upon previously learned principles of pharmacotherapeutics.

6. Protect the patient from harm and provide empathetic nursing care.

7. Complete patient education and discharge instructions to safely discharge the patient home for further recovery.

Student Assignment

1. The student will perform ongoing assessments until the patient is awake and physiologically stable.

2. The student will analyze assessment data to promote homeostasis.

3. The student will formulate nursing diagnosis from the NANDA patterns including Exchanging, Communicating, Relating, Moving, Feeling, and Perceiving.

4. The student will implement medical orders to promote patient recovery, safety, and welfare.

5. The student will give ordered medications correctly based upon previously learned principles of pharmacotherapeutics.

6. The student will protect the patient from harm and provide empathetic nursing care.

7. The student will complete patient education and discharge instructions.

Student Testing

1. The student will successfully complete the above assignment, on a beginning practice level, during the postoperative experience.

Index

Page numbers in italics indicate figures.

ISBN 0-397-54799-4

90000

9 780397 547999